BASIC ORTHOPAEDIC SCIENCES

SECOND EDITION

Edited by MANOJ RAMACHANDRAN

with illustrations by Tom Nunn

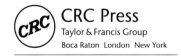

CRC Press
Taylor & Francis Group
Boca Raton London New York

CRC Press is an imprint of the
Taylor & Francis Group, an **informa** business

CRC Press

Taylor & Francis Group

6000 Broken Sound Parkway NW, Suite 300

Boca Raton, FL 33487-2742

© 2017 by Taylor & Francis Group, LLC

CRC Press is an imprint of Taylor & Francis Group, an Informa business

No claim to original U.S. Government works

Printed in the UK by Severn, Gloucester on responsibly sourced paper

 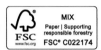

International Standard Book Number-13: 978-1-4441-2098-1 (Pack – Book and Ebook)

Dedication (First edition)

For Joanna.
Everything I do, I do is for you and you only.

Dedication (Second edition)

As always, for my gorgeous wife Joanna but now also for my three
beautiful children, Isabel, Mia and Zac.

Contents

Contributors

Pramod Achan
Consultant Orthopaedic Surgeon
and Clinical Director
Royal London Hospital
London, UK

Paul Allen
Consultant Orthopaedic Surgeon
Princess Alexandra Hospital
Essex, UK

Amit Amin
Consultant Foot and Ankle Surgeon
St George's University Hospital
London, UK

Nick Aresti
Specialty Registrar in Trauma &
Orthopaedic Surgery
Royal London Hospital
London, UK

Will Aston
Consultant Orthopaedic Surgeon
and Honorary Senior Lecturer
Royal National Orthopaedic Hospital
Middlesex, UK

Rajiv Bajekal
Consultant Orthopaedic Surgeon
Barnet Hospital
Herts, UK

Marcus Bankes
Consultant Orthopaedic Surgeon
Guy's Hospital
London, UK

Toby Baring
Consultant Shoulder and Elbow
Surgeon
Homerton University Hospitals NHS
Trust
London, UK

Peter Bates
Consultant Orthopaedic Surgeon
and Honorary Senior Lecturer
Royal London Hospital
London, UK

Professor George Bentley
Emeritus Professor and Director,
Institute of Orthopaedics and
Musculoskeletal-Skeletal Science,
University College London
Consultant Orthopaedic Surgeon
(retired),
Royal National Othopaedic Hospital
Middlesex, UK

Rej Bhumbra
Consultant Trauma and
Orthopaedic Surgeon
Royal London Hospital
London, UK

Professor Rolfe Birch
Consultant Orthopaedic Surgeon
(retired)
Royal National Orthopaedic Hospital
Middlesex, UK

Gurdeep Biring
Consultant Orthopaedic Surgeon
Wycombe Hospital
Bucks, UK

Professor Gordon Blunn
Professor of Biomedical Engineering
Royal National Orthopaedic Hospital
Middlesex, UK

Richard Brown
Consultant Orthopaedic Surgeon
Cheltenham General Hospital
Gloucester, UK

Peter Calder
Consultant Orthopaedic Surgeon
Royal National Orthopaedic Hospital
Middlesex, UK

Steve Cannon
Consultant Orthopaedic Surgeon
(retired)
Royal National Orthopaedic Hospital
Middlesex, UK

Richard Carrington
Consultant Orthopaedic Surgeon
and Joint Reconstruction Unit Lead
Royal National Orthopaedic Hospital
Middlesex, UK

Subhamoy Chatterjee
Consultant Spinal Surgeon
Chase Farm Hospital
Enfield, UK

Daud Chou
Specialty Registrar in Trauma &
Orthopaedic Surgery
Royal London Hospital
London, UK

Paul Culpan
Consultant Orthopaedic Surgeon
(Lower Limb and Pelvic and
Acetabular Service)
Royal London Hospital
London, UK

Jo Dartnell
Consultant Paediatric Orthopaedic
Surgeon
Maidstone and Tunbridge Wells
NHS Trust
Kent, UK

Deborah Eastwood
Consultant Paediatric Orthopaedic
Surgeon
Great Ormond Street Hospital
for Children and Royal National
Orthopaedic Hospital
Middlesex UK

David Evans
Consultant Hand Surgeon
The Hand Clinic
Berks, UK

Mark Falworth
Consultant Orthopaedic Surgeon
Royal National Orthopaedic Hospital
Middlesex, UK

Michael Fox
Consultant Orthopaedic Surgeon
Royal National Orthopaedic Hospital
Middlesex, UK

Fares Haddad
Consultant Orthopaedic Surgeon
Divisional Clinical Director - Surgical
Specialties
University College London Hospitals
London, UK

Alister Hart
Consultant Orthopaedic Surgeon and
Professor of Orthopaedic Surgery
Royal National Orthopaedic Hospital
Middlesex, UK

Sam Heaton
Specialty Registrar in Trauma &
Orthopaedic Surgery
Royal London Hospital
London, UK

Nima Heidari
Consultant Foot, Ankle and Limb
Reconstruction Surgeon
Royal London Hospital
London, UK

Caroline Hing
Consultant Orthopaedic Surgeon
St George's University Hospitals NHS
Trust
London, UK

Harish Hosalkar
Attending Orthopedic Surgeon,
Director, Centre for Hip Preservation
and Children's Orthopedics
California, USA

Brian Hsu
Consultant Spinal Surgeon
Children's Hospital at Westmead
Sydney, Australia

James Hui
Head, Senior Consultant and
Professor
Division of Paediatric Orthopaedics
Department of Orthopaedic Surgery
National University Hospital
Singapore

Kyle James
Medical Director and Orthopaedic
Surgeon
Beit Cure International Hospital
Malawi
and Honorary Senior Lecturer,
Trauma Sciences MSc Programme
Queen Mary University of London,
UK

Chetan Jayadev
Specialty Registrar in Trauma &
Orthopaedic Surgery
Royal London Hospital
London, UK

Prakash Jayakumar
Specialty Registrar in Trauma &
Orthopaedic Surgery
Royal London Hospital
London, UK

Steve Key
Specialty Registrar in Trauma &
Orthopaedic Surgery
Royal London Hospital
London, UK

Vikas Khanduja
Consultant Orthopaedic Surgeon
and Associate Lecturer
Addenbrookes Hospital
Cambridge, UK

Dennis Kosuge
Consultant Orthopaedic Surgeon
Princess Alexandra Hospital NHS
Trust
Essex, UK

Simon Lambert
Consultant Shoulder and Elbow
Surgeon
University College Hospital
London, UK

Joshua Lee
Consultant Orthopaedic Surgeon
(Lower Limb Service)
Royal London Hospital
London, UK

Paul Lee
Consultant Orthopaedic Surgeon
(Lower Limb Service)
Royal London Hospital
London, UK

David Little
Senior Staff Specialist
Department of Orthopaedics
The Children's Hospital at
Westmead, Australia
Conjoint Professor
Paediatrics and Child Health
University of Sydney, Australia

Rohit Madhav
Consultant Orthopaedic Surgeon
London Orthopaedic Surgeons Ltd
The Princess Grace Hospital
London, UK

Linda Marks
Consultant in Rehabilitation
Medicine (retired)
Royal National Orthopaedic Hospital
Middlesex, UK

Nimal Maruthainar
Consultant Orthopaedic Surgeon
Royal Free Hospital
London, UK

Livio diMascio
Consultant in Upper Limb
and Hand Surgery
Royal London Hospital
London, UK

Iain McNamara
Consultant Orthopaedic Surgeon
and Honorary Professor
The Norfolk and Norwich University
Hospitals NHS Trust
Norwich, UK

Jay Meswania
Department of Biomechanical
Engineering
Royal National Orthopaedic Hospital
Middlesex, UK

Lisa Mitchell
Clinical Specialist Orthotist
Great Ormond Street Hospital for
Children
London, UK

Bjarne Moller-Madsen
Consultant and Professor
Department of Children`s
Orthopaedics
Aarhus University Hospital NBG
Denmark

Fergal Monsell
Consultant Paediatric Orthopaedic
Surgeon
Bristol Royal Hospital for Children
Bristol, UK

Alexander Montgomery
Consultant Spinal
Orthopaedic Surgeon
Royal London Hospital
London, UK

Mark Mullins
Consultant Orthopaedic Surgeon
Morriston Hospital
Swansea, UK

Amir Ali Narvani
Consultant Orthopaedic Surgeon
Ashford and St Peter's Hospitals
NHS Trust
Surrey, UK

Aresh-Hashemi Nejad
Consultant Orthopaedic Surgeon
Royal National Orthopaedic Hospital
Middlesex, UK

Ali Noorani
Consultant Orthopaedic and Trauma
Surgeon (Upper Limb Service)
Royal London Hospital
London, UK

Tom Nunn
Consultant Trauma and Orthopaedics
Surgeon
Royal Alexandra Hospital
Glasgow, UK

Natasha Rahman
Consultant Orthopaedic Surgeon
Royal Sussex County Hospital
Brighton, UK

Manoj Ramachandran
Consultant Orthopaedic Surgeon
and Honorary Reader
Royal London Hospital
London, UK

Navin Ramachandran
Consultant Radiologist and Honorary
Senior Lecturer
University College London Hospitals
NHS Trust
London, UK

Anil Ranawat
Associate Attending Orthopedic
Surgeon and Associate Professor of
Orthopedic Surgery
Hospital for Special Surgery
New York, USA

Vijai Ranawat
Senior Medical Practitioner
Department of Orthopaedics
The Repatriation General Hospital
Adelaide, Australia

Arun Ranganathan
Consultant Orthopaedic and Spinal
Surgeon
Royal London Hospital
London, UK

Mark Paterson
Consultant Paediatric Orthopaedic
Surgeon (ex)
Royal London Hospital
London, UK

Dan Perry
Senior Lecturer in Orthopaedic
Surgery and Honorary Consultant
Orthopaedic Surgeon
Alder Hey Children's NHS Trust
Liverpool, UK

Andrew Price
Consultant Orthopaedic Surgeon
and Professor
Nuffield Orthopaedic Centre
Oxford, UK

Asif Saifuddin
Consultant Radiologist
Royal National Orthopaedic Hospital
Middlesex UK

Anish Sangrajka
Consultant Paediatric Orthopaedic
Surgeon
The Norfolk and Norwich University
Hospitals NHS Trust
Norwich, UK

Nicholas Saw
Consultant Orthopaedic Surgeon
Princess Alexandra Hospital
Essex, UK

Patrick Schottel
Orthopedic Surgeon and Assistant
Professor
The University of Vermont Medical
Center
Vermont, USA

Imad Sedki
Consultant in Rehabilitation
Medicine
Royal National Orthopaedic Hospital
Middlesex, UK

Dishan Singh
Consultant Orthopaedic Surgeon
Royal National Orthopaedic Hospital
Middlesex, UK

Sertazniel SinghKang
Consultant Trauma & Orthopaedic
Surgeon and Associate Lecturer
Cambridge University Hospitals NHS
Foundation Trust
Cambridge, UK

John Skinner
Consultant Orthopaedic Surgeon
Royal National Orthopaedic Hospital
Middlesex, UK

John Stammers
Specialty Registrar in Trauma &
Orthopaedic Surgery Royal London
Hospital
London, UK

Cheh-Chin Tai
Hip & Knee Orthopaedic Surgeon
Department of Orthopaedic Surgery
University of Malaya
Malaysia

Tim Waters
Consultant Orthopaedic Surgeon,
Clinical Director for Trauma &
Orthopaedics
West Hertfordshire Hospitals NHS
Trust
Herts, UK

Alan White
Consultant Orthopaedic Surgeon
Southend University Hospital
Westcliff-on-Sea, UK

Andrew Williams
Consultant Orthopaedic Surgeon
Chelsea and Westminster Hospital
NHS Trust
London, UK

Lester Wilson
Consultant Spinal Surgeon
Royal National Orthopaedic Hospital
Middlesex, UK

Andrea Yeo
Consultant Paediatric Orthopaedic
Surgeon
St George's University Hospital NHS
Trust
London, UK

Thomas Youm
Clinical Assistant Professor and
Director of Hip Arthroscopy
NYU Hospital for Joint Diseases
New York, USA

Preface to the second edition

I am extremely proud to be able to bring you, the reader, the second edition of the Basic Orthopaedic Sciences book. It has been another labour of love but this time, I have had constant and incredible help from Tom Nunn who has kept me going through this process but has also signficantly enhanced the book with his amazing illustrations. Thanks Tom!

I've tried to correct any and all the mistakes from the first edition but if any creep through, do let me know. There are new chapters and updated concepts throughout and I hope this book continues to be as comprehensive as the first was.

You may have noticed that the title of the second edition has been shortened to Basic Orthopaedic Sciences. This is for two reasons. The first is that all the new contributors (each chapter has had at least one new contributor added whose job was to refresh the text, approaching it with new eyes) came from institutions around the world, which made this book a truly global effort. Therefore, I wanted to stay away from a title that implied parochialism. Secondly, I have been a Consultant Orthopaedic Surgeon for more than ten years now, primarily at the Royal London and Barts and The London Children's Hospitals, Barts Health NHS Trust in London, England and although the concepts for the second edition matured during my time here, I still wanted to keep the title general and not allied to any particular institution.

Finally, I want to thank all the contributors, new and old, for making this book what it has become and I hope you, the reader, find it helpful for building the solid foundations of your orthopaedic knowledge and practice.

Manoj Ramachandran

manojorthopod@gmail.com

London 2017

The first edition of this book is legendary, the sacred text of orthopaedic basic science. I am convinced it is the reason I, and many like me, passed the FRCS(Tr&Orth).

In the preface to that edition, as here, Manoj suggests the reader send any feedback they may have in order that he may improve upon the edition. This is not mere editorial rhetoric. He means it. In 2009 I met Manoj at what was then the pre-exam revision course based upon his book. I gave my "feedback" on the diagrams, and a few emails and years later, I found myself entrusted with reconceptualising and producing pretty much every image in the book.

I am not a formally trained illustrator, I am an orthopaedic surgeon just like many of you. I do however know the importance of a good diagram and have an enthusiasm for them and the role they have in the learning process. The English idiom "a picture paints a thousand words" may often be over used, but here I feel it is entirely appropriate. Drawings have three main uses as I see it: to aid in the understanding of a concept, to help in the recollection of that information, and to allow one to relay that same information quickly and easily when needed (to an examiner for example). The diagrams I have produced will hopefully deliver on the first two and I would implore you to not shy away from using them for the third.

I hope you enjoy this book as much as I have enjoyed helping produce it, and do send your feedback. Who knows, in another few years, it could be you sitting here writing an entry for a future edition!

Tom Nunn

tom@nunngeo.com

Glasgow 2017

Preface to the first edition

How many times have you heard a colleague say, "I once knew everything about articular cartilage/hip biomechanics/statistics (*substitute any orthopaedic basic science topic here*) but I seem to have forgotten the exact details. Anyway, you're the one sitting the exam, not me!" Oh, how trainees love to hear those dulcet tones of encouragement . . .

I like to think that learning orthopaedic basic sciences is somewhat similar to learning anatomy at medical school. It is certainly better to have learnt once than not at all. Equally, it is better to have understood concepts than to have committed facts to rote memory. Having spouted all these wise words though, I still feel that there is an awful lot to learn in orthopaedic basic sciences. The aim of this book is to tease out the pertinent points that are relevant both to exam situations and day-to-day clinical practice. Although originally conceived with postgraduate orthopaedic exams in mind, the final text has evolved into a primer in basic sciences for all health professionals with an interest in orthopaedics, mainly as a result of the input from all the contributors.

This first edition has drawn from and expanded on the popular "Stanmore Basic Sciences course" run at the Royal National Orthopaedic Hospital in Middlesex, UK. The book's scope and focus were determined by feedback from candidates on the course and from field-testing at its various stages of development (which makes it sound much more impressive than it really was!). Ideas such as bold highlighting of key words and concepts, and the use of only five key references for further reading, were added along the way. Diagrams have been kept simple for ease of reproduction as and when required. Although the book is not exhaustive, and indeed does not claim to be, a working knowledge of the text should serve the readers well in their journey through the quagmire that is basic sciences.

Finally, a personal note. I wanted to put together a text that doesn't insult the reader by aiming too low and omitting key information. Equally, aiming too high (as some books do) would be disastrous. I've settled for a happy medium. I urge you, the reader, having read this book, to rest safe in the knowledge that you are at the higher end of the orthopaedic basic science Gaussian curve. And from this vantage position, from where you can attack any exam-related or basic science query, I urge you to send me feedback so I can improve upon this edition and perhaps even invite you onto the panel of authors on the next one.

Now all you have to do is start by learning how exactly a Gaussian curve is defined . . .

Manoj Ramachandran

manojorthopod@gmail.com

London 2006

Foreword to the first edition

Knowledge of basic science is an essential platform on which to build an understanding of orthopaedics. It is necessary for day-to-day clinical work, research, publications and examinations. This book has been developed to cover the major areas of basic science required by orthopaedic surgeons and all those associated with musculoskeletal function and dysfunction.

Although it would be impossible to cover every facet of basic science, the sections are wide-ranging, from statistics to biomechanics and from pharmacology to gait analysis. Sections on all the musculoskeletal tissues have been included, together with sections on the functions of all the joints. Relevant areas of biomaterials, friction and lubrication, together with the basic tools of research, including statistics, have also been included in a form that provides the essence of knowledge required of the trainee.

The majority of the chapters have a junior and senior author. Each senior author has an expertise in the area covered, while the junior author has provided the focus required for postgraduate orthopaedic examinations. Each section is well organized and easy to read and contains a wealth of information essential to the reader. The viva questions are useful in assessing the reader's understanding of the section with an added essential reading section for the examination candidate.

Basic Orthopaedic Sciences: The Stanmore Guide has been ably edited by Manoj Ramachandran, Paediatric and Young Adult Fellow on the Stanmore Rotation, who is to be congratulated in bringing together such a disparate group of topics, along with the contributors for making many difficult topics so understandable.

I am sure this book will become a necessary addition to any library for those requiring information on orthopaedic basic sciences in a concise and readable form.

George SE Dowd MD MCh(Orth) FRCS

Consultant Orthopaedic Surgeon (ex),

Royal Free Hospital, London, UK

Acknowledgements in the first edition

I'd like to start by thanking all the authors for putting up with my constant nagging about deadlines. I hope you all think it was worth the effort. The senior reviewers did a great job too. I must single out Dishan Singh as the book's catalyst during its embryonic stages. The conversations we had back in 2002 are the reason why this book even came into being. In addition, Deborah Eastwood worked tirelessly (as always!) in the latter stages of the book's development to ensure that deadlines were met and people were chased up.

I'd also like to thank and congratulate the team at Hodder Arnold for making this book happen. Finally, I must thank everyone in my personal life for putting up with me during my multiple projects. My deepest gratitude though goes to my wife, Joanna.

Abbreviations

5-ASA 5-aminosalicylic acid

A&E Accident & Emergency

AA atlantoaxial, abduction/adduction

AAOS American Academy of Orthopedic Surgeons

AbDM abductor digiti minimi

ABS amniotic band syndrome

AC alternating current

ACh acetylcholine

AChR acetylecholine receptor

ACI autologous chondrocyte implantation

ACL anterior cruciate ligament

ACR American College of Rheumatology

ADAMT a disintegrin and metalloproteinase

ADI atlantodens interval

AER apical ectodermal ridge

AFO ankle–foot orthosis

AL annular ligament

ALCL accessory lateral collateral ligament

ALVAL aseptic lymphocyte vasculitis-associated lesions

AML acute myeloid leukaemia

(c)AMP (cyclic) adenosine monophosphate

ANA antinuclear antibody

ANOVA analysis of one-way variance

AOFAS American Orthopaedic Foot and Ankle Society

AOL anterior oblique ligament

AP adductor pollicis, anteroposterior

APB abductor pollicis brevis

APL abductor pollicis longus

APTT activated partial thromboplastin time

ARDS acute respiratory distress syndrome

AS ankylosing spondylitis

ASA American Society of Anesthesiologists

ASTM American Standard Testing and Materials

ATP adenosine triphosphate

BCG bacillus Calmette–Guèrin

BCP bacteria-carrying particles

BMD bone mineral density

BMI body mass index

BML bone marrow oedema-like lesion

BMP bone morphogenetic protein

BOA British Orthopaedic Association

BR brachioradialis

BRU bone remodelling unit

CA community acquired

CAS Crk-associated substrate

CCP citrullinated cyclic peptide

CFU colony-forming units

CI confidence interval

CIA carpal instability adaptive

CIC carpal instability complex

CID carpal instability dissociative

CIND carpal instability non-dissociative

CKD chronic kidney disease

CMAP compound muscle action potential

CMC carpometacarpal

CMGP cartilage matrix glycoprotein

CMP cartilage matrix protein

CN cranial nerve

CNS central nervous system

COMP cartilage oligometric matrix protein

COPD chronic obstructive pulmonary disease

COR centre of rotation

COX cyclo-oxygenase

coxib cyclo-oxygenase-2 inhibitor

CPON C-flanking peptide of neuropeptide Y

CROW Charcot restraint orthotic walker

CRP C-reactive protein

CS chondroitin sulphate

CSF cerebrospinal fluid

CT computed tomography

CTEV congenital talipes equinovarus

CTS carpal tunnel syndrome

CTX carboxy-terminal

DAF decay accelerating factor

DAFO dynamic ankle–foot orthosis

DAMP distal-anterior and medial proximal

DBM demineralized bone matrix

DCO damage control orthopaedics

DDH developmental dysplasia of the hip

DDP direct dynamic problems

DEXA dual energy X-ray absorptiometry

DHFR dihydrofolate reductase

DIMS Digital Image Management System

DIO dorsal interosseous

DIP distal interphalangeal

DISI dorsal intercalated segmental instability

DMARD disease modifying antirheumatoid drug

DMD Duchenne's muscular dystrophy

DMOAD disease-modifying osteoarthritis drug

DMPT dimethyl-p-toluidine

DNA deoxyribonucleic acid

DOF degrees of freedom

DOMS delayed onset muscle soreness

DR digital radiography

DRUJ distal radioulnar joint

DTI direct thrombin inhibitor

DVT deep vein thrombosis

ECG electrocardiography

ECM extracellular matrix

ECRB extensor carpi radialis brevis

ECRL extensor carpi radialis longus

ECU extensor carpi ulnaris

EDC extensor digitorum communis

EDS Ehlers–Danlos' syndrome

EGF epidermal growth factor

EHD elastohydrodynamic

EIP extensor indicis

EM electromagnetic field

EMG electromyography

EPB extensor pollicis brevis

EPL extensor pollicis longus

ESR erythrocyte sedimentation rate

FBC full blood count

FCR flexor carpi radialis

FCU flexor carpi ulnaris

FDA Food and Drug Administration

FDG fluorodeoxyglucose

FDP flexor digitorum profundus

FDS flexor digitorum superficialis

F/E flexion/extension

FGF fibroblast growth factor

FGFR fibroblast growth factor receptor

FN false negative

FP false positive

FPB flexor pollicis brevis

FPL flexor pollicis longus

FPP farnesyl pyrophosphate

FR fluoroscopic receptor

GABA gamma aminobutyric acid

GAG glycosaminoglycan

G-CSF granulocyte colony-stimulating factor

GCT giant-cell tumour

GFR glomerular filtration rate

GHJ glenohumeral joint

GI gastrointestinal

G/M-CSF granulocyte/macrophage colony-stimulating factor

GnRH gonadotrophin releasing hormone

GRAFO ground reaction ankle–foot orthosis

GRF ground reaction force

HA hospital acquired/hyaluronic acid

HD hydrodynamic

HEPA high-efficiency particulate air

HGPRT hypoxanthine–guanine phosphoribosyltransferase

HIP hot isostatic press(ing)

HIT heparin-induced thrombocytopenia

HIV human immunodeficiency virus

HKAFO hip–knee–ankle–foot orthosis

HLA human leucocyte antigen

HMO hereditary multiple osteochondromatosis

HR heart rate

HRT hormone replacement therapy

IC initial contact

IDP inverse dynamic problems

IFSSH International Federation of Societies Surgery of the Hand

Ig immunoglobulin

IGF insulin-like growth factor

IGHL inferior glenohumeral ligament

II image intensifier

IL interleukin

IM intramedullary

INF interferon

INR international normalized ratio

IP interphalangeal

IRMER Ionizing Radiation (Medical Exposure) Regulations

ISO International Standards Organization

ISW initial swing

ITAP intraosseous trans-cutaneous amputation prosthesis

ITU Intensive Therapy Unit

JRF joint reaction force

KS keratan sulphate

LCL lateral collateral ligament

LFA low friction arthroplasty

LIA local infiltration analgesia

LIPUS low-intensity pulsed ultrasound

LL lumbar lordosis

LM lateral meniscus

LMWH low-molecular weight heparin

LR loading response

LTL lunotriquetral ligament

LUCL lateral ulnar collateral ligament

MACI matrix-induced autologous chondrocyte implantation

MCI mid-carpal instability

MCL medial collateral ligament

MCP metacarpophalangeal, monocyte chemoattractant protein

M-CSF monocyte colony-stimulating factor

MDR multi-drug resistant

MED multiple endocrine neoplasia

MEHD micro-elastohydrodynamic

MEN multiple endocrine neoplasia

MGHL middle glenohumeral ligament

MIP macrophage inflammatory protein

MIPO minimally invasive plate osteosynthesis

MM medial meniscus

MMP matrix metalloproteinase

MMTV mouse mammary tumour virus

MOFS multiple organ failure syndrome

MPFL medial patellofemoral ligament

MPS mucopolysaccharidoses

MR magnetic resonance

MRC Medical Research Council

MRI magnetic resonance imaging

MRSA methicillin-resistant *Staphylococcus aureus*

MS mid-stance

MSC mesenchymal stem cell

MSW mid-swing

MT metatarsal

MTP metatarsaophalangeal

MUAP motor unit action potential

MW molecular weight

NAC N-acetylcysteine

NAP nerve action potential

NAPQI N-acetyl-p-benzoquinone imine

NCS nerve conduction studies

NF neurofibromatosis

NICE National Institute for Health and Care Excellence

NJR National Joint Registry

NMDA N-methyl-D-aspartate

NPV negative predictive value

NSAID non-steroidal anti-inflammatory drug

NSF nephrogenic systemic fibrosis

NSU non-specific urethritis

NTD neural tube defect

OA osteoarthritis

OI osteogenesis imperfecta

ON osteonecrosis

OP opponens pollicis

OR odds ratio

PACS Patient Archiving and Communications System

PBP penicillin-binding protein

PCA patient controlled analgesia

PCL posterior cruciate ligament

PCP peri-meniscal capillary plexus

PCR polymerase chain reaction

PDGF platelet-derived growth factor

PDS polydioxanone

PET positron emission tomography

PF platelet factor

PFL popliteofibular ligament

PG prostaglandin/proteoglycan

PHP pseudo-parathyroidism

PI pelvic incidence

PIN posterior interosseous nerve

PIP proximal interphalangeal

PIVKA proteins in vitamin K absence

PL phospholipase/palmaris longus

PMA polar moment area

PMC posteromedial complex

PMMA polymethyl-methacrylate

PMN polymorphonucleocyte

PNET primitive neuroectodermal tumour

PNS peripheral nervous system

POL popliteal oblique ligament/posterior oblique ligament

PPAMaid pneumatic post-amputation mobility aid

PPV positive predictive value

PQ pronator quadratus

PROM patient-related outcome measure

PRP platelet-rich plasma

PSA prostate specific antigen

PT pronator teres, parathyroid

PTB patella tendon-bearing

PTFE polytetrafluoroethylene

PTH parathyroid hormone

PVL Panton Valentine Leukocidin

PZ progress zone

RA rheumatoid arthritis

RCL radial collateral ligament

RCT randomized controlled trial

RDA recommended daily allowance

RF radiofrequency

RhF rheumatoid factor

RGO reciprocating gait orthosis

RMM relative molecular mass

RNA ribonucleic acid

RNS reactive nitrogen species

ROS reactive oxygen species

RR relative risk

SACH solid ankle cushioned heel

SCD sickle cell disease

SD standard deviation

SE standard error

SED spondyloepiphyseal dysplasia

SERM selective oestrogen receptor modulator

SFR screen film radiography

SGHL superior glenohumeral ligament

SHH sonic hedgehog homologue

SI Systéme International (d'Unitès)/sacral inclination

SIJ sacroiliac joint

SIRS systemic inflammatory response syndrome

SLAC scapholunate advanced collapse

SLAP superior labrum anterior and posterior

SLE systemic lupus erythmatosus

SLL scapholunate ligament

SMA second moment area

SNAC scaphoid non-union advanced collapse

SNAP sensory nerve action potential

SORL spiral oblique retinacular ligament of Landsmeer

SPECT single photon-emission computed tomography

SSEP somatosensory evoked potential

TAR thrombocytopaenia-absent radius syndrome/total ankle replacement

TB tuberculosis

TEL trans-epicondylar line

TES total elastic suspension

TFCC triangular fibrocartilage complex

TG trochlear groove

TGF transforming growth factor

Th T-helper

THKAFO trunk–hip–knee–ankle–foot orthosis

THR total hip replacement

TIMMP tissue inhibitor of matrix metalloproteinase

TKA trochanter–knee–ankle

TKR total knee replacement

TL transverse ligament

TLO thoracolumbar orthosis

TLSO thoracolumbar sacral orthosis

TN true negative

TNF-α tumour necrosis factor-alpha

TP true positive

TRAFO tone-reducing ankle–foot orthosis

TRAP tartrate-resistant isoenzyme of acid phosphatase

TS terminal stance

TSE transmissible spongiform encephalopathy

TSH thyroid stimulating hormone

TSW terminal swing

TT tibial tuberosity

UCBL University of California at Berkeley Laboratory

UHMWPE ultra-high-molecular weight polyethylene

US ultrasound

UV ultraviolet

VACTERL vertebral anomalies, anal atresia, cardiac abnormalities, tracheoesophageal fistula, oesophageal atresia, renal disorders, limb abnormalities

VCAM vascular cell adhesion molecule

VDDR vitamin D-dependent rickets

VDR vitamin D receptor

VEGF vascular endothelial growth factor

VISI volar intercalated segmental instability

WHO World Health Organization

WWC white cell count

ZPA zone of polarizing activity

1 Statistics

Manoj Ramachandran, Dan Perry, David Little and Fares Haddad

Introduction

A working knowledge of statistics is essential for any healthcare professional working within the sphere of orthopaedics. At its most basic, statistics involves the handling of data, best thought of in three ways:

- **Data collection**, e.g. surveys.
- **Data presentation,** e.g. graphs, tables.
- **Data interpretation**, e.g. hypothesis testing, confidence intervals.

In well-designed studies, statisticians work in conjunction with orthopaedic surgeons from the outset, to maximize the methodological and statistical strength of a research study. All orthopaedic surgeons should have an awareness of the principles of study design, and be able to interpret the results of a study objectively.

Data type

Types of data are summarized in *Table 1.1*.

Table 1.1 Data types

Discrete → Continuous			
	Nominal	Categories without order, e.g. eye colour	Non-parametric
	Binomial	2 possible outcomes, e.g.dead/alive, success/failure, heads/tails	Non-parametric
	Ordinal	Categories with order, e.g. small/medium/large	Non-parametric
	Integer	Ordered scale of whole numbers (no fractions or divisions), e.g. screw lengths (22 mm, 24 mm, 26 mm…)	Non-parametric or parametric
	Interval	Ordered numerical measurement with subdivisions, e.g. height, weight, volume	Parametric

Data presentation

Plotting of data allows determination of **central tendency** and **spread** (or variability/variance). The familiar symmetrical bell-shaped curve of a **normal (or Gaussian) distribution** (**Figure 1.1a**) allows for the use of the mean as a measure of central tendency and is common throughout medicine.

Bell-shaped curves, when asymmetrical, are not distributed normally. A **skewed distribution** is asymmetrical and has a tail, which is either positive or negative. If data distribution is skewed, then the median or mode has to be used to measure central tendency. By assuming that the mode of the distribution represents the 'zero point', then positive skews have the long tail on the positive side, and negative skews have the long tail on the negative side. If there is doubt about the normality of a distribution, then it is best to assume that any given distribution is not normal. The easiest examples of skewed distributions concern age, i.e. positive skew – age at which anterior cruciate ligament (ACL) surgery occurs; negative skew – age at which total hip replacement (THR) surgery occurs.

Transformation is the method by which non-normal data can be mathematically normalized in order to allow parametric testing. This is most commonly achieved using logarithmic transformations.

Measures of central tendency

- **Mean**: the average of the data, measured by dividing the sum of all the observations by the number of observations.
- **Median**: the central value of the data; used for ordinal data.
- **Mode**: the data value with the most frequency; used for nominal data.

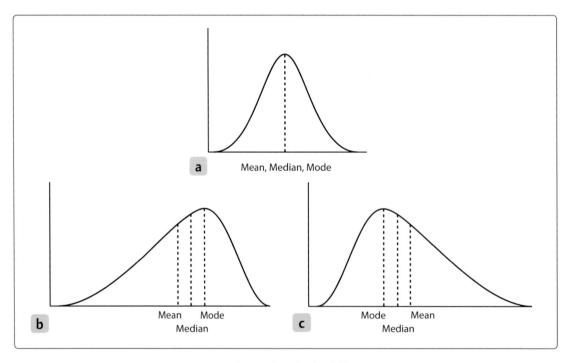

Figure 1.1 Mean, median and modes for different data spreads.
(a) normal distribution (b) negative skew (c) positive skew.

For perfectly normally distributed data, the mean, median and mode are the same. This does not hold true for skewed data (**Figure 1.1b,c**). In skewed distributions the median (i.e. middle) is always in between the mode and mean on a graph.

Measures of spread/variability

- **Range:** the lowest and highest values of the data. The range does not give much information about the spread of the data about the mean.
- **Percentiles:** groupings of data into brackets. Commonly this is groupings of 25% (known as quartiles), from which the interquartile range can be calculated.
- **Variance:** the measure of the spread where the mean is the measure of the central tendency. Variance is the corrected sum of squares about the mean $[\sigma(x-\text{mean})^2/(n-1)]$.
- **Standard deviation (σ):** the square root of the variance (the use of the square root gives the same dimension as the data). For reasonably symmetrical bell-shaped data, one standard deviation (SD) contains roughly 68% of the data, two SD contains roughly 95% of the data and three SD contains around 99.7% of the data (**Figure 1.2**). A normal distribution is defined uniquely by two parameters, the mean and the SD of the population. Other features of a normal distribution include that it is symmetrical (mean = mode = median) and that the data are continuous.
- **Standard error (SE) of the mean:** defined as the SD divided by the square root of the sample size. Used in relation to a sample rather than the population as a whole. It can be thought of as being equivalent to the SD for the true mean, i.e. 68% confidence that the population mean lies within one SE of the calculated (sample) mean, 95% confidence that population mean lies within two SEs of the sample mean, 99.7% for three SEs. The formula does not assume a normal distribution.

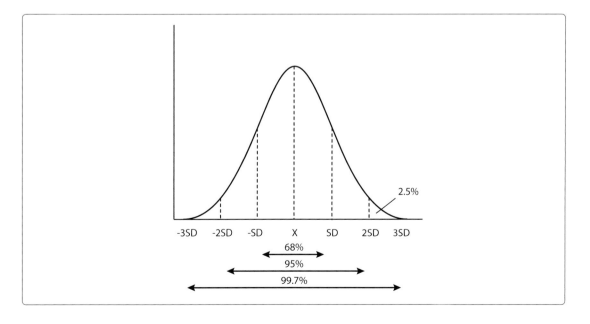

Figure 1.2 Standard deviations (SDs) of normally distributed data.

- **Confidence interval (CI):** two SEs either side of the sample mean determines the 95% CI of the mean (i.e. we are confident that the true population mean lies within this range of values). Confidence intervals are preferred to *P* values (see below) because:
  - CIs relate to the sample size;
  - a range of values is provided;
  - CIs provide a rapid visual impression of significance;
  - CIs have the same units as the variable.

Data interpretation

All good studies test hypotheses. When statistics are used to examine data concerning hypotheses, the key concept is that of the **null hypothesis**, where a primary assumption is made that any difference seen occurred purely by chance. The collected data are then tested to disprove the null hypothesis; if the result is statistically significant, then the hypothesis is rejected on the basis that it is wrong. The difference, therefore, must be real and did not occur by chance.

It is possible to calculate the probability that any difference seen did occur by chance. Orthopaedic surgeons are usually willing to accept a 5% probability that the difference seen was due to chance ($P=0.05$). If *P* is less than 0.05, then this suggests that the probability of the difference seen being due to chance is less than 5% (for $P<0.001$, the probability is less than 0.1%).

Errors

Errors may arise when accepting or rejecting the null hypothesis. A type I (α) error occurs when a difference is found, but in reality there is not a difference (i.e. a false-positive result, and therefore the null hypothesis is rejected incorrectly). This is one of those 5% of cases where the difference occurred by chance. A good analogy is convicting an innocent person of a crime. We can protect against type I errors by reducing significance levels, although this increases the risk of a type II error occurring. Note that the risk of a type I error decreases as the acceptable *P* value is lowered, but then bigger study samples are needed in order to protect against a type II error.

A type II (β) error occurs when no difference is found but in reality a difference does exist (i.e. a false-negative result, and therefore the null hypothesis is accepted incorrectly). A good analogy here is failing to convict a person who is guilty of a crime. Type II errors are usually the result of a small sample size; therefore, it is important to perform a power analysis before undertaking a study. We can protect against type II errors with statistical power. Note that type I and type II errors are related inversely. Type II errors are common in orthopaedic studies.

A type III (γ) error occurs rarely when the researcher correctly rejects the null hypothesis but incorrectly attributes the cause. In other words, the researcher misinterprets cause and effect. Type III error is also used facetiously to refer to the mistake of switching the definitions of type I and type II errors.

Power analysis

A **statistical power analysis** is a method of determining the number of subjects needed in a study in order to have a reasonable chance of showing a difference if one exists. The statistical power is the probability of demonstrating a true effect or statistically significant difference and is defined by $1 - \beta$ expressed as a percentage. The statistical power is therefore the probability that the test will correctly reject the null hypothesis. Power analysis must be performed before a study commences; without power analysis, it is difficult to know whether any lack of statistical significance is due to the lack of a real difference or due to a small sample size. When reviewing a study that lacks a statement about power, a post-hoc power analysis can be useful in estimating the probability of type II error.

Factors affecting power analyses

- Size of the difference between the means (the larger the difference, the easier it is to detect a difference and the greater the power).
- Spread/variability of the data (the larger the spread, the less likely a difference will be detected).
- Acceptable level of significance (i.e. the *P* value that is set).
- Sample size (power increases with increasing sample size).
- Experimental design (e.g. within subjects versus between subjects).
- Type of data (parametric versus non-parametric).

If the power of an experiment is low, then there is a good chance that the experiment will be inconclusive or give a type II error; thus, it is important to consider power in the design of experiments. As a general rule, if the clinically relevant difference approximates one SD of the measured variable, then 17 (or about 20) subjects are required in each group.

Study design

The first decision is whether the study is to be **observational** or **experimental**. In an observational study, the investigator observes rather than alters events. A review of the prevalence of pulmonary emboli after total hip replacement is an example of an observational or descriptive study. In an experimental study, the investigator applies a manoeuvre and then observes the outcome. For example, a surgeon may conduct a randomized trial comparing the effects of warfarin and heparin on the prevalence of deep venous thromboses in patients managed with total hip replacement. The investigator must also decide on the timeline of the study.

Study timelines

- **Retrospective study:** the outcome of interest has already occurred and the patient or cohort (group of patients) is followed forward in time from a point in the past. This is most typically a case–control study with the study participants divided based on outcome (i.e. disease or no disease).
- **Prospective study:** follows the patient or cohort forward in time; stronger than a retrospective study. This is most typically a cohort study with the study participants divided based on exposure (i.e. exposure to a chemical or no exposure to a chemical – to have surgery or not to have surgery).
- **Cross-sectional study:** examines patients or events at one point in time without follow-up; used, for example, when looking at the prevalence of a condition or describing the distribution of variables.

The next step is the generation of a null hypothesis. Following this, a power calculation is required in order to estimate the sample size. Value judgements are made regarding the risks of type I and type II errors acceptable, based on the clinical and financial consequences of such a result. Typically, **the type I (α) error is set at 0.05** and the **type II (β) is set at 0.20, i.e. a power of 80% (1 – β)**. Calculation of the sample size also requires knowledge of the **effect size** (i.e. the difference expected between the means) and an estimation of the variance.

When performing multiple tests, each test carries a 5% risk of type I error, therefore multiple tests have a cumulative effect. To accommodate this the P value may have to be decreased. An example of correcting for this is the Bonferroni correction, which states simply that if one is testing "n" independent hypotheses, then one should use a significance level of 0.05/n. For example, if there are two independent hypotheses, then a result would be declared significant only if P is less than 0.025. Note that although tests are rarely independent, the Bonferroni correction is a very conservative procedure that is unlikely to reject the null hypothesis. Other corrections are available, e.g. Tukey's least significant difference procedure.

Significance testing

It is important to note that there may be a difference between clinical and statistical significance.

To test for statistical significance, think about the following:

- What type of data have been used in the study?
- What is the sample size?
- Are the groups distributed normally?
- Do the data need to be transformed so that we can make a normality assumption?
- Are the groups interdependent? (Is a paired test required?)
- Is a single- or two-tailed P value necessary? (Two-tailed tests are most common, though if looking for a unidirectional association then a single-tailed test may be used.)

Always remember that statistical significance and clinical significance are not the same. For example, a 5% change in callus size is unlikely to be relevant clinically, but a 25% change may be relevant. The P value does not relate to clinical significance but merely tells us how certain we are that the difference we are considering is real.

Next, the type of test to be used is considered. Tests can be **parametric** or **non-parametric**. Parametric tests assume that data were sampled from a normal distribution; non-parametric tests make no such assumption.

Features of parametric tests

- Assumes the data were sampled from a normal population.
- Observations must be independent.
- Populations must have the same variance.
- Can use absolute difference between data points.
- Increased power for a given sample size (n).

Features of non-parametric tests

- No assumptions are made about the origins of the data.
- No limitations on types of data.
- Rank order of values.
- Less likely to be significant.
- Decreased power for a given n.
- Cannot relate back to any parametric properties of the data.

It is best to use non-parametric tests if the outcome is a rank or score and the population is clearly not Gaussian, or if some of the values are off the scale (too high or low to measure). *Table 1.2* indicates which tests to use in which situation. It is worth knowing a little about the following tests:

Table 1.2 Tests for data types

	Normally distributed (from Gaussian population)	Not normally distributed (e.g. rank, score or measurement)	Nominal data (binomial outcome)
Describing one group	Mean, SD	Median, interquartile range	Proportion
Two treatments in different groups	Unpaired t-test	Mann-Whitney U test (rank test)	Chi-squared test (Fisher's for small samples)
Two treatments in same or matched group(s)	Paired t-test	Wilcoxon signed rank test	McNemar's test
More than two treatments in different groups	ANOVA	Kruksal-Wallis test	Chi-squared test
More than two treatments in same or matched group(s)	Repeated measures ANOVA	Friedman test	Cochrane Q test
Quantify association between two variables	Pearson correlation	Spearman correlation	Contingency coefficents
Predict value from another measured variable	Simple linear or nonlinear regression	Nonparametric regression	Simple logistic regression
Predict value from several measured or binomial variables	Multiple linear or nonlinear regression		Multiple logistic regression

ANOVA: analysis of one way variance; SD: standard deviation.

Paired t-test

This should be used when there is a pair of observations on a single subject, e.g. blood pressure before and after application of a tourniquet. If there are multiple observations, then analysis of one-way variance (ANOVA) should be used. Note that the t-test is also known as Student's t-test (it was developed by WS Gosset, writing under the pseudonym Student, who developed it whilst working for the Guinness brewery to monitor the quality of stout!).

Unpaired t-test

This can be used to compare two random samples provided they both follow a normal distribution. Samples can be of differing size but should be independent, i.e. there must be no chance that a subject could appear in both of the groups being compared.

Analysis of one-way variance

ANOVA determines the probability that two or more samples were drawn from the same parent population. ANOVA can be subclassified by secondary or grouping variables (two-way ANOVA), e.g. blood pressure before and after two different antihypertensive drugs. If some of the measurements were made in the same subjects, then the data can be corrected for repeated measures. Note that comparison of two samples with one-way ANOVA is very similar to performing an unpaired t-test.

Chi-squared test

The chi-squared (X^2) test can be used for qualitative data. It is used only on actual numbers of occurrences (i.e. frequencies), but not proportions, percentages, means or other derived statistics. The test compares distribution of a categorical variable in a sample with the distribution of a categorical variable in another sample. It assesses whether the observed data fit the expected pattern using the equation $\chi^2 = \sigma(O - E)^2/E$, where O is observed data and E is expected data. The test is unreliable if any of the expected values is less than five (in which case, use Fisher's exact test instead). If the number of subjects is small (fewer than 30), Yates' continuity correction has to be made in order to avoid individual values having an overly significant effect on the end result. Note that McNemar's test is a variant of the χ^2 test and is used for paired nominal data.

Correlation and regression

Correlation measures the degree of association between two parameters, with the correlation coefficient (r) being anywhere between −1 and +1. For the association between two continuous measures, **Pearson's correlation coefficient** is usually used, as a measure of association. If one parameter increases as the other does, then the correlation coefficient is positive (and vice versa). The data are always represented on a scatter plot. If a curved line is needed to express the relationship, then more complicated measures of correlation should be considered or **Spearman's rank correlation coefficient** may be used (which is also useful for demonstrating interdependence using ordinal data).

Once correlation is established, regression is the line drawn over the scatter plot using a regression equation $y = a + b_x$ with the regression coefficient being the direction coefficient of the regression line. Regression shows how one variable changes with another and can be used to find out what one variable is likely to be when the other is known. Regression relationships may be linear, multiple or logistic. The regression function r^2 indicates what amount of variance in the dependent variable is related to variance in the independent variable. For example, if knee pain correlates with walking distance by $r^2 = 0.6$, then 60% of the variation in walking distance can be explained by variation in knee pain. The remaining 40% of variability is not explained.

Data collection

In orthopaedics, there has been a drive to categorize different types of study according to the levels of evidence that they provide (*Table 1.3*).

Table 1.3 Level of evidence provided by types of trial

Types of studies				
	Therapeutic studies (investigating results of treatment)	Prognostic studies (investigating outcome of disease)	Diagnostic studies (investigating a diagnostic test)	Economic and decision analyses (developing an economic or decision model)
Level I	1 Randomized controlled trial (RCT) a. Significant difference b. No significant difference but narrow confidence intervals 2. Systematic reviews of Level-I RCTs (studies homogeneous)	1. Prospective study 2. Systematic review of Level-I studies	1. Testing of previously developed diagnostic criteria in series of consecutive patients (with universally applied reference "gold" standard) 2. Systematic review of Level-I studies	1. Clinically sensible costs and alternatives; values obtained from many studies; multiway sensitivity analyses 2. Systematic review of Level-I studies
Level II	1. Prospective cohort study 2. Poor-quality RCT (e.g. 80% follow-up) 3. Systematic review a. Level-II studies b. Non-homogeneous Level-I studies	1. Retrospective study 2. Study of untreated controls from a previous RCT 3. Systematic review of Level-II studies	1. Development of diagnostic criteria on basis of consecutive patients (with universally applied reference 'gold' standard) 2. Systematic review of Level-II studies	1. Clinically sensible costs and alternatives; values obtained from limited studies; multiway sensitivity analyses 2. Systematic review of Level-II studies
Level III	1. Case-control study 2. Retrospective cohort study 3. Systematic review of Level-III studies		1. Study of non-consecutive patients (no consistently applied reference "gold" standard) 2. Systematic review of Level-III studies	1. Limited alternatives and costs; poor estimates 2. Systematic review of Level-III studies
Level IV	Case series (no, or historical, control group)	Case series	1. Case-control study 2. Poor reference standard	No sensitivity analyses
Level V	Expert opinion	Expert opinion	Expert opinion	Expert opinion

Expert opinions

What an expert in the field has to say on a given subject.

Case series

With case series, the outcomes of a group are reported, but there is no comparison group. Case series are very weak in terms of causation. They should act as a stimulus for more powerful studies.

Case–control studies

Case-control studies are studies where individuals with a certain outcome (cases) are compared to individuals without the outcome (controls). A historic analysis of 'exposures' (i.e. the things that may have triggered the disease outcome) is then made. These studies are quick and cheap to perform and, if constructed carefully, can yield clinically relevant information, e.g. odds ratios (see below). They are particularly useful in trying to identify the causes of uncommon diseases. Unfortunately, case–control studies have many methodological biases.

Cohort studies

In a cohort study, two groups, one of which has been exposed to a factor of interest (i.e. a possible aetiological determinant – an intervention or a treatment), are followed up over time in order to compare outcomes such as onset of disease or adverse events. These studies are useful for identifying the incidence of the outcome within the defined population, and establishing relative risk. Problems with cohort studies include lengthy follow-up (i.e. a disease may only become apparent after many years following exposure), expense and the difficulty in examining rare diseases/outcomes as the practicalities of the study limit the initial size of the cohort.

Randomized controlled trials

Randomized controlled trials (RCTs) are intervention studies that are considered the gold standard. Groups of patients are randomized to either receive or not receive an intervention, and the outcomes are compared in a prospective manner. The aim of the study and the hypothesis to be tested are stated clearly.

Study design features

Important features of RCTs, and other types of study design, include the following:

- **Randomization:** this ensures that all prognostic variables, both known and unknown, will probably be distributed equally among the treatment groups. This avoids bias in treatment assignment. Types of randomization include the following:
  - **simple:** treatment allocations are assigned by computer-generated tables. This method may not be appropriate in small or multicentre trials. Note that dates of birth and days of the week are not appropriate methods of randomization.
  - **stratified:** if there are prognostic variables that are extremely important, then stratification ensures equal distribution between treatment groups. The computer programme also takes into account previously identified confounding factors. Generally, only two or three variables are stratified. Stratification is practical only in large trials and should be performed by each centre in multicentre trials.

- **block**: treatment is allocated by blocks of set size. This ensures that an equal number of patients is assigned to each treatment. For example, if the block size is six, then three receive treatment A and three receive treatment B.
- **Generalizability**: it is important to know to what or whom the results of the study apply (e.g. patients, surgeons) and also what the clinical implication of the results will be.
- **Sample selection: inclusion** and **exclusion criteria** should be decided upon and stated clearly in advance.
- **Outcome selection:** measures of outcome should be valid, reproducible and responsive to change. The choice of outcome should be clinically relevant. Note that objective outcomes, although measured more easily than subjective outcomes, may not always be the best choice. It is also worth considering **primary** and **secondary outcome measures**. Analysis is best made on an **intention-to-treat** basis, i.e. if a subject drops out during the study or changes treatment, that subject should still be included in the analyses. Another way of looking at this is to analyse according to the treatment that the subject was assigned to rather than the treatment that the subject actually underwent. The opposite of intention-to-treat analysis is **analysis per protocol** or on study.
- **Bias:** this refers to a flaw in impartiality that introduces systematic error into the methodology and results of a study. Bias can be reduced in a number of ways, including randomization, masking (previously known as blinding), and meticulous attention to the study protocol. Types of bias include the following:
  - **selection bias:** an individual may, or may not be included in the study if the investigator believes that one particular treatment would favour the individual over the other. This is particularly a concern if the investigator has awareness of the randomization sequence, and may therefore chose to include/exclude patients based on knowledge of their randomization allocation. This can be overcome by allocation concealment.
  - **ascertainment bias:** knowledge of the intervention (by either the researcher or the participant) may distort the results, because a belief is held that one treatment is better than the other. This can be overcome by masking/blinding.
  - **recall bias:** a person's recall may change based on the presence of disease (i.e. if a child is diagnosed with transient synovitis, then the parents are likely to have tried to rationalize the cause, and are more likely to remember that the child had a cough last week, compared with parents whose child doesn't have the condition). This is best overcome by prospective data collection, and/or biological measures where possible to validate results.
  - **publication bias:** higher publication success amongst those studies with positive findings.
- **Confounding factors:** when a variable is independently associated with both the outcome and the exposure, such that false conclusions are reached. One example may be that grey hair is associated with osteoarthritis (OA), which of course is confounded by age (age is associated with grey hair and OA). Confounding can be reduced by matching or measuring (i.e. stratification can be done looking at people at different ages with and without grey hair to see if hair colour really is independently associated with OA).
- **Masking/blinding:** this protects against ascertainment bias. Blinding can be single (only the patient is blinded) or double (both the patient and the investigator are blinded).
- **Ethics:** consent from an ethics committee (usually local or regional) is required for RCTs.

- **Publication:** it is important to know a target for publication from the outset of a study, so it can be focused towards the readership.
- **Equivalence study:** this is a RCT in which two treatments are expected to have the same outcome. The research hypothesis is that there is a difference between the two groups (known as the **alternative hypothesis,** as opposed to the null hypothesis). Studies such as this are used, for example, to compare prophylactic methods for preventing deep vein thromboses.

Meta-analyses and systematic reviews

Meta-analyses are becoming increasingly popular with the advent of evidence-based medicine. They are also termed 'secondary research'. The aim is to find the relevant evidence from several studies in an unbiased manner and to appraise each paper, including all randomized trials, for methodological quality. The results are reported as a common estimate with its confidence interval. Meta-analyses are at the top of the evidence hierarchy, but they may vary in their methodologies, may be heterogeneous in their results, may paint a overly rosy picture because of publication bias (i.e. reporting positive more often than negative results) and may duplicate data. The results are usually presented in the form of a forest plot (**Figure 1.3**), The left hand column includes the studies reviewed, and the right has a measure of the effect size for each study with a CI. The area of each 'square' indicates the weight of the study (i.e. fatter squares are from bigger studies, and the CI is usually narrower). A vertical line indicates the line of no effect i.e. odds ratio = 1, so if the CIs cross this line then the study demonstrated no significant effect. An overall effect size is denoted by a diamond, the size of which is determined by the overall 95% CI.

Systematic reviews are different from meta-analyses, in that no common estimate or CIs are given. The Cochrane Collaboration organizes and publishes highly detailed systematic reviews in its database and maintains a register of all published RCTs. The Cochrane Collaboration also maintains a prospective register of RCTs as they commence.

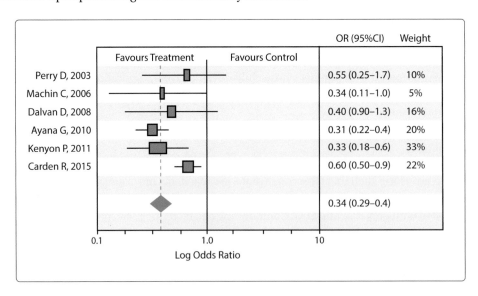

Figure 1.3 Example of a forest plot.

Screening and epidemiology

It is worth knowing a little about screening – who to screen and why should we screen people. In orthopaedics the most commonly encountered screening situation is that for developmental dysplasia of the hip, which causes lots of controversy regarding who and how to screen. The Wilson–Jungner criteria (published by the World Health Organization, 1968) form a framework on which to consider the optimal criteria for screening. The mnemonic '**IATROGENIC**' is a useful aide-memoire.

Screening criteria

- The condition should be an **I**mportant health problem with known incidence.
- There is an **A**ccepted and effective treatment.
- **T**reatment and diagnostic facilities should be available.
- **R**ecognizable latent and early symptomatic stage(s) should be present, and consideration should be given to whether early pick-up at the latent stage leads to intervention and to whether intervention improves outcome.
- **O**pinions on who to treat are agreed.
- There is **G**uaranteed safety, sensitivity and specificity of the test.
- Examination and/or treatment are acceptable to the patient.
- The **N**atural history of the condition should be known.
- Tests are **I**nexpensive and simple to perform.
- The screening programme should be **C**ost-effective, with a policy drawn up on whom to treat, and it should be continuously rolled out and repeated at intervals.

In orthopaedics the screening programme to be most aware of is that for developmental dysplasia of the hip in childhood, although some authorities have termed the programme 'surveillance' rather than true screening.

Epidemiology is the study of the patterns, causes and effects of disease in a population. The following definitions are important to remember:

- **Incidence**: incidence is in the number of new cases of disease in a defined population in a given time period. The rate is found by dividing the number of new cases in the study period by the population at risk.
- **Prevalence**: prevalence is the number of cases of a disease at a given time. Prevalence is found by dividing the number of patients with the disease by the total population (i.e. sum of the number of the patients with the disease and the number of patients at risk).
- **Sensitivity**: sensitivity is the ability of a test to identify true cases of disease. The sensitivity is found by dividing the number of true positives (TPs) by the sum of all the patients with the condition (TP + FN) = [TP/(TP + FN)], i.e. true positive/disease positive. *Table 1.4* helps when working this and other test-related values out.
- **Specificity**: the specificity is the ability of a test to exclude false positives (FPs), i.e. to exclude the disease. Specificity is found by dividing the number of true negatives (TNs) by the sum of all the patients without the condition [TN/(TN + FP)], i.e. true negative/ disease negative.

Table 1.4 Standard contingency table

	Disease positive	Disease negative
Test positive	True positive (TP)	False positive (FP)
Test negative	False negative (FN)	True negative (TN)

- **Positive predictive value:** the positive predictive value (PPV) is the probability that a subject who tests positive is truly positive, i.e. the PPV indicates the significance of a positive test. The PPV is found by dividing all positive test results in patients with the disease by the total number of positive test results [TP/(TP + FP)], i.e. true positive/test positive.
- **Negative predictive value:** the negative predictive value (NPV) is the probability that a subject who tests negative is truly negative, i.e. the NPV indicates the significance of a negative test. The NPV is found by dividing all negative test results in patients without the condition by the total number of negative test results [TN/(TN + FN)], i.e. true negative/test negative.
- **Accuracy:** the accuracy gives an idea of how often a test is correct [TP + TN)/(TP + TN + FP + FN)].
- **Odds ratio and relative risk:** both of these terms are used to compare the likelihood of an event between two groups. However, the results can be very different, and it is best shown by example. *Table 1.5* shows the results of a fictional cohort study that looked at the risk of OA in a group of runners, compared to non-runners. It is evident that 2/3 of runners developed OA, and only 1/3 of non-runners – the relative risk (RR) in runners is therefore 2, as runners are twice as likely to get OA. However, in runners the odds of OA were 2:1 in favour of OA, and in non-runners were 1:2 (more correctly described as 2:1 against OA). The odds ratio (OR) (simply the ratio of the odds) is therefore (2/1 divided by 1/2) = 4. ORs are generally less logical and always overstate an association. Odds ratios are necessary in some study designs, such as case–control studies, when the sample is selected based on outcome rather than exposure, which artificially alters the proportion of disease in the sample, relative to the normal population.

Table 1.5 Relative risk and odds ratio

	Osteoarthritis	No osteoarthritis
Runners	30	15
Non-runners	15	30

Outcome measures

There are several properties required of an outcome measure, which is especially important of patient-related outcome measures (PROMs).

Validity

The validity is the extent to which a test or outcome measure actually measures what it purports to measure. Tests have to be **precise** (consistency of repeated measures) and **accurate** (represent what they mean to represent). The different types of validity include:

- **Construct validity:** the extent to which a measure corresponds to theoretical concepts or constructs concerning the phenomenon of interest.
- **Content validity:** the extent to which a measure represents the domain of interest.
- **Criterion or concurrent validity:** correlating scores on a new instrument or test with external criteria known or believed to measure the attribute.

Responsiveness to change

The test has to be able to reflect the positive or negative effects of any interventions. This has to be tested in a clinical setting.

Reliability

The reliability assesses the random error of a measure. It is important to consider reliability within the same assessor (**intraobserver**) and with different assessors (**interobserver**). Clinical disagreement is ubiquitous in medicine, e.g. classification systems have come under a great deal of scrutiny. If two clinicians do not agree, then the classification cannot be accurate. In general, most systems show at best slight to moderate agreement. Sources of disagreement may arise from the following:

- The examiner:
  - understanding of classification;
  - prior expectation;
  - level of expertise and experience.
- The classification:
  - vague;
  - complex;
  - inaccurate.
- The tool:
  - inaccurate;
  - imprecise.

When measuring agreement, one must be aware that, as a result of the law of averages, there is bound to be agreement by chance. **Kappa analysis** involves adjusting the observed proportion of agreement in relation to the proportion of agreement expected by chance. Kappa analysis is used for categorical data. A value of 1.0 indicates complete agreement, a value of 0 indicates that the agreement can be explained purely by chance, and a negative value suggests systematic disagreement. Generally the following subclassification for kappa is used: 0–0.2, slight agreement; 0.2–0.4, fair agreement; 0.4–0.6, moderate agreement; 0.6–0.8, substantial agreement; 0.8–1.0, almost perfect agreement.

Correlation coefficients (or modifications thereof) are used when testing reliability of continuous data.

Survival analysis

Survival analysis is a study in which the outcome of an intervention is plotted over time, which allows for variable dates of entry and different lengths of follow-up. Data can be analysed at fixed intervals (**actuarial life-table method**) or at times of failure (**Kaplan–Meier product-limit method**) (**Figure 1.4**). The **definition of failure** must be clear from the outset, as must the treatment of loss to follow-up and death.

In order to construct a life table for joint replacements, the endpoint needs to be defined, which is usually 'revision' when investigating joint replacements. The number of joints being followed and the number of failures are determined for each year after operation. For each time period, the number of patients **at risk**, the number of **failures** and the number of **withdrawals** are recorded. The latter includes patients who have died, patients who have reached the end of the trial and patients lost to follow-up. Patients who complete the trial and deaths are treated as **successful withdrawals** – also known as censored data or non-endpoints; they do not count as failures and affect only the number of patients at risk. Losses to follow-up can be treated as **unsuccessful or successful withdrawals**, but this must be clarified in the methodology.

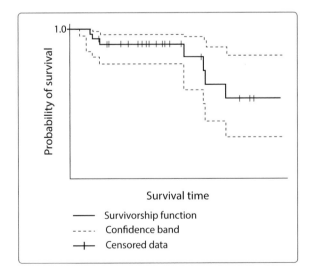

Figure 1.4 An example of Kaplan–Meier survival analysis.

The number of individuals at risk during each time period is calculated as the number of patients at the beginning of the period less half the number of withdrawals. The percentage failure rate for each period is determined from the number at risk and the number of failures (by dividing the number of failures during the interval by the number of patients at risk); from this, the percentage success rate is calculated. **Cumulative estimate of survival** is calculated as: (100% – cumulative probability of failure).The **annual survival rate** is calculated by cumulating the success rate for all previous years and the year in question.

Calculations are performed at intervals according to the method used, and graphs are drawn with steps at each time point or failure. **The survivorship curve is the cumulative estimate of survival plotted with 95% CIs (Figure 1.4)**. Upward blips or solid circles are used to represent censored data on graphs. Typically, very small numbers remain at the latest time interval, and such data are the least reliable with the widest CIs. One must not extrapolate the results beyond the defined time periods, and only specific hard endpoints must be used.

Measuring performance

Funnel plots are increasingly used in surgery to describe variations in performance between surgeons and/or centres, and identify outliers. They are **scatter plots, with superimposed control limits (typically 2 SD, 3 SD or 4 SD)**. The smaller the size of the sample, the wider the control limits (increased variability). As the sample increases the certainty increases and the 'funnel' is formed. Data within the control limits are consistent with common cause variation or natural variation, whereas those outside these limits indicate unexpected good or bad results.

Figure 1.5 from the National Joint Registry (NJR) of England and Wales represents hip revision procedures at a unit level. The estimated rate of revision is calculated based on the number of primary procedures undertaken, with adjustment for patient factors (i.e. age, sex, diagnosis). The standardized revision rate is a proportion of the observed revision rate divided by the expected revision rate. Control limits are set at 4 SD. Units above the control limit are achieving

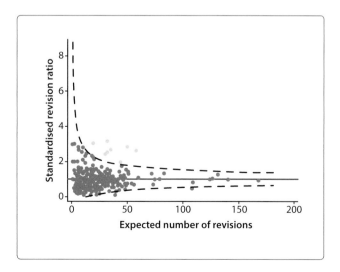

Figure 1.5 From the National Joint Registry (NJR) of England and Wales (2012 report) reproduced with permission.

unexpectedly poor results, and those below are achieving unexpectedly good results. The outliers with poor results in this analysis were generally centres using a high volume of metal-on-metal articulations.

Viva questions

1. What do you understand by sensitivity, specificity, positive predictive value and negative predictive value?

2. Name a condition suitable for screening in orthopaedics. What are the essential criteria for screening?

3. What are the differences between interventional and observational studies, and can you give examples?

4. What do we mean by survival analysis?

5. Can you draw a funnel plot and explain the key features?

Further reading

Bland JM. *An Introduction to Medical Statistics.* Oxford: Oxford University Press, 2000.

Greenhalgh T. *How to Read a Paper: The Basics of Evidence Based Medicine.* London: BMJ Publishing Group, 1997.

Griffin D, Audige L. Common statistical methods in orthopaedic clinical studies. *Clin Orthop Relat Res* 2003;**413**:70–79.

Kocher MS, Zurakowski D. Clinical epidemiology and biostatistics: a primer for orthopaedic surgeons. *J Bone Joint Surg Am* 2004;**86**:607–20.

Murray DW, Carr AJ, Bulstrode C. Survival analysis of joint replacements. *J Bone Joint Surg Br* 1993;**75**:697–704.

2 Genetics

Peter Calder, Harish Hosalkar and Aresh Hashemi-Nejad

Introduction

Our understanding of genetics has advanced greatly since 1953, when Watson and Crick first deduced the structure of **deoxyribonucleic acid** (DNA). Conditions once grouped by phenotype have been shown to have similar genotypes. Knowledge of the genes responsible for specific diseases can lead to more accurate classifications, prognosis and possibly improved treatment techniques.

A basic knowledge of disease inheritance and relevant genetic musculoskeletal disorders is required by the orthopaedic surgeon. Learn to draw a family pedigree of single-gene inheritance and know the gene mutations of the more common conditions.

Chromosomal structure and function

Chromosomes are structures found within the cell nucleus. The karyotype of a normal human somatic cell is 46 chromosomes (the diploid number). This includes 22 autosomal pairs and two sex chromosomes (**Figure 2.1**).

Chromosomes are composed of DNA, **ribonucleic acid** (RNA), **polysaccharides** and **histone** and **non-histone proteins**. Normally chromosomes cannot be seen under a light microscope, but during cell division they become condensed, allowing visualization at 1000× magnification. Chromosomes are thin thread-like structures that have a **short p arm** and a **long q arm** separated by a constriction known as the **centromere** (**Figure 2.1**). The chromosomes have three basic shapes depending on the centromere location. **Metacentric** chromosomes have p and q arms of approximately equal length, e.g. chromosome 1. **Submetacentric** chromosomes have p and q arms of differing lengths, e.g. chromosome 6. In **acrocentric** chromosomes, the centromere is near one end and, therefore, there is a very small p arm and a correspondingly longer q arm, e.g. chromosome 13.

Deoxyribonucleic acid

DNA sequences are arranged in a specific order to form genes. About 100,000 genes make up the human genome. DNA is a polymer of **deoxyribonucleotides** composed of a **nitrogenous base**, a **sugar** and a **phosphate group**. The bases contain the genetic information and are derived from **purines** or **pyrimidines**. The purine bases are **adenine** and **guanine**; the pyrimidine bases are **thymine** and **cytosine**. Watson and Crick deduced the double-helical structure of DNA with paired bases in the centre. Hydrogen bonds between the bases hold the two chains together. Adenine is always paired with thymine, and guanine with cytosine (**Figure 2.2**).

Growth and division of somatic cells is via the process of mitosis. Replication of DNA involves unwinding of the double helix, allowing a complementary DNA daughter strand to be formed using the original strand as a template. This is a semi-conservative process, as each new helix contains one of the original chromosomal strands.

Genes code for protein synthesis. During the process of **transcription**, templates are produced from the DNA in the form of messenger ribonucleic acid (**mRNA**). The mRNA exits the nucleus into the cellular cytoplasm. By combining with other RNA molecules, such as transfer RNA (tRNA) and ribosomal RNA (rRNA), **protein synthesis (translation)** takes place at the **ribosomes**. Proteins have many different biological functions: mechanical tissue strength seen in skeletal tissues is due to the presence of collagen; muscle contraction occurs with the interaction of actin and myosin protein filaments; proteins act as transport molecules and enzymes during biological reactions; and the immune system relies on complex proteins in the form of antibodies.

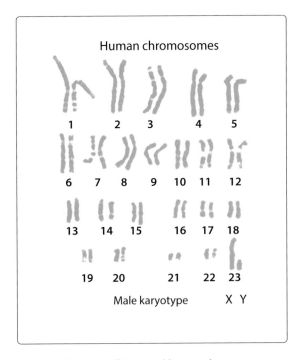

Figure 2.1 Diagram of 23 paired human chromosomes.

Inheritance

In normal somatic cells, females have two X chromosomes and males have one X and one Y chromosome. During the process of **meiosis**, the chromosomes separate to form a **haploid** number, including one copy of each **autosome** and a single sex chromosome. A child inherits one-half of his or her autosomal pair and one sex chromosome from each parent. The mother can contribute only an X chromosome, but the father can contribute either an X or a Y sex chromosome.

Chromosomal abnormalities

Chromosomal abnormalities can involve whole chromosomes or result from structural changes of one or more chromosomes (**Table 2.1**).

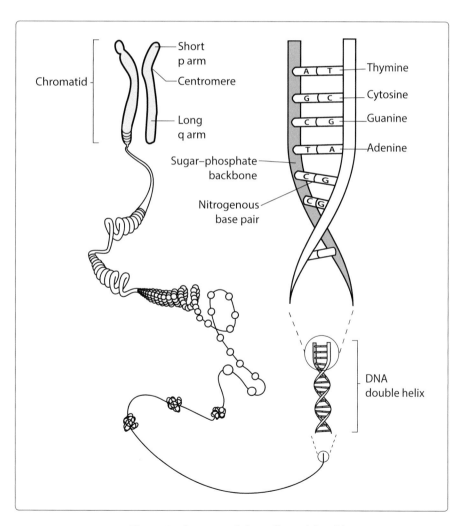

Figure 2.2 Structure of deoxyribonucleic acid.

Table 2.1 Examples of chromosomal abnormalities

Whole chromosome	
Monosomy, e.g. Turner's syndrome	Trisomy, e.g. Klinefelter's syndrome
Structural abnormalities	
Point mutations, deletions, inversions, translocations	

Whole-chromosome abnormalities

Whole-chromosome anomalies include the loss and/or gain of a whole chromosome, referred to as **aneuploidy**. This can affect the autosomes or the sex chromosomes. In general terms, the loss of a chromosome has a greater effect on an individual than the loss of a gene due to the loss of more genetic information.

Monosomy

Monosomy, the loss of one chromosome, occurs less often than an increase in number of chromosomes. Survival does not occur with the loss of one-half of an autosome, but it is possible to lose one X chromosome. This is documented as XO and is known as **Turner syndrome**. The incidence is approximately 1 in 2000 live births, although Turner's syndrome is more commonly seen in miscarried fetuses. The syndrome is exclusively found in females.

Clinically, Turner syndrome is seen as a short female with skeletal abnormalities, including cubitus valgus, medial tibial exostosis and a short fourth metacarpal/metatarsal. The condition is inherited. The paternal X chromosome is more likely to be missing, usually as a sporadic event. The diagnosis is usually made on the basis of a delay in puberty. Other physical features are webbed neck, flat chest with widely spaced nipples, low hairline, low-set ears, and a high-arched palate. It is associated with anomalies of the urinary tract system and coarctation of the aorta. No treatment is usually required for the increased cubitus valgus angle and short fourth and fifth metacarpals. Idiopathic scoliosis should be treated in the standard fashion. Malignant hyperthermia is common with anaesthetic use.

Trisomy

In **trisomy**, the cells have an **extra chromosome**. The most common trisomy compatible with life is **trisomy 21**, or **Down's syndrome**. The incidence of trisomy 21 is around 1 in 660 live births, with an increased risk in mothers over the age of 35 years. The aetiology in 94% of cases is the failure of separation of the autosomal pair during meiosis. This produces a gamete with two homologous chromosomes, which, when joined with a normal gamete during fertilization, produces trisomy. In 3.5% of case, chromosomal rearrangement occurs following **translocation** of one of the autosomes. The remaining 2.5% of cases occur due to **mosaicism**, ain which some of the body cells have a normal complement of 46 chromosomes but others have 47 chromosomes. Mosaicism occurs following defects in mitosis during formation of the zygote.

These patients have typical facies with a wide forehead, flat nose, widely spaced eyes, flat occiput and learning difficulties. Other medical and surgical issues are coeliac disease, Hirschsprung disease, gastroesophageal reflux, epilepsy, xerosis, blood disorders (acute myeloid leukaemia [AML]), abnormal thyroid function and cardiac anomalies (endocardial cushion defects). Orthopaedic problems are scoliosis, hip instability, slipped capital femoral epiphysis, patellar instability, flat foot, metatarsus primus varus and most importantly, atlantoaxial instability. The atlantodens interval (ADI) is measured on flexion–extension lateral radiographs of the cervical spine. An ADI between 5 and 10 mm with no neurological symptoms is observed with yearly radiographic and neurological examinations. Surgical stabilization is indicated in asymptomatic ADI of more than 10 mm or symptomatic ADI between 5 and 10 mm. All children with trisomy 21 should have cervical spine clearance before they participate in sports. Asymptomatic children with instability should avoid contact sports, diving and gymnastics.

The addition of an extra X sex chromosome is seen in **Kleinfelter's syndrome** (XXY). The incidence of this syndrome is 1 in 1000 male births and results in a tall, thin male with infertility and hypogonadism.

Structural abnormalities

Changes in the structure of the chromosomes may involve one or both copies of a gene. The **genotype** is the inherited genetic code that produces the physical appearance known as the **phenotype**. Disorders occur at specific alleles on one or both individual autosomes. An **allele** is defined as one or two alternative forms of a gene that can have the same locus on homologous chromosomes and are responsible for alternative traits. If both alleles are similarly involved, then there is a homozygous trait; if the alleles differ, then there is a heterozygous trait.

The alteration in chromosomal structure may occur at specific nucleotide bases, known as **point mutations**, or may involve larger parts of the chromosome. Examples include **deletions**, where part of the chromosome is removed, with a consequent loss of genetic material; **inversions** of part of the chromosome by 180°, which results in misreading of the genetic code as the DNA is out of the correct sequence; and **translocations** of genetic material from one chromosome to another.

Noonan syndrome. Present only in boys, Noonan syndrome is characterized by short stature, droopy and wide-set eyes, low hairline, blue or grey eyes and chest deformities. Cubitus valgus does not require any intervention. The incidence is reported to be 1 in 1000–2500 children. It is similar in presentation to Turner's syndrome, except there is normal gonadal development, learning difficulties and more severe scoliosis.

Prader-Willi's syndrome. This syndrome is caused by abnormalities in genes located in 15q11q13 (partial chromosome 15 deletion from father) and has an incidence of 1 in 12,000–15,000 newborns. The major clinical criteria are neonatal and infantile hypotonia, dolicocephaly (head length is longer than expected compared to the width, leading to a narrow face), almond-shaped eyes, hypogonadism and mild to moderate learning difficulties. Patients with Prader-Willi's syndrome have hyperphagia, food foraging and an obsession with food. Hip dysplasia and scoliosis is also observed.

Single-gene inheritance

Gene defects may be inherited by autosomal chromosomal transmission or may be linked to X chromosomes. Defects can be either dominant or recessive. The **penetrance** of a genetic disorder relates to the probability that the phenotype will be expressed.

The **severity** of the phenotypic expression may alter between individuals with the same genotype; this is known as **variable expressivity**. An example is Marfan's syndrome, an autosomal dominant condition that results in a defect in collagen formation.

Marfan's syndrome. Mutation in the gene fibrillin-1 (which acts as a Chinese finger trap around collagen) causes a defect in scaffolding for elastic tissues in the body. Clinical features include myopia, lens dislocation (superiorly), retinal detachment, aortic regurgitation, dissecting aortic aneurysm and mitral valve prolapse. Prominent skeletal issues are joint laxity, protrusio acetabuli and scoliosis. Bracing is recommended for progressive curves, many of which will require surgical fusion. Early echocardiogram and eye examination are part of routine care.

Ehlers–Danlos syndrome (EDS). At least nine different types of EDS have been identified. Types I and II are most common and present with soft fragile skin, easy and severe bruising, eye problems, near sightedness, joint laxity, double jointedness and frequent dislocations in shoulder, knee and hip. The other types have gum disease, weak blood vessels, easy rupture of intestine and uterus, clotting problems and scoliosis. Physical therapy and bracing are helpful in the majority of patients. Spinal arthrodesis is required for progressive scoliosis. Soft tissue procedures are avoided if possible due to the risk of complications and recurrence of deformities.

Incomplete penetrance is defined as inheritance of the mutant gene without expression of the phenotype of the disorder. This is in contrast to **variable expressivity**, in which the patient always expresses some of the symptoms.

Examples of single-gene inheritance

- **Autosomal dominant**: achondroplasia, osteogenesis imperfecta, neurofibromatosis.
- **Autosomal recessive**: mucopolysaccharidoses (except Hunter syndrome), sickle cell anaemia.
- **X-linked dominant**: hypophosphataemic rickets.
- **X-linked recessive**: Duchenne's muscular dystrophy, haemophilia A.

Autosomal dominant inheritance

Affected individuals are heterozygous for the mutation (**Figure 2.3**). Homozygous individuals of the allele usually are more severely affected and usually do not survive to term (**Figure 2.3a**). There is a 50% chance of inheritance from one heterozygous parent (**Figure 2.3b**). Males and females are affected equally. Examples of autosomal dominant conditions include achondroplasia, osteogenesis imperfecta (OI) and neurofibromatosis type 1 (NF-1).

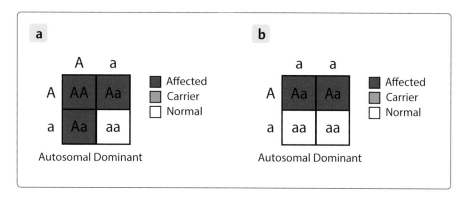

Figure 2.3a,b Punnett square showing inheritance of an autosomal dominant trait (a) two heterozygous parents (b) one heterozygous and one unaffected parent.

Achondroplasia

This is the most common form of **short-limb** or **disproportionate rhizomelic dwarfism** with a prevalence of approximately 1 in 30,000–50,000. It is inherited as complete penetrance. Eighty-seven per cent of cases are as a result of a new mutation. The gene is encoded on chromosome 4, locus p16.3. The mutation affects the gene for **fibroblast growth factor receptor 3** (FGFR3).

Short stature is caused by rhizomelic shortening of the limbs, and there are characteristic facies with frontal bossing and mid-face hypoplasia, as well as limitation of elbow extension, genu varum, and trident hand. The primary defect is abnormal endochondral bone formation in the cartilaginous proliferative zone of the physis. Increased risk of having a child with achondroplasia is directly proportional to paternal age after 36 years. Trunk height tends to be normal, but arm span and standing height are diminished. Radial heads may be subluxated. Developmental motor milestones are frequently delayed, although normal motor coordination is achieved in later childhood. Many children do not walk independently until 2–3 years of age. Hypotonic ligamentous laxity, relatively large head, and disproportionate trunk and limbs may contribute to the problem. Obesity is common. Patients have normal intelligence, but early speech maybe difficult because of tongue thrust; this difficulty usually resolves by school age.

Kyphosis at the thoracolumbar junction usually improves spontaneously. Ligamentous laxity is present in most patients, and the knees are most commonly in varus alignment but may be in excessive valgus. Facial bones, skull base and foramen magnum are underdeveloped. Cranial bones are normal. Foramen magnum stenosis is common. Significant respiratory problems develop in 10% of affected individuals because of an abnormal thoracic cage configuration, mid-facial hypoplasia, upper airway obstruction or spinal cord compression at the foramen magnum. Three percent of affected individuals have hydrocephalus, and detection is difficult because head size may run above the 97th percentile. In the lumbar spine, spinal stenosis is common. Interpedicular distance decreases from L1 to L5. The vertebral bodies have a scalloped appearance. The pelvis characteristically appears broad and flat, with squared iliac wings (champagne glass pelvis). The long bones are short and thick with metaphyseal flaring. Angulation is common at both the distal femoral and the proximal tibial metaphyses. Lumbar spinal stenosis is the most common and disabling problem.

Onset of symptoms is typical in the third decade. Spinal decompression may be indicated in these circumstances. Because instability rarely develops, primary fusion is generally not indicated. Between 10% and 15% of patients retain kyphosis, which can increase the risk of symptomatic stenosis. Bracing is indicated if the deformity is accompanied by significant and progressive structural changes in the anterior vertebral bodies. Failed bracing needs posterior spinal fusion. The treatment of genu varum usually involves surgical correction by proximal tibiofibular realignment osteotomy.

Hypochondroplasia has a milder phenotype than achondroplasia and is caused by mutation of other regions of the FGFR3 gene.

Osteogenesis imperfecta

This is a generalized disease of connective tissue due to a quantitative or qualitative **defect of type I collagen**. It has marked clinical and genetic heterogeneity. Sillence in 1981 classified the condition into types I–IV, with subgroups A and B in types I and IV, where B represents dentinogenesis imperfecta. Initially, inheritance of types I and IV was thought to be autosomal dominant, and that of types II and III autosomal recessive. However, it is now accepted to be an autosomal dominant condition, with cases from unaffected parents being due to mosaicism rather than recessive genes.

Type I collagen is the major extracellular protein in bone, skin and tendons. It is a heterotrimer made of two α1 chains (tropocollagen) and one α2 chain in a triple helix structure. The pro-α1 chain is encoded by the *COL1A1* gene on chromosome 17 and the pro-α2 chain is encoded by the *COL1A2* gene on chromosome 7.

In **common type I** OI, the clinical features include osteopenia, mild bone fragility, grey/blue sclera and ligament laxity. The *COL1A1* mutant allele results in failure of production of the pro-α1 chain due to a premature stop codon. The mRNA remains within the nucleus, resulting in only 50% production of normal α1 chain. Other epidemiological and genetic factors affect the disease process, as there is a spectrum of severity.

In **more severe types** of OI, there are mutations of either the *COL1A1* or the *COL1A2* gene, resulting in a mixture of normal and abnormal collagen chains. The α1 chains are long molecules consisting of 338 repeating triplet amino acid sequences, usually glycine, proline and hydroxyproline. The most common mutation is the substitution of the small glycine molecule with a larger amino acid. This results in 50% of abnormal α1 and α2 chains being formed. These abnormal chains bind to form an abnormal collagen molecule that interferes with the extracellular matrix formation by impairing the function of the normal α1 chains.

Neurofibromatosis type 1

NF1 is inherited as complete penetrance, but it has a high variable expressivity. Fifty per cent of patients have a fresh gene mutation. The gene is encoded on chromosome 17, locus q11.2. The gene encodes the protein neurofibromin and acts as a tumour-suppressor gene.

Autosomal recessive inheritance

Affected individuals are homozygous for the genetic mutation (**Figure 2.4**). Heterozygous individuals are known as carriers. There is a 25% chance of producing an affected individual from two parental carriers.

Males and females are affected equally. Most autosomal recessive conditions produce errors of metabolism due to the deficiency of specific enzymes. This can result in an accumulation of substrate or product, or both. Examples of autosomal recessive disorders include sickle cell anaemia, mucopolysaccharidoses and diastrophic dysplasia.

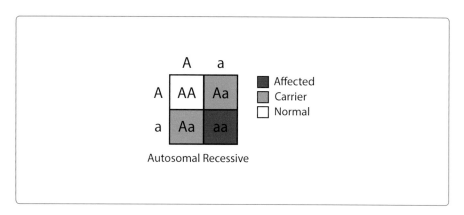

Figure 2.4 Punnett square showing inheritance of an autosomal recessive trait (two carrier parents).

Sickle cell anaemia

Sickling of red cells occurs as a result of an inherited autosomal recessive single-gene mutation, leading to substitution of glutamine for valine at position 6 of the beta-globin chain of haemoglobin.

Sickle cell disease (SCD) is a heterogeneous disorder, with clinical manifestations including chronic haemolysis, an increased susceptibility to infections and vasoocclusive complications. Early manifestations are splenic sequestration and dactylitis. Sickle cell crisis presents with severe pain in abdomen, chest or bones. Treatment is analgesia, fluids, oxygen and in severe cases, exchange transfusion. Bone infarcts cause osteonecrosis of the femoral and humeral heads. Biconcave 'fish' vertebrae and septic arthritis are common. Although *Salmonella* osteomyelitis is associated with SCD (encapsulated bacteria due to asplenia), *Staphylococcus aureus* is the more common causative organism. Radiographs demonstrate osteoporosis, bone thinning and infarcts. Hydroxyurea has been used to increase the fetal haemoglobin and decrease the incidence of painful crisis.

Mucopolysaccharidoses

Mucopolysaccharidoses (MPS) are a group of inherited metabolic disorders caused by deficiency of specific lysosomal enzymes, which results in intracellular accumulation of partially degraded glycoaminoglycans (*Table 2.2*). Incidence of the MPS is 1 in 25,000 live births.

Table 2.2 Mucopolysaccharidoses (MPS) and specific enzyme deficiencies

Mucopolysaccharidoses (MPS)	Enzyme deficiency	Gene locus	Urinary excretion
MPS I (Hurler syndrome)	α-L-iduronidase	Chromosome 4 (AR)	Dermatan/heparan sulphate
MPS II (Hunter disease)	Iduronate-2-sulphatase	X chromosome	Dermatan/heparan sulphate
MPS III (Sanfilippo syndrome)	Heparan sulphatase	Chromosome 12 (AR)	Heparan sulphate
type A	α-N-acetylglucosaminidase	SGSH gene	
type B	Acetyl CoA:α-glucosaminide-N- acetyltransferase	NAGLU gene	
type C	N-acetyl-glucosaminide-6- sulphatase	HGSNAT gene	
type D		GNS gene	
MPS IV (Morquio syndrome)	Galactosamine-6- sulphatase	(AR)	Keratan sulphate
type A	β-galactosidase		
type B			
MPS V (polydystrophic dysplasia)	Arylsulphatase B	Chromosome 5	

Adapted from Erol B, Moroz LA, Dormans JP. Skeletal dysplasia. In: Dormans JP (ed). Core *Knowledge in Orthopaedics*. Philadelphia: Elsevier Mosby, 2005.

The MPS are subdivided on the basis of their enzyme deficiency and the type of substance that accumulates. Although there is phenotypic variability, these disorders share some common clinical features, such as facial dysmorphism, short stature, organomegaly, cardiac problems and joint contractures.

Most of the MPS show similar changes in the cartilage; resting cartilage consists of uniformly stained matrix, with chondrocytes that are larger than normal and stain positively for glycosaminoglycans. Biochemical analysis of the urine can lead to the diagnosis of the specific MPS. Identification of the MPS is also possible through skin fibroblast culture. The fibroblasts are assayed for specific enzyme activity known to be abnormal in the different MPS. Molecular genetic research determines the specific mutations that result in MPS.

The clinical diagnosis of MPS is usually made between 6 months and 10 years of age, depending on the type. A flat nasal bridge, hypertelorism and corneal clouding are typical facial features seen in children with MPS. Short stature, short neck and joint contractures occur in most types. Cervical instability and thoracolumbar kyphoscoliosis are common spinal problems. Dysplasia of the pelvis and broadening and shortening of the long bones may be seen. Generalized joint laxity is a feature of Morquio syndrome (most common), making it distinctly different from the other MPS, in which joint stiffness is the rule. The patients with MPS I (Hurler syndrome) and MPS IV (Morquio syndrome) are usually more severely affected than the other types.

Radiographic changes are commonly seen in the skull; the skull is enlarged, with a thick calvarium. The clavicles are broad, especially medially. The ribs are oar-shaped and broader anteriorly than posteriorly. The vertebral bodies are ovoid when immature. Scoliosis and kyphosis are frequently present. The iliac wings are flared, and the acetabulae are dysplastic. Coxa valga is common, and the long bones often have thickened cortices. There is delay in ossification of the carpal bones. It is difficult to differentiate the various types of MPS on the basis of radiographic findings alone.

Genetic counselling is essential for all children diagnosed with MPS. Orthopaedic treatment usually consists of symptomatic corrective measures: fusion of cervical spine instability and conservative or surgical treatment of spinal curvatures and joint contractures.

Diastrophic dysplasia

The Greek root of the term diastrophic means distorted, which aptly describes the ears, spine, joints and feet of patients with diastrophic dysplasia. Diastrophic dysplasia was described by Lamy and Maroteaux in 1960. It is inherited as an autosomal recessive trait and is rare except in Finland. The defect is on chromosome 5 in the gene that codes for a sulphate transporter protein called diastrophic dysplasia sulphate transporter. Histopathology reveals that chondrocytes appear to degenerate prematurely and collagen is present in excess.

Facial characteristics include prominent cheeks (cherubic), flattened nasal bridge and cauliflower ears. Spinal features include bifid posterior arches of the cervical spine, cervical kyphosis and scoliosis. Because of rhizomelic shortening, the hands are short, broad and ulnarly deviated. The Z-shaped deformity of the thumb ('hitchhiker's thumb') results from a short, proximally placed, often-triangular first metacarpal that may be hypermobile.

The hips maintain a persistent flexion contracture. The proximal femoral epiphyses progressively deform and may subluxate. Epiphyseal flattening and hinge abduction develop in many patients. Arthritic changes develop by early to middle adulthood. The knees usually have flexion contractures. Excessive valgus is also common. One-fourth of patients have a dislocated patella. Although patients with diastrophic dysplasia are described as having clubfoot, many foot complications exist in these patients. The great toe may be in additional varus, beyond the degree commonly occurring in idiopathic clubfoot. The great toe in varus is analogous to the Z-shaped deformity of the thumb. These foot complications cause stiffness, bony malformations and contracture, and are as difficult to correct as clubfoot. Approximately 8% of patients die in infancy from respiratory causes or during childhood from cervical myelopathy.

X-linked dominant inheritance

Either sex can be affected. The phenotype is dominant when a heterozygous female expresses the phenotype.

From **Figure 2.5**, all daughters will inherit the affected gene from an affected male, but no sons will be affected.

From **Figure 2.6,** 50% of sons and 50% of daughters risk inheriting the mutated gene from an affected mother.

An example of an X-linked dominant disorder is **hypophosphataemic rickets.** Males express the disease fully, but females have variable expressivity in the heterozygous genotype.

X-linked recessive inheritance

The phenotype is recessive when expressed by a homozygous female. All males are affected, as they possess only one X chromosome. Heterozygous females are carriers.

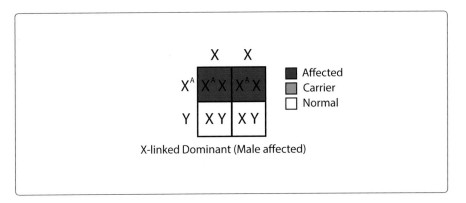

Figure 2.5 Punnett square showing inheritance of an X-linked dominant trait (normal mother and affected father).

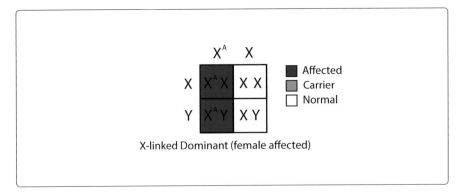

Figure 2.6 Punnett square showing inheritance of an X-linked dominant trait (affected mother and normal father).

From **Figure 2.7**, with a carrier mother and normal father, there is a 25% chance of producing a normal male and equally a normal female. There is a 25% risk of producing an affected male and equally a female carrier.

In **Figure 2.8**, with a carrier mother and affected father, the affected male transmits the affected gene through all his daughters. As the female is also a carrier, then there is a 25% risk of producing an affected female, an affected male, a female carrier or a normal male.

Examples of X-linked recessive disorders include Duchenne's muscular dystrophy, a deficiency of the protein dystrophin, and haemophilia A, which produces a deficiency in clotting factor VIII.

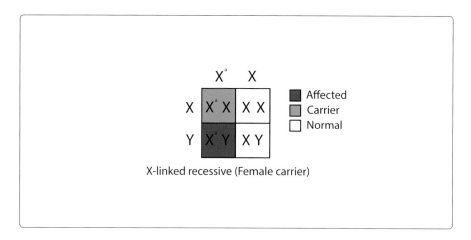

Figure 2.7 Punnett square showing inheritance of an X-linked recessive trait (carrier mother and normal father).

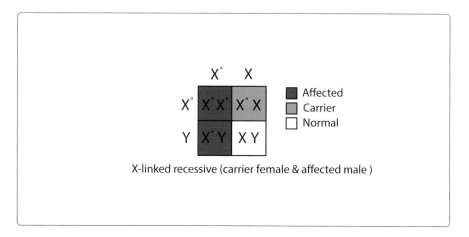

Figure 2.8 Punnett square showing inheritance of an X-linked recessive trait (carrier mother and affected father).

Duchenne's muscular dystrophy (DMD) is the most common form of muscular dystrophy, and is an X-linked recessive myopathy affecting only males. The incidence ranges from 13 to 33 per 100,000 live births, of which one-third arise from new mutations. This progressive disease results in the infiltration of muscle with fibrofatty tissue, resulting in progressive loss of muscle power and contractures. Typically, proximal muscles such as those around the shoulder and hip girdles are involved initially, followed by more distal muscle groups. Corticosteroids have been demonstrated to slow the rate of progression of weakness in DMD and may also transiently improve strength in some cases.

In DMD joint contractures develop as weakness progresses, and are commonly observed at the ankle (equinus, equinovarus), the knee (flexion), and the hip (flexion/abduction). With progressive weakness around the hip girdle and lower extremity, coupled with equinus or equinovarus deformities, walking becomes difficult and could result in frequent falls. The muscles responsible for standing upright, particularly the extensors of the hips and knees become weak early, and compensatory mechanisms during gait include hyperlordosis of the lumbar spine to maintain upright balance. More than 90% of patients will develop a progressive scoliosis, usually within 1–2 years after losing the ability to ambulate, and an instrumented posterior spinal fusion is offered for progressive curves greater than 20°. Ideally, the procedure is performed early, before any significant decline in cardiopulmonary function.

Haemophilia. Haemophilia is the oldest known hereditary bleeding disorder with an X-linked recessive inheritance. Haemophilia A has abnormal factor VIII and haemophilia B (Christmas disease) has abnormal factor IX. Because of deficiency of the clotting factor, patients present with abnormal bleeding spontaneously or following trauma. Typically, bleeds occur deep within muscles and in joints. The iliacus is the most commonly involved muscle, presenting with abdominal or hip pain, flexion deformity and swelling (pseudotumour) of the hip. Ultrasonography is very helpful in delineating the cause. Haemarthrosis presents with pain, swelling and restricted motion (most commonly in the knee). Acute medical management of the disease often includes factor replacement and splinting of the affected joints. It is important to determine the factor inhibitor level so that factor levels can be raised to at least one-fourth of the baseline in major bleeds. Some of the radiological features include osteopenia, thinning of the bones, overgrowth of bones and squaring of the patella.

Recurrent bleeds cause deposition of haemosiderin in the synovium and the articular cartilage, leading to early destruction of joints and causing chronic haemophilic arthropathy. Surgical interventions include arthroscopic or open synovectomy, arthrodesis or joint replacement. Factor replacement is necessary before any surgical procedure, and the presence of antibody inhibitors is no longer a contraindication for elective surgery.

Many of the gene defects for common musculoskeletal disorders have now been characterized (*Table 2.3*).

Multifactorial inheritance

Many orthopaedic conditions are derived from multiple gene defects and environmental factors. Examples include developmental dysplasia of the hip, talipes equinovarus and neural tube defects. These conditions demonstrate familial inheritance but do not behave like single-

Table 2.3 Musculoskeletal disorders and their genetic defects

Musculoskeletal disorder	Genetic mutation
Achondroplasia/hypochondroplasia	FGF receptor 3
Diastrophic dysplasia	Sulphate transporter
Duchenne's muscular dystrophy	Dystrophin
Jansen metaphyseal chondrodysplasia	PTH/PTHrP receptor
Marfan's syndrome	Fibrillin
Multiple epiphyseal dysplasia	COMP or type IX collagen (COL9A2)
Multiple hereditary exostoses	EXT1, EXT2 genes
Osteogenesis imperfecta	Type I collagen
Pseudoachondroplasia	COMP
Schmid metaphyseal dysplasia	Type X collagen
Spondyloepiphyseal dysplasia	Type II collagen
Thanatophoric dysplasia	FGF receptor 3
X-linked hypophosphataemic rickets	PEX (cellular endopeptidase)

Adapted from Erol B, Moroz LA, Dormans JP. Skeletal dysplasia. In: Dormans JP (ed). Core *Knowledge in Orthopaedics*. Philadelphia: Elsevier Mosby, 2005.

gene disorders. The risk of the condition being inherited in subsequent relatives increases compared with the population but decreases in subsequent-degree relatives. An example is talipes equinovarus, which has an incidence of 1 in 1000 births. In first-degree relatives of an affected parent, there is a 25 times increased risk of the condition; this risk decreases in second-degree relatives to a 5 times higher risk.

Genetic counselling

The aim of genetic counselling is to provide information to allow informed decisions to be made on the risk of inheritable disease being transmitted in future pregnancies. Parents need to be made aware that the risk documented for any condition – one in four for autosomal recessive conditions, one in two for autosomal dominant conditions – refers to each specific pregnancy, i.e. if one child is affected, the next pregnancy cannot be guaranteed to produce a normal child as one of the other possible outcomes for the original pregnancy. Subsequent pregnancies carry the original risk of inheritance. Prenatal diagnosis can be achieved by various methods, including amniocentesis, chorionic villous biopsy and fetal-imaging techniques such as ultrasound.

Viva questions

1. What are chromosomes composed of? What is the basic structure of DNA?

2. What chromosomal abnormalities are you aware of?

3. Draw an inheritance table for an autosomal dominant condition of your choice.

4. Do you know of any X-linked dominant conditions? What is the risk of future offspring developing the condition?

5. Osteogenesis imperfecta (OI) is an example of single-gene inheritance. What are the different types of OI? What are the clinical manifestations?

Further reading

Cole WG. Genes and orthopaedics. *J Bone Joint Surg Br* 1999;**8**:190–2.

Cole WG. Advances in osteogenesis imperfecta. *Clin Orthop Relat Res* 2002;**401**:6–16.

Dietz FR, Mathews, KD. Update on the genetic bases of disorders with orthopaedic manifestations. *J Bone Joint Surg Am* 1996;**78**:1583–98.

Econs MJ. New insights into the pathogenesis of inherited phosphate wasting disorders. *Bone* 1999;**25**:131–5.

Horton WA. Fibroblast growth factor receptor 3 and the human chondrodysplasias. *Curr Opin Pediatr* 1997;**9**:437–42.

3 Skeletal Embryology and Limb Growth

Rick Brown, Anish Sanghrajka and Deborah Eastwood

Limb development

During the early stages of development, the embryo has a laminar structure consisting of three different germ cell layers, from which specific systems will develop (*Table 3.1*). The **limb buds** first appear at the end of the **fourth week** of development, with the forelimbs preceding the hindlimbs by 1–2 days. The limb bud consists of a mesenchymal chondrogenic core (from the lateral plate mesoderm) covered by a layer of ectoderm (**Figure 3.1**).

The ectoderm covering the distal tip of the limb bud, under the influence of bone morphogenetic protein (BMP), thickens to form the **apical ectodermal ridge** (AER). The AER is essential for growth and development of the limb, particularly its **width and dorsoventral axis**. Beneath the AER is the **progress zone** (PZ), in which undifferentiated mesenchymal cells rapidly proliferate resulting in **longitudinal outgrowth** of the limb (**proximodistal axis**). The anteroposterior axis (thumb to little finger) is regulated by the **zone of polarizing activity** (ZPA), a mass of cells within the posterior aspect of the limb bud. The **dorsoventral** axis (dorsal to volar) is regulated by a complex interaction between Wnt (dorsal) and engrailed (ventral) proteins.

Table 3.2a summarizes the various molecular controls over limb development and *Table 3.2b* the three axes of growth and influences on their development.

The major **neural plexuses** and **peripheral nerves** develop by **the fifth week**, at which time mesenchymal cells from the somitic mesoderm migrate into the limb buds to produce the limb musculature. **Most muscles** are identifiable and sufficiently developed to produce movement during the **eighth week**.

By the **sixth week** of development, the terminal limb bud flattens to form a **hand-shaped paddle**. Cells of the **AER undergo apoptosis**, separating the AER of each limb into five segments, from which develop the digits. During this period, the central mesenchymal cells of the core differentiate into chondrocytes, which produce the hyaline cartilage anlage of the entire upper limb.

During the **seventh week**, the upper limbs **rotate 90° laterally** (extensors posterior, thumb lateral), whilst the **lower limbs rotate approximately 90° medially** (extensors anterior, hallux medial).

Endochondral ossification of the extremities begins by the **eighth week** (Figure 3.2). All long bones have developed a **diaphyseal primary ossification centre by the 12th week**, from which enchondral ossification progresses outwards. By birth, every long bone diaphysis is usually completely ossified, with the secondary ossification centres in every epiphysis only just beginning to develop. The **distal femoral epiphysis usually is the first to ossify** shortly after birth and is an indicator of fetal maturity.

Table 3.1 Structure of the embryo

Germ cell line	Products of development
Ectoderm	Skin epidermis, nervous system
Mesoderm	Cartilage, bone and muscle
Endoderm	Viscera including lungs and gastrointestinal system

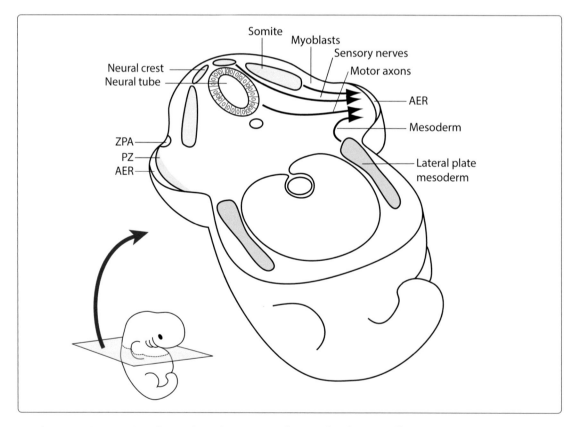

Figure 3.1 Cross section of an embryo showing contribution of embryonic cells to the developing limb. bud. AER: apical ectodermal ridge; PZ: progress zone; ZPA: zone of polarizing activity.

Table 3.2a Molecular influences on embryogenesis

Protein	Function
T-Box transcription factor (tbx)	Early limb bud development
FGF-2, -4, -8, -10	Development of limb bud Maintenance of PZ by AER Controls proximodistal growth
Wingless type MMTV integration site family (Wnt-7a) and engrailed-1 (En-1)	Maintenance of AER Controls dorsoventral axis
Sonic hedgehog homologue (SHH)	Secreted at ZPA Controls AP axis
Homeobox transcription Factors (HOX-A and HOX-D)	Regulate limb position and shapes of bone

AER: apical ectodermal ridge; AP: anteroposterior; FGF: fibroblast growth factor; MMTV: mouse mammary tumour virus; PZ: progress zone; ZPA: zone of polarizing activity.

Table 3.2b Influences on axes of growth

Axis of growth	Zone of control	Important molecules
Proximodistal	AER	FGF-2, -4, -8 and -10
Radioulnar (anteroposterior)	ZPA	SHH
Dorsoventral	Dorsal ectoderm Ventral ectoderm	Wnt-7a via LMX-1b (dorsal) En-1 (ventral)

AER: apical ectodermal ridge; FGF: fibroblast growth factor; SHH: sonic hedgehog homologue; ZPA: zone of polarizing activity.

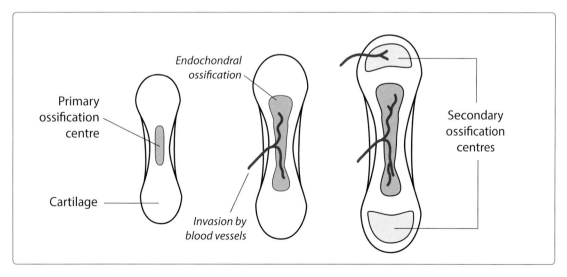

Figure 3.2 Diagrammatic representation of an early fetal bone with a primary ossification centre alone, a mid-term fetal bone showing the site of enchondral ossification and a late fetal bone with addition of the secondary ossification centres.

Synovial joints form during the **sixth week** when cellular apoptosis creates joint cavities in areas of cartilaginous condensation (interzones). **Noggin**, an inhibitor of BMP, is essential for the normal formation of joints; if uninhibited, BMP results in a jointless skeleton. Intrauterine fetal movement is also essential for normal joint development.

The menisci of the knee differentiate from mesenchymal tissue, achieving their mature anatomical morphology by the 14th week. It has long been believed that the discoid meniscus is secondary to failure of absorption of the central portion of the 'normal' discoid shape of meniscus in early embryological development. However, no embryological meniscal specimen has ever shown a discoid shape during normal development. The more popularly held 'congenital' theory suggests that hypermobility secondary to separation of the meniscus from the capsule allows repetitive microtrauma, resulting in the discoid morphology.

Limb abnormalities

Limb deficiencies occur in about 6 per 1000 live births, half of which will be associated with other malformations. Although these deficiencies can arise from genetic or environmental factors (*Table 3.3*), an identifiable cause will not be found in the majority of cases.

Many congenital anomalies are believed to be secondary to a vascular disturbance in the embryo, such as the subclavian artery supply disruption sequence. Disruption of the supply

Table 3.3 Causes of limb abnormalities

Cause	Example	Anomalies
Genetic	P63	Ectrodactyly
	HOX	Brachydactyly or synpolydactyly
	GLI-3	Polydactyly
	LMX-1b	Nail–patella syndrome
Vascular	Subclavian artery disruption sequence	Klippel–Feil's syndrome, Poland's anomaly, Sprengel's deformity, Terminal transverse limb deficiency
Environmental	Infection	
	Hyperthermia	
	Hypoxia	
	Vasculitis	
	Drug effect	Thalidomide, valproate
	Amniotic band syndrome	

from this artery, either by intrinsic occlusion (e.g. thromboembolism), extrinsic compression (e.g. cervical rib, amniotic bands) or environmental insult results in one of a number of different congenital deformities of the upper limb girdle (*Table 3.3*). The magnitude and nature of the deficiency are determined by the extent, location and timing of the resultant ischaemia.

Amniotic band syndrome (ABS) is a congenital disorder believed to result from the entrapment of fetal limbs or organs within intrauterine fibrous amniotic bands, produced by partial rupture of the amniotic sac. These bands, which are often multiple, become constricting because they do not grow as the fetus does. The depth of the ring determines whether the limb distal to the ring becomes engorged (congenital lymphoedema) or amputated (secondary to ischaemia). The high rate of associated congenital malformations (up to 50% have cleft lip and/or palate and congenital talipes equinovarus [CTEV]), has led some to suggest that ABS must be associated with some element of intrinsic circulatory abnormality.

Classification of congenital limb deformity

Originally proposed by Swanson, the International Federation of Societies has adopted a comprehensive classification of congenital upper limb malformations for surgery of the hand (IFSSH). Although originally conceived for the hand, it lends itself to use for the entire upper limb as well as the lower limb (*Table 3.4*).

Failure of formation is divided into either transverse or longitudinal deficiencies. **Transverse deficiencies** are congenital amputation stumps, beyond which the limb has completely failed to develop. Any limb deficiency other than the transverse type is classified as a **longitudinal deficiency**; as well as pre- or post-axial deficiencies of the limbs, it includes phocomelia, in which there may be complete absence of the arm and forearm, but the presence of a hand.

Pre-axial deficiency in the upper limb ranges from minor abnormalities of the thenar muscles to complete absence of all pre-axial structures. Most common is the **radial club hand**, which is frequently associated with a syndrome. It is bilateral in 50% of cases, and over 75% of these are associated with a syndrome. That figure is 40% when unilateral. *Table 3.5* lists the syndromes commonly associated with radial deficiency.

Ulnar deficiencies are 10 times less common than radial deficiencies, and rarely associated with syndromes. Most demonstrate autosomal dominant patterns of inheritance.

Fibular hemimelia/dysplasia is the most common long bone deficiency, and is the most common skeletal deficiency in the lower limb. In addition to the fibular dysplasia, associations include femoral shortening, lateral femoral condyle hypoplasia, anterior cruciate ligament (ACL) deficiency, tarsal coalition resulting in a ball-and-socket ankle joint and lateral ray deficiencies in the foot.

Tibial hemimelia/dysplasia is 20 times less common than fibular hemimelia. It has an autosomal dominant inheritance pattern and is associated with pre-axial polydactyly in the foot and cleft hand.

Polydactyly is the most common congenital anomaly of the upper limb. Post-axial polydactyly is transmitted in an autosomal dominant pattern in most cases, and is most common in people of African origin.

Table 3.4 Swanson's classification of congenital upper limb malformations

I	Failure of formation	Transverse arrest		Most commonly at proximal third forearm level
		Longitudinal arrest	Preaxial	Radial club hand Tibial hemimelia/dysplasia
			Postaxial	Ulna clubhand Fibula hemimelia/dysplasia
			Central	Cleft hand
			Intercalary	Phocomelia
II	Failure of differentiation (separation)	Soft tissue		Simple syndactyly
				Trigger thumb
		Skeletal		Synostoses
				Coalitions
				Complex syndactyly
III	Duplication			Polydactyly
				Mirror hand
IV	Overgrowth			Hemihypertrophy
V	Undergrowth			Radial dysplasia, brachydactyly, fibular dysplasia
VI	Constriction band syndromes			Amniotic band syndrome
VII	Generalized skeletal abnormalities			Marfan's syndrome, achondroplasia

Table 3.5 Syndromes associated with radial clubhand

Holt–Oram's syndrome (cardiac defects)
Thrombocytopaenia-absent radius syndrome (TAR)
VACTERL (**V**ertebral anomalies, **A**nal atresia, **C**ardiac abnormalities, **T**racheoesophageal fistula, o**E**sophageal atresia, **R**enal disorders, **L**imb abnormalities)
Fanconi's anaemia (aplastic anaemia developing around age 6 years)

Developmental anatomy of the vertebral column

The vertebral column develops from the **notochord** and **somites**. The notochord is a solid rod, which forms from cranial to caudal (see Chapter 15).

The **ectoderm** forms the **neural tube** by a process called **neurulation**. In the midline, ectodermal cells become elongated, causing a relative thickening in that region (the **neural plate**). The two edges of the neural plate thicken to form the neural groove and neural folds. The neural tube forms by the fusion of the edges of these folds, which begins near the anterior end of the embryo and proceeds in anterior and posterior directions. The neural groove closes by the third week, except at its ends (the anterior and posterior **neuropores**), which normally close by the end of the fourth week. Failure of the **anterior neuropore** to close results in **anencephaly**, whilst **neural tube defects** (NTDs) are most commonly thought to arise from a failure of the **posterior neuropore** to close.

The cells at the dorsal-most portion of the neural tube form the neural crest, from which cells will migrate throughout the embryo to give rise to several cell populations including neurons and supporting glial cells of sensory, sympathetic and parasympathetic nervous systems and epidermal melanocytes.

The **mesoderm** on either side of the midline divides into complex structured, repeating blocks (**somites**) along the axis of the embryo. *Table 3.6* summarizes the outcome of development of the various parts of the somite.

Spinal abnormalities

Table 3.7 summarizes the different types of NTD, which are widely believed to result from a **failure of closure** of the neural tube. Another hypothesis suggests that the pathogenesis is **overdistension** and rupture of a closed neural tube. There is a genetic predisposition to NTDs, with some families demonstrating an increased incidence, and a variation in prevalence among different ethnic groups (highest in the Hispanic population). Mutations in the *PAX-3* gene in a mouse model have been shown to result in NTDs.

Various **teratogens** have been found to interfere with neurulation including vinblastine, calcium channel blockers, retinoic acid and valproate. Hypothermia has also been implicated as a cause of NTDs. **Folate** supplementation (400 µg daily), if commenced prior to, and for the first month after, conception is significantly protective against neural tube defects, by an unknown mechanism.

Table 3.6 Products of development from the somite

Sclerotome	Vertebral bodies and arches
Central cavity	Intervertebral discs and ribs
Dermatome	Dermis
Myotome	Muscles, tendons, fascia

Table 3.7 Types of neural tube defect

Neural tube defect	Features
Meningocoele	Cyst involves only the meninges, not neural elements
Myelomeningocoele	Abnormal neural elements as part of the sac
Lipomeningocoele	Sac contains a lipoma closely associated with the sacral nerves
Rachischisis	Complete absence of skin and sac, with dysplastic spinal cord exposed

The neural arch of the vertebra develops from ventral to dorsal; **spina bifida occulta** is a failure of complete neural arch formation, without neurological compromise. It is most common in the lumbosacral region, and can be found in approximately 20% of adults.

Disorders of somatogenesis can result in variations in numbers, shape and position of vertebrae (e.g. hemivertebrae, block vertebrae, vertebral bars, lumbarization and sacralization). The **Klippel–Feil** sequence is due to a defect in cervical segmentation resulting in multiple vertebral abnormalities.

Diastematomyelia is a longitudinal splitting of the spinal cord by a bony or fibrocartilaginous spicule arising from the vertebral body, which is believed to be a remnant of the early connection to the primitive gut or amniotic cavity.

Bone formation

Intra-membranous ossification

This is the process by which **mesenchymal tissue transforms directly into bone**. Mesenchymal cells proliferate and condense into packed nodules, with some cells becoming osteoid-secreting osteoblasts. Once surrounded by calcified matrix, the cells become osteocytes. Only the clavicle and flat-bones of the calvarium are formed by intramembranous ossification during embryological development. Regenerate from **distraction osteogenesis** and **blastema bone on amputation stumps** form via this process.

Endochondral ossification

Mesenchymal cells condense and proliferate, with cells developing into chondroblasts (**chondrification**). A cartilaginous extracellular matrix is laid down (**anlage**) forming the template for bone formation. The matrix is resorbed, and osteoblasts brought into the area by newly formed capillary networks begin ossification. This process begins within the centre of the diaphysis (primary ossification centre), and proceeds outward from the medullary cavity and inward from the periosteum. This sequence of events then occurs at the epiphyseal centres of ossification.

The physis

The physis is a structure consisting of **chondrocytes** arranged in a highly ordered, layered fashion within an extracellular matrix in line with the longitudinal axis of the bone (**Figure 3.3**). Within it are several histologically distinct zones:

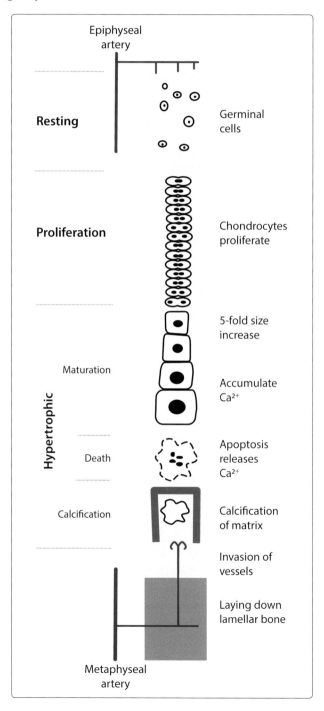

Figure 3.3 Layers of a physis.

- The **resting zone** lies immediately beneath the secondary ossification centre. It comprises germinal cells of stem cell origin widely dispersed throughout a mechanically strong thick layer of matrix in relatively low oxygen tension.
- The **proliferative zone** is characterized by longitudinal columns of flattened cells parallel to the long axis of the bone. This zone has the highest rate of matrix turnover with high oxygen tension.
- The **hypertrophic zone** is subdivided into the **zones of maturation, degeneration and calcification**. The cells increase in size fivefold, but because of the constraint provided by the **perichondrial ring of LaCroix**, the resultant volume changes of the physis are expressed largely in the longitudinal direction. The chondrocytes accumulate calcium, which is released into the matrix when they undergo apoptosis. In **rickets**, failure of calcification results in a widened, flared physis due to persistence of cartilage.

In the **metaphysis**, the mineralized cartilage is removed, and **primary spongiosa** laid down by osteoblasts. This is then remodelled into **lamellar bone** to produce the secondary spongiosa.

The physis is circumferentially surrounded by the **groove of Ranvier**, which consists of active proliferative cells. The **perichondrial ring of LaCroix** is a fibro-osseous structure that provides a strong supporting girdle around the periphery of the physis. Additional stability of the physis is provided by its large and small undulations (**lappet formation** and **mammillary processes**, respectively).

Longitudinal bone growth occurs by enchondral ossification at the physis. Circumferential growth of the physis occurs at the groove of Ranvier, whilst appositional ossification in the osteogenic layer of the periosteum is responsible for diaphyseal widening. The secondary centre of ossification has a hemispherical physis that contributes to longitudinal growth of the bone, as well as the contour of the articular surface.

There are a number of key physes relevant to orthopaedic practice. In the arm, 80% of humeral growth occurs at the proximal physis, while 75% of the growth of the radius occurs distally. The sequence of appearance of the distal humeral physis is important in understanding paediatric elbow injuries (**Figure 3.4**).

The first is the **c**apitellum (2 years), followed approximately every 2 years by the **r**adial head, medial (**i**nternal) epicondyle, **t**rochlear, **o**lecranon and **l**ateral (external) epicondyle (use the mnemonic **CRITOL** to remember the order). Thus, no secondary centres are visible in an infant, making interpretation of trans-physeal fractures difficult. In a trans-physeal fracture, the relationship of the radius to the ulna is preserved, unlike a dislocation around the elbow or a displaced intraphyseal fracture.

Two-thirds of lower limb growth occurs around the knee, with 70% attributable to the distal femoral physis. For the last 4–6 years of skeletal growth, one can estimate that the distal femur grows at 9 mm/year and the proximal tibia at 6 mm/year. The proximal femur and distal tibia account for only a few millimetres (3–4 mm) each per year.

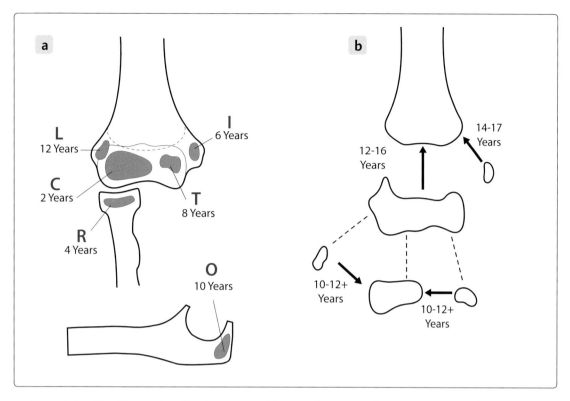

Figure 3.4 a: Distal humeral ossification centres with approximate age of appearance. C: capitelar; I: internal epicondyle; L: lateral epicondyle. O: olecranon; R: radial; T: trochlear; b: Approximate age of fusion of the distal humeral ossification centres.

Vascular anatomy of the growth plate

Table 3.8 summarises the three main vascular systems supplying the growth plate. As no blood vessels traverse the growth plate after the neonatal period, the epiphyseal and metaphyseal systems do not have any direct communication. The resultant extensive metaphyseal capillary loops are believed to be the cause of the preponderance of metaphyseal osteomyelitis in children.

Table 3.8 Vascular supply of the physis

Arterial system	Features
Epiphyseal arteries	Enter secondary ossification centre Supplies resting and uppermost proliferative layers
Nutrient artery of diaphysis	Supplies the capillary loop network at junction of metaphysis and physis
Perichondrial arteries	Supplies the groove of Ranvier and ring of LaCroix Anastomoses with epiphyseal and metaphyseal systems

Blood vessels supplying epiphyses that are entirely intracapsular (e.g. proximal femur, radial head) must enter around the periphery of the physis. They are therefore very susceptible to damage during physeal separation, which can result in avascular necrosis of the epiphysis.

Clinical significance

Estimating skeletal maturity

Many treatments in paediatric orthopaedics depend on the child's bone age, which may differ significantly from chronological age in about 50% of children.

Most physes close in a predictable fashion, enabling radiological assessment of bone age. The **Greulich and Pyle** atlas, based on a hand and wrist radiograph, is probably the most commonly employed method in the UK. The **Sauvegrain** method employs the anteroposterior (AP) and lateral views of the elbow, and is said to be more useful during puberty. The **Risser sign** is based upon the lateral to medial ossification of the iliac apophysis, and is commonly used when making decisions about the management of childhood spinal deformity.

Guiding growth

Altering the forces acting upon the physis affects its activity, with compression retarding growth (**Hueter–Volkmann principle**). In tibia vara, the medial proximal tibial physis is subjected to increasing compressive forces, resulting in progressive worsening of the deformity. Many treatments employed in children's orthopaedics also rely on this phenomenon to correct deformity (e.g. splinting for developmental dysplasia of the hip [DDH], Ponseti method for CTEV correction, plaster jackets for spinal deformity). Implants such as staples or plate–screw constructs have also been used to reversibly and differentially restrain part of the physis, allowing the natural correction of angular deformities, especially about the knee.

Physeal fractures

Laboratory experiments have demonstrated that the zone of hypertrophy is the weakest area within the physis. However, fractures are usually not limited to this layer, traversing longitudinally through the various layers, up to and including the resting zone. The metaphysis is the most susceptible to compressive forces, explaining why the Thurston–Holland fragment of type II injuries occurs on the compression side of the fracture.

Skeletally immature bone has excellent remodelling potential, which should be appreciated when managing fractures in a paediatric population. Although some remodelling occurs at the fracture site (**Wolff's law**), most occurs at the adjacent physes (Hueter–Volkmann principle). *Table 3.9* summarizes the factors affecting remodelling potential.

Physeal arrest

Growth arrest after fracture can be a consequence of:

- Compromised vascularity of the physis.
- Damage to resting zone.
- Bone bridge formation between epiphysis and metaphysis.
- Or a combination of these factors.

Table 3.9 Factors affecting fracture remodelling potential

Patient age
Degree of angulation
Distance of fracture from physis
Activity of the adjacent physis (e.g. proximal vs. distal humerus)
Deformity in plane of joint movement

When complete, growth arrest may result in limb length discrepancy. Partial arrests can be further classified according to the location of the bony bar into:

- Peripheral (produces angular deformity).
- Central (tethers the central physis, distorting the articular surface).
- Linear, which involves portions of both central and peripheral physis (often resulting from a malunited Salter–Harris type 4 fracture).

Resection of the bony bar, with interposition of fat or cement (**Langenskiold procedure**), is advocated if the bar involves less than 50% of physeal area, and the physis has over 2 years of growth remaining. It is advisable to follow-up high-risk physeal fractures to exclude growth arrest. The appearance of parallel Harris growth arrest lines is reassuring in this situation.

Skeletal dysplasias

Skeletal dysplasias are a diverse group of developmental disorders of bone and/or cartilage that result in altered limb growth. **Rubin's classification** categorizes these conditions according to the location of the defect and relative activity (*Table 3.10*).

Achondroplasia, an autosomal dominant genetic defect in the production of fibroblast growth factor receptor 3 (**FGFR3**), is the most common dysplasia. Eighty per cent of cases are due to spontaneous mutations. A disorder of enchondral ossification in the proliferative zone of the physis results in reduced longitudinal growth of the long bones. The skull and clavicle are spared as intramembranous ossification is relatively unaffected.

There are two types of **spondyloepiphyseal dysplasia** (SED), congenita and tarda. The **congenita** type is due to a defect in the *COL2 A1* gene, with an autosomal dominant pattern of inheritance. The **tarda** subtype is most often due to an abnormality in the *SEDL* gene, which is inherited in an **X-linked recessive** pattern of inheritance.

Multiple epiphyseal dysplasia (MED), a defect in ossification of the epiphysis, occurs in both autosomal and recessive forms. Both types affect the hips and knees, but the recessive type is commonly associated with scoliosis and deformities of the hands and knees. 70% of the dominant forms are due to mutations in the gene coding the **cartilage oligometric matrix protein** (COMP).

Table 3.10 Rubin's classification of skeletal dysplasias

Epiphysis	Hyperplasia	Trevor's disease
	Hypoplasia	SED, MED, pseudoachondroplasia
Physis	Hyperplasia	Enchondromatosis
	Hypoplasia	Achondroplasia
Metaphysis	Hyperplasia	Hereditary multiple exostoses
	Hypoplasia	Osteopetrosis
Diaphysis	Hyperplasia	Diaphyseal dysplasia
	Hypoplasia	Osteogenesis imperfecta

MED: multiple epiphyseal dysplasia; SED: spondyloepiphyseal dysplasia.

Trevor's disease (dysplasia epiphysealis hemimelica) is a rare condition in which an osteochondroma occurs within one side of the epiphysis. It is more common on the medial side, and usually affects the distal femur, distal tibia or talus. No genetic cause has yet been identified.

Ollier's disease, or multiple enchondromatosis, is characterized by lesions of hyaline cartilage extending from the physis into the metaphysis and into the medullary canal. The lesions can be bilateral, but are more often found unilaterally. The risk of malignant transformation is about 30%. **Maffucci's syndrome** is characterized by multiple enchondromata with **haemangiomas** and occasionally **lymphangiomas**. The risk of malignant transformation of the enchondromata is similar to Ollier's, but the condition has an increased risk of non-skeletal malignancy (including liver and ovarian). Neither Ollier's nor Maffucci's are inherited, and no genetic defect has yet been identified.

Hereditary multiple osteochondromatosis (HMO, diaphyseal aclasia) is the most common skeletal tumour-like dysplasia, with an incidence of 1 in 50,000. It is characterized by the growth of cartilage-capped benign bone tumours arising from the metaphysis towards the diaphysis. HMO is an **autosomal dominant** disorder, with 96% penetrance, linked to mutations in the *EXT1* and *EXT2* genes (the *EXT1* gene is associated with greater involvement). The risk of sarcomatous transformation has been reported as 0.57%.

All these tumour-like dysplasias cease growth after physeal closure.

Osteogenesis imperfecta (OI) has been described as a diaphyseal hypoplasia, where defective collagen production results in weakened, soft, deformed bones. In the most common form (Sillence type I), only 50% of the normal collagen is produced; in the other forms, there is both a qualitative and a quantitative reduction in the amount of normal collagen. Despite possessing a weak bone matrix, these patients are able to heal bone well.

Conclusion

The activity of the physis is central to the understanding of paediatric orthopaedics. Development of the physis starts in utero however, where, along with the developing limb, it can be affected by a variety of insults that may be detectable antenatally on ultrasound scan or may become apparent only with further growth in infancy and childhood. After birth, the physis again may be affected by injury and disease.

Viva questions

1. When does the limb bud of the embryo first appear?
2. What is a secondary ossification centre?
3. Draw a sketch of a physis.
4. Through which layer of the physis do fractures occur?
5. How is the physis affected by rickets?

Further reading

Jones DH, Barnes J, Lloyd-Roberts G. Congenital aplasia and dysplasia of the tibia with intact fibula: classification and management. *J Bone Joint Surg Br* 1978;**60**:31–9.

Rivas R, Shapiro, F. Structural stages in the development of the long bones and epiphyses. *J Bone Joint Surg Am* 2002;**84**:85–100.

Rubin P. *Dynamic Classification of Bone Dysplasias.* Chicago, IL: Year Book Medical Publishers, 1964.

Salter RB, Harris WR. Injuries involving the epiphyseal plate. *J Bone Joint Surg Am* 1963;**45**:587–622.

Swanson AB. The classification of congenital limb malformations. *J Hand Surg Am* 1976;**1**:8–22.

Al-Qattan MM, Kozin SH. Update on embryology of the upper limb. *J Hand Surg Am* 2013;38(**9**):1835–44.

4 Orthopaedic Pharmacology

Manoj Ramachandran, Daud Chou and Natasha Rahman

Introduction

Orthopaedic surgeons should have a sound working knowledge of the indications for, and the actions and adverse effects of, any therapeutic drug that they prescribe on a regular basis. This chapter provides an overview of the common classes of drugs encountered by orthopaedic surgeons. Antibiotics are discussed in Chapter 5.

Analgesic and anti-inflammatory drugs

The choice and route of analgesic drug administration depends on the nature and duration of the pain. A **progressive approach** is used, starting with **simple analgesics** such as paracetamol and non-steroidal anti-inflammatory drugs (NSAIDs), supplemented first by **weak opioid** analgesics and later by **strong opioids**. As a general rule, severe acute pain (e.g. trauma, post-operative pain) is treated with strong opioid drugs given by injection. Patient controlled analgesia (PCA) with morphine can be an effective method of post-operative pain management. Mild inflammatory pain (e.g. rheumatoid arthritis) is treated with NSAIDs supplemented by weak opioids given orally. Severe chronic pain (e.g. severe rheumatoid arthritis, back pain) is treated with strong opioids given orally, subcutaneously or epidurally.

There are three main classes of analgesic drug:

- Centrally acting non-opioid drugs, e.g. paracetamol.
- NSAIDs.
- Opioid analgesics.

Paracetamol (acetaminophen)

Essentials

Paracetamol is generally considered to be a **weak inhibitor of the synthesis of prostaglandins**. Its mechanism of action may be via the production of reactive metabolites by the peroxidase function of cyclo-oxygenase (**COX-2**), which could deplete glutathione, a cofactor of enzymes such as PGE synthase. The central action of paracetamol may also be due to activation of **descending serotonergic pathways**. **COX-3**, an isoenzyme of COX-1 found in the central nervous system (CNS), has been suggested to be the site of action of paracetamol, but this selective interaction may not be clinically relevant. Other pathways that may be involved include **opiodergic** systems, **eicosanoid** systems, **nitric oxide** containing pathways and **endocannabinoid** signaling. Paracetamol has analgesic and antipyretic actions but only weak anti-inflammatory effects. It is well absorbed orally and does not cause gastric irritation.

Adverse effects

In recommended doses, the side-effects of paracetamol are mild to non-existent.

- Analgesic-associated nephropathy: may occur following long-term high doses of paracetamol.
- Hepatotoxicity: paracetamol is metabolized by the liver and can cause fatal hepatotoxicity in overdose. Under normal conditions, the highly-reactive metabolite, N-acetyl-p-benzoquinone imine (NAPQI), is detoxified by conjugation with glutathione. Saturation of the normal conjugating enzymes in overdose causes accumulation of NAPQI which reacts with cell proteins, causing hepatocyte necrosis. Therapeutic replenishment of glutathione is achieved by the administration of N-acetylcysteine (NAC).

Non-steroidal anti-inflammatory drugs

Examples

- **Salicylic acid derivatives**: aspirin (rarely used for analgesia).
- **Propionic acid derivatives**: ibuprofen, naproxen (first line treatment in inflammatory arthropathies).
- **Acetic acid derivatives**: diclofenac (also available for topical application), indomethacin, ketorolac.
- **Selective COX-2 inhibitors**: celecoxib (reduced gastrointestinal effects).
- **Oxicams**: piroxicam (long half-life, but associated with high incidence of gastrointestinal bleeding in elderly people).
- **Pyrazolones**: azapropazone (potent, but high incidence of side-effects).

Essentials

Although NSAIDs are a chemically diverse group, they **all inhibit COX**, resulting in inhibition of **prostaglandin and thromboxane synthesis** (**Figure 4.1**). Most NSAIDs reversibly and non-selectively inhibit both the COX-1 and COX-2 isoenzymes. In the process of inflammation, prostaglandins sensitize nociceptive nerve endings to inflammatory mediators, promote vasodilatation and oedema, and elevate the hypothalamic set point for temperature control.

Thus the inhibition of prostaglandins produces the analgesic, anti-inflammatory and antipyretic properties of NSAIDs. Inhibition of COX-1 by NSAIDs results in gastrointestinal damage (dyspepsia, nausea, gastritis) due to a loss of the gastroprotective effects of **prostaglandins E2** (PGE2) and **I2** (PGI2), which normally inhibit gastric acid secretions, increase blood flow through the gastric mucosa and act in a cytoprotective manner.

Aspirin is an **irreversible inactivator** of COX, acting by acetylating a serine residue in the active site of the enzyme. It is increasingly being thought of as a cardiovascular drug rather than an NSAID due to its antiplatelet effects through suppression of **thromboxanes**.

Selective COX-2 inhibitors are more selective in their action, resulting in fewer gastrointestinal side-effects, but they may be associated with an increased risk of cardiovascular morbidity.

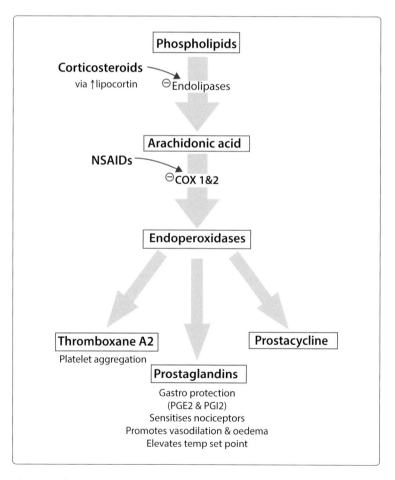

Figure 4.1 Mechanism of action of non-steroidal anti-inflammatory drugs (NSAIDs) (and corticosteroids). COX: cyclo-oxygenase; PG: prostaglandin.

Adverse effects

- Gastrointestinal: due to inhibition of PGE2 and PGI2 (see above). A proton pump inhibitor should be co-prescribed with all oral NSAIDs.
- Renal: renal haemodynamics, sodium and water excretion are ordinarily mediated by prostaglandins, which cause vasodilatation of the afferent arterioles of the glomeruli. By inhibiting renal prostaglandin synthesis, NSAIDs cause unopposed constriction of the afferent arterioles and decreased renal perfusion pressure, resulting in renal insufficiency. This is especially important in patients with heart failure and cirrhosis, who already have high levels of circulating vasoconstrictors.
- Pulmonary: bronchospasm in aspirin-sensitive asthmatic patients (the triad of aspirin sensitivity, asthma and nasal polyposis is known as Samter's syndrome).
- Minor effects: rash, urticaria, photosensitivity reactions.

Miscellaneous facts

The APPROVe trial showed an increased relative risk of adverse thrombotic cardiovascular events in patients taking rofecoxib (selective COX-2 inhibitor) compared to a placebo. This resulted in the worldwide withdrawal of rofecoxib in October 2004.

Opioid analgesics

Examples

- **Strong**: morphine, diamorphine, fentanyl, pethidine, buprenorphine.
- **Weak**: codeine, dihydrocodeine, dextropropoxyphene.

Essentials

Opioid analgesics **mimic endogenous opioid peptides** by causing prolonged activation of opioid receptors, usually mu (μ) receptors. Opioid receptors are distributed widely throughout the CNS and are concentrated most highly in areas involved in nociception, such as the **dorsal horn of the spinal cord** and the **thalamus**. At the cellular level, opioid receptors are G-protein-coupled receptors and inhibit adenylate cyclase, so reducing the intracellular cyclic adenosine monophosphate (cAMP) content. Opioid agonists reduce neuronal excitability by **increasing potassium conductance** causing hyperpolarization; and inhibit neurotransmitter release, by **decreasing calcium influx**. The clinical effects of these drugs are **analgesia**, **sedation** and **euphoria** and have many therapeutic applications.

Adverse effects

- **Respiratory depression**: due to its action on brainstem respiratory centres. This can be reversed with naloxone (short-acting) or naltrexone (long-acting), although reversal is more difficult with overdoses of partial μ-agonists, such as dextropropoxyphene (found in coproxamol) and buprenorphine.
- **Nausea and vomiting**: due to stimulation of the chemoreceptor trigger zone; necessitating an antiemetic when administering strong opioids.
- **Constipation**: due to reduced gut motility via action on the myenteric plexus; often requiring laxatives.

- **Tolerance and dependence**: to strong opioids in addicts.
- **Postural hypotension**: due to depression of the vasomotor centre and release of histamine.
- **Biliary spasm, constriction of the sphincter of Oddi**: particularly with morphine.
- **Pruritus**: due to histamine release; can be managed with chlorphenamine.
- **Bronchoconstriction**: due to histamine release.

Miscellaneous facts

- Diamorphine (also known as heroin) is more lipid-soluble than morphine and so has a faster onset of action than morphine.
- Fentanyl can be given transdermally (patches) for chronic pain.
- Buprenorphine is an effective analgesic when given sublingually but can be associated with prolonged vomiting.

Glucocorticoids

In orthopaedics, glucocorticoids are used for a variety of different indications: intraarticular injections for arthritis, peri-operative dosing for patients on long-term steroids, symptom relief in rheumatoid arthritis and for spinal cord injuries.

Examples

- **Mildly potent (class I)**: hydrocortisone.
- **Moderately potent (class II)**: triamcinolone.
- **Potent (class III)**: methylprednisolone.
- **Very potent (class IV)**: betamethasone dipropionate.

Essentials

Glucocorticoids have **anti-inflammatory** and **immunosuppressive** effects. They act on all phases of the inflammatory response, from the early changes of acute inflammation to the later proliferative changes of chronic inflammation. Glucocorticoids interact with intracellular receptors, forming **steroid–receptor complexes** that **modify gene transcription** at the DNA level, resulting in either **induction or inhibition of protein synthesis**. Examples include inhibition of gene transcription for COX-2, phospholipase A2 (PLA2; an endolipase) and cytokines such as the interleukins. Glucocorticoids' primary anti-inflammatory mechanism is increased synthesis of **lipocortin 1**, which exerts its anti-inflammatory actions by inhibiting endolipases (Figure 4.1). Glucocorticoids also directly **depress monocyte/macrophage function, decrease circulating T-cell levels**, and directly **inhibit lymphocyte transport** to the site of antigenic stimulation and antibody production.

Glucocorticoids are bound to corticosteroid-binding globulin in the blood and enter cells by diffusion, eventually being metabolized in the liver.

Adverse effects

The adverse effects of glucocorticoids are best remembered using the mnemonic 'I WAS HOPPING MAD':

- **Infection** (including reactivation of nascent infections, e.g. tuberculosis).
- **Wasting of muscles** (due to protein loss).
- **Adrenal insufficiency.**
- **Sugar disturbances** (hyperglycaemia, diabetes).
- **Hypotension.**
- **Osteoporosis** (due to increase in bone catabolism; one mechanism is the inhibition of vitamin D3-mediated induction of the osteocalcin gene in osteoblasts).
- **Peptic ulcer.**
- **Pancreatitis.**
- **Proximal myopathy** (due to protein loss).
- **Incidental** (moon facies, 'orange-on-stick' appearance due to central obesity, easy bruising, hirsutism).
- **Necrosis**, e.g. of the femoral and humeral heads.
- **Glaucoma, cataracts.**
- **'MAD'** (psychological changes, e.g. euphoria, depression, psychosis, emotional lability).

Anaesthetics

- Local anaesthetics.
- General anaesthetics:
  - inhalation;
  - intravenous.
- Neuromuscular blockers.

Local anaesthetics

Examples

- **Esters**: cocaine, procaine.
- **Amides**: lignocaine, bupivacaine, prilocaine.

Essentials

Local anaesthetics **block action potential initiation and propagation** in neurons by physically plugging the trans-membrane pore of sodium channels. Local anaesthetics are **amphiphilic** molecules with a hydrophobic aromatic group linked by an ester or amide bond to a basic amine group. Their activity is strongly pH-dependent, being increased at alkaline pH when the proportion of unionized molecules is high, which allows them to penetrate the nerve sheath and axonal membrane as the unionized form is more membrane-permeant.

Local anaesthetics block conduction in the following order: small myelinated axons, unmyelinated axons, large myelinated axons. Therefore, nociceptive and sympathetic transmission in Aδ and C fibres is blocked first. Local anaesthetics may be given topically, by direct infiltration, intravenously, as nerve blocks, or by spinal (subarachnoid space) or epidural (extradural space) administration. Esters are rapidly hydrolyzed by plasma cholinesterases, and amides are metabolized in the liver.

Adverse effects

- **Central nervous system**: agitation, confusion, tremors progressing to convulsions, respiratory depression.
- **Cardiovascular**: myocardial depression and vasodilation, leading to a drop in blood pressure.
- **Hypersensitivity reactions**.

Miscellaneous facts

Local infiltration analgesia (LIA) following joint arthroplasty is gaining popularity; however, the outcomes of this method with respect to analgesic and adverse effects have not yet been fully evaluated.

General anaesthetics

General anaesthetic agents induce a reversible state of amnesia, analgesia, loss of responsiveness, loss of skeletal muscle reflexes or decreased stress response, or all simultaneously. At a cellular level it is thought that anaesthetic agents inhibit **synaptic transmission** by inhibiting the release of excitatory transmitters or the response of post-synaptic receptors through the **gamma aminobutyric acid (GABA)** and **N-methyl-D-aspartate (NMDA)** systems. Although all parts of the nervous system are affected the main targets appear to be the thalamus, cortex and hippocampus.

INHALATION ANAESTHETICS

Inhalation anaesthetics are volatile liquids or gases that **depress the CNS**. Rapid induction and recovery are important properties that are determined by the agents solubility in blood (blood: gas partition coefficient) and solubility in fat (lipid solubility).

Examples

- Gases – nitrous oxide (N_2O).
- Volatile liquids – isoflurane, sevoflurane, desflurane.

Essentials

Isoflurane and sevoflurane are ethers used for induction and maintenance of general anaesthesia. Isoflurane is a halogenated ether, while sevoflurane is a sweet-smelling, highly fluorinated methyl isopropyl ether. Therapeutic N_2O (Entonox or Nitronox) is normally administered as a mixture with 50% N_2O and 50% oxygen. Depending on the concentration and length of administration, N_2O can cause various levels of sedation; paraesthesia, euphoria (laughing), sleepiness and difficulty opening the eyes. Inhalation of N_2O is frequently used to relieve pain associated with trauma and fracture reduction in Accident & Emergency (A&E).

Adverse effects

- Increases cerebral blood flow – should be avoided in polytrauma patients with a possible head injury and raised intracranial pressures.
- Malignant hyperthermia – a rare life-threatening condition in susceptible individuals, which induces a drastic and uncontrolled increase in skeletal muscle oxidative metabolism.

INTRAVENOUS ANAESTHETICS

Examples

- Midazolam.
- Ketamine.
- Propofol.

Essentials

Midazolam is a short-acting benzodiazepine with anxiolytic, amnesic, hypnotic, muscle relaxant, and sedative properties. Midazolam increases the efficiency of **GABA neurotransmitter** action on **GABAA receptors**, resulting in **chloride channels opening more frequently** and therefore causing neural inhibition. Intravenous midazolam is commonly used for pre-operative sedation and induction of general anaesthesia as well as a procedural sedative in A&E.

Ketamine is a **NMDA receptor antagonist**. At high doses, it also binds to opioid μ receptors and sigma receptors as well as interacting with muscarinic receptors, descending monoaminergic pain pathways and voltage-gated calcium channels. It has hypnotic, analgesic and amnesic effects and produces a state of **dissociative anaesthesia**. Primarily it is used for the induction and maintenance of general anesthesia, but other uses include sedation and analgesia in A&E.

Propofol is the most widely used intravenous anaesthetic. It is a short-acting hypnotic used for induction and maintenance of general anaesthesia in adults and children, but it is not commonly used in neonates. Several mechanisms of action have been proposed, both through potentiation of **GABAA receptor** activity, thereby slowing the channel-closing time, and also acting as a **sodium channel blocker**. Propofol is rapidly metabolized in the liver and therefore is associated with rapid recovery and less 'hangover' effect.

Adverse effects

- Midazolam – causes hypotension and respiratory depression and therefore an antagonist such as **flumazenil** should be available in case of overdose.
- Ketamine – causes a rise in intracranial pressure and should not be used in patients who have sustained a recent head injury. Common short-term adverse effects include nausea, hallucinations, irrational behaviour and nightmares. The use of **benzodiazepines as pre-medication**, as well as allowing the patient an undisturbed recovery, helps to reduce some of these unpleasant side-effects.

- Propofol – aside from low blood pressure (mainly through vasodilation) and transient apnoea following induction doses, one of propofol's most frequent adverse effects is **pain on injection**, especially in smaller veins. A more serious but rarer side-effect is dystonia. Mild myoclonic movements are common, as with other intravenous hypnotic agents.

NEUROMUSCULAR BLOCKERS

Examples

- Non-depolarizing: atracurium, pancuronium.
- Depolarizing: suxamethonium.

Essentials

Non-depolarizing agents **competitively block the binding of acetylcholine (ACh) receptors** at the post-synaptic membrane. This leaves fewer receptors available for ACh to bind to and initiate channel opening, resulting in paralysis of the affected skeletal muscles.

Suxamethonium **depolarizes the post-synaptic plasma membrane** of the muscle fibre, similar to ACh, but as these agents are more resistant to degradation it can more persistently depolarize the muscle fibres. There are two phases to the depolarizing block. During the initial **depolarizing phase**, it causes fasciculations whilst the muscle fibres are depolarized. Eventually, after sufficient depolarization has occurred, the **desensitizing phase** sets in and the muscle is no longer responsive to neurotransmitter released by the motor neurones. Full neuromuscular block is achieved at this point.

Adverse effects

Neuromuscular blockade promotes **histamine release**, which can cause transient hypotension, flushing, and tachycardia. Suxamethonium may trigger a transient release of large amounts of potassium from muscle fibres, which may cause hyperkalaemia and cardiac arrhythmias.

Anticoagulants

Anticoagulants are used in the prophylaxis and treatment of thromboembolism. There are several classes of these drugs:

- **Vitamin K antagonists** (coumadins): warfarin.
- **Heparin and derivative substances**: unfractionated heparin, low-molecular weight heparin (enoxaparin, dalteparin), fondaparinux.
- **Direct thrombin inhibitors**: dabigatran, apixaban, rivaroxaban.

Warfarin

Essentials

Warfarin is a coumarin derivative with a structure similar to vitamin K. It **blocks vitamin K-dependent γ-carboxylation of glutamate residues** on clotting factors II, VII, IX and X, resulting in the production of modified factors known as **PIVKA** (proteins in vitamin K absence).

These modified factors cannot bind calcium and therefore become inactive in coagulation (**Figure 4.2**). Warfarin is orally active and takes **2–3 days** to achieve its full anticoagulant effect, as the modified, inactive factors slowly replace those originally present. The effects of warfarin are monitored with the prothrombin time, which is expressed as an international normalized ratio (INR). Warfarin has a **long half-life** (around 40 h), and it takes as long as 5 days for the INR to return to normal after cessation of treatment. Warfarin is metabolized by hepatic microsomal enzymes to inactive 7-hydroxywarfarin.

Adverse effects

- **Haemorrhage**: in overdose can be reversed acutely with clotting factor concentrates or fresh frozen plasma; if severe, consider intravenous vitamin K (phytomenadione).
- **Drug interactions**: drugs that induce (e.g. barbiturates, carbamazepine) or inhibit (e.g. ethanol, metronidazole) hepatic microsomal enzymes may have an effect on the action of warfarin; either leading to reduction or enhancement of anticoagulant effect respectively.
- **Teratogenicity**: absolute contraindication in pregnancy.

Heparins

Essentials

Heparin is a **naturally occurring glycosaminoglycan** of varying molecular weight (5000–15,000 Daltons). It is given by subcutaneous or intravenous injection and is **short acting**. Heparin forms a 1:1 complex with antithrombin III, a protease inhibitor that **inactivates thrombin** when bound to heparin. As thrombin enables fibrinogen conversion to fibrin during the coagulation cascade, inactivating it prevents thrombus development (**Figure 4.2**). The heparin–antithrombin III complex also inactivates factor Xa (among others). When heparin is given intravenously, its effects need to be monitored with the activated partial thromboplastin time (APTT). Heparin has a short duration of action (4–6 h).

Low-molecular weight heparins (LMWHs) are defined as heparin salts having an average molecular weight of less than 8000 Daltons. The LMWH–antithrombin III complex **inhibits factor Xa only**, thereby preventing thrombin synthesis. LMWHs have **longer half-lives** and therefore require only **single daily dosing**. They are given by subcutaneous injection and prophylactic doses do not require monitoring.

Adverse effects

- **Haemorrhage**: less with LMWHs than with heparin. Bleeding with heparin can normally be controlled by stopping its administration, but in severe cases protamine sulphate (a basic peptide that combines with the acidic heparin) may be required.
- **Heparin-induced thrombocytopenia** (HIT): caused by heparin-dependent immunoglobulin G (IgG) antibodies binding to platelet factor 4 (PF4). The heparin–PF4–IgG immune complex binds to platelets causing platelet activation, which accelerates coagulation reactions and generates thrombin.
- **Osteoporosis**: when used long term.
- **Allergic reaction, bruising** at the injection site.

Miscellaneous facts

Fondaparinux is a pentasaccharide that precisely inhibits factor Xa and has been shown to reduce venous thromboembolism more effectively than LMWHs in hip and knee arthroplasty and fractures of the hip. Another potential advantage is the **reduced risk of HIT**. It is given at least 6 h after surgery and at least 12 h after removal of the spinal/epidural catheter in order to avoid the risk of surgical or neuraxial bleeding.

The use of LMWHs may need to be monitored closely in patients at extremes of weight or in-patients with renal dysfunction. An **antifactor Xa assay** may be useful for monitoring LMWH anticoagulation.

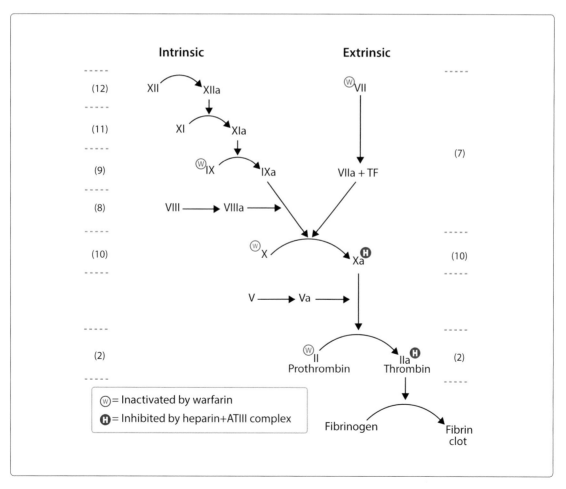

Figure 4.2 Sites of action of anticoagulants on the coagulation cascade. ATIII: antithrombin III; TF: tissue factor (factor III). (Arabic notation of factors in each step are in parentheses.)

Direct thrombin inhibitors

Essentials

Direct thrombin inhibitors (DTIs) act as anticoagulants by competitively and directly inhibiting the enzyme **thrombin** (**Figure 4.2**). They are taken orally, require no therapeutic drug monitoring and have no reported significant drug interactions. A phase III study, comparing dabigatran with enoxaparin, confirmed their equal efficacy in preventing thrombosis, with a similar risk profile. **Dabigatran** has been authorised for use as thromboprophylaxis following hip and knee arthroplasty. Ximelagatran was discontinued in 2006 due to fears of increased hepatotoxicity and myocardial infarctions.

Adverse effects

- Gastritis, hypersensitivity, rash.
- Haemorrhage: similar to LMWHs but less than warfarin.

Drugs acting on bone metabolism

Bone remodelling

Remodelling of bone occurs continuously throughout life (see Chapter 13). To summarize, the cycle commences with osteoclast recruitment by cytokines, e.g. interleukin 6 (IL-6). The osteoclasts adhere to areas of trabecular bone and dig pits by secreting hydrogen ions and proteolytic enzymes (**Figure 4.3**). This action leads to liberation of factors that are embedded in bone, such as insulin-like growth factor 1 (IGF-1). These in turn recruit and activate osteoblasts, which have been primed to develop from precursor cells by parathyroid hormone (PTH) and 1, 25-dihydroxycholecalciferol (calcitriol). Osteoblasts invade the pits and synthesize and secrete osteoid, the organic matrix of bone. The osteoid is then mineralized, i.e. complex calcium phosphate crystals (hydroxyapatites) are deposited. Osteoblasts and their precursors secrete IGF-1 (which becomes embedded in the osteoid) and other cytokines, such as IL-6, which in turn recruit osteoclasts (a return to the start of the cycle). Bone metabolism and mineralization therefore involves the action of PTH, the vitamin D family, cytokines and calcitonin.

BISPHOSPHONATES

Examples

- **Non-nitrogenous:** etidronate.
- **Nitrogenous:** pamidronate, alendronate, risedronate, zoledronate.

Essentials

Bisphosphonates are used clinically to treat post-menopausal and glucocorticoid-induced osteoporosis, Paget's disease of bone and malignant hypercalcaemia. They are also used in paediatrics for the treatment of decreased bone mineral density and pain in conditions such as osteogenesis imperfecta and fibrous dysplasia.

Bisphosphonates are enzyme-resistant analogues of pyrophosphate, which normally inhibits mineralization in bone. They are characterized by a **P–C–P backbone, resistant to phosphatases**, in contrast to pyrophosphate, which has a P–O–P backbone. No known enzymes can metabolize the P–C–P backbone of bisphosphonates, resulting in considerable longevity of these drugs once administered. Around 50% of a dose accumulates at sites of bone mineralization, where it remains until the bone is absorbed.

Bisphosphonates inhibit recruitment and promote apoptosis of osteoclasts as well as indirectly stimulating osteoblastic activity. Nitrogenous bisphosphonates **directly inhibit the action of osteoclasts** (via the mevalonate pathway through inhibition of farnesyl pyrophosphate (FPP) synthase), preventing prenylation (formation of brush border) and functioning of signalling proteins required for osteoclast formation. Older, non-nitrogenous bisphosphonates, such as etidronate, have less specific osteoclastic activity. Bisphosphonates also **directly stabilize the hydroxyapatite crystal**, making it more resistant to resorption.

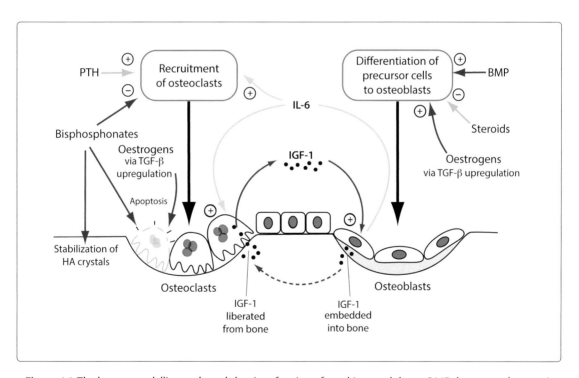

Figure 4.3 The bone-remodelling cycle and the site of action of cytokines and drugs. BMP: bone morphogenetic protein; IGF: insulin-like growth factor; HA: hydroxyapatite; IL: interleukin; PTH: parathyroid hormone. Note that oestrogens are thought to exert their anti-osteoporotic effects by upregulating transforming growth factor-β (TGF-β), which results in apoptosis of osteoclasts and their precursors.

Adverse effects

- Oral intake must be on an empty stomach, which can cause **gastric pain** and **oesophagitis**.
- Rarer adverse effects include **transient leucopenia** and ophthalmic changes, such as **scleritis**.

Miscellaneous facts

- Atypical low-energy subtrochanteric **fractures** of the femur have been reported in patients treated with long-term bisphosphonates. Concomitant use of glucocorticoids and proton pump inhibitors are important risk factors but the exact pathogenesis is unknown. As yet there is no rationale to withhold bisphosphonate therapy from patients with osteoporosis.

VITAMIN D DERIVATIVES

Examples

- Ergocalciferol (vitamin D2) – used in vitamin D deficiency (rickets, osteomalacia).
- Cholecalciferol (vitamin D3) – used in vitamin D deficiency and osteoporosis.
- Calcitriol (1,25-OH-vitamin D3) – used in renal osteodystrophy.
- Alphacalcidiol (1α-hydroxycholecalciferol) – used in renal osteodystrophy.

Essentials

A variety of vitamin D derivatives are commonly used in the treatment of metabolic bone diseases such as rickets and osteomalacia. Vitamin D promotes calcium absorption in the intestines, bone resorption by osteoclasts and maintains serum calcium and phosphate levels for bone formation (see Chapter 13). The biologically active **calcitriol** mediates its effects by binding to the **vitamin D receptors** (VDRs), which are located in the nuclei of cells in the intestines, bones, kidneys and parathyroid glands. The bound VDR acts as a transcription factor that modulates the gene expression of transport proteins that are involved in calcium haemostasis. Vitamin D derivatives are fat-soluble and can be given orally or intravenously. Bile salts are essential for absorption via the intestines.

Adverse effects

Excessive intake leads to **hypercalcaemia**, the symptoms of which can be remembered by the mnemonic '**bones, stones, abdominal groans and psychiatric moans**' – osteitis fibrosa cystica, renal stones, abdominal symptoms such as constipation, and CNS side-effects such as depression. Toxicity is treated by discontinuing supplementation and restricting calcium intake.

CALCITONIN

Essentials

Calcitonin is a **polypeptide hormone** that directly inhibits osteoclasts (see Chapter 13). Natural porcine calcitonin may contain traces of thyroid hormones and can lead to antibody production. Synthetic or recombinant salmon calcitonin (salcalcitonin) can be administered by subcutaneous or intramuscular injection or intranasally. It is used clinically to treat **Paget's**

disease of bone (for pain relief and to reduce neurological complications), **hypercalcaemia** and as part of combination therapy for **post-menopausal and glucocorticoid-induced osteoporosis**.

Adverse effects

- **Nausea and vomiting**.
- **Facial flushing**.
- **Tingling sensation** in the hands.
- **Unpleasant taste** in the mouth.

Disease modifying antirheumatoid drugs

Disease modifying antirheumatoid drugs (DMARDs) are a chemically and pharmacologically very heterogeneous group of drugs; however, they all act to ameliorate symptoms and arrest the disease process in rheumatoid arthritis and other inflammatory arthritides.

Examples

- Methotrexate .
- Sulfasalazine.
- Leflunomide.
- Intramuscular gold (sodium aurothiomalate).
- Tumour necrosis factor alpha (TNF-α) inhibitors (adalimumab, etanercept and infliximab).

Essentials

Methotrexate is an **antimetabolite**, and acts by **inhibiting the metabolism of folic acid** by competitively inhibiting dihydrofolate reductase (DHFR), an enzyme that participates in tetrahydrofolate synthesis. Methotrexate also inhibits the enzymes involved in purine metabolism, leading to accumulation of adenosine, or the inhibition of T-cell activation and **suppression of intercellular adhesion molecule expression by T-cells**. This is thought to reduce inflammation and retard the progression of rheumatoid arthritis.

Sulfasalazine is a combination of sulphonamide with a salicylate. In the colon, sulfasalazine is reduced by the bacterial enzyme azoreductase to sulfapyridine and 5-aminosalicylic acid (5-ASA). It is thought that the **5-ASA scavenges the toxic oxygen metabolites** produced by neutrophils thereby retarding disease activity.

Leflunomide is an antimetabolite and **inhibits dihydroorotate dehydrogenase**, an enzyme involved in pyrimidine synthesis. This has a relatively specific inhibitory effect on activated T-cells.

Sodium aurothiomalate is administered by deep intramuscular injection and the maximum effect is seen after 3 months. The exact mechanism of action is unknown; however, it is proposed that it is able to **inhibit macrophage activation**.

TNF-α inhibitors interfere with the inflammatory cascade in rheumatoid arthritis by binding to TNF-α receptors. Adalimumab is a human-sequence antibody that binds specifically to TNF-α and neutralizes its biological function by blocking its interaction with cell-surface TNF-α receptors. Etanercept is a recombinant human TNF-α-receptor fusion protein, while infliximab is a chimeric monoclonal antibody that binds with high affinity to TNF-α.

Adverse effects

- Common – rash, ulcerative stomatitis, nausea, abdominal pain, diarrhoea and dizziness. Folic acid supplements may help prevent some of the minor side-effects.
- Rare – leucopenia and predisposition to infection, pulmonary fibrosis, hepatic, renal and bone marrow toxicity, necessitating regular blood monitoring.

Miscellaneous drugs

Tranexamic acid

Tranexamic acid is an **antifibrinolytic that competitively inhibits the activation of plasminogen to plasmin**. Plasmin is a molecule responsible for the degradation of fibrin, which is vital for the formation of a blood clot (**Figure 4.4**). The use of tranexamic acid in elective lower limb arthroplasty reduces blood loss and the need for blood transfusions post-operatively. In patients with traumatic haemorrhage, tranexamic acid has been shown to reduce all-cause mortality and is now routinely used at many trauma centres worldwide (multinational CRASH-2 trial).

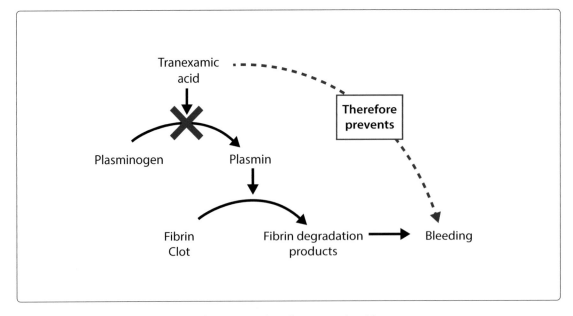

Figure 4.4 Action of transexamic acid.

Botulinum toxin

Botulinum toxin is a protein produced by *Clostridium botulinum*, which can be used as a very potent therapeutic neurotoxin causing muscle weakness. The toxin enters the axon terminals and degrades the **SNAP-25 protein**, a type of SNARE protein required for vesicle fusion. This prevents neurosecretory vesicles from docking with the nerve synapse plasma membrane and releasing their neurotransmitters. In orthopaedics, botulinum toxin is used in the treatment of movement disorders associated with injury or disease of the CNS including cerebral palsy and trauma.

Teriparatide

Teriparatide is a recombinant fragment of PTH used in the treatment of post-menopausal osteoporosis, osteoporosis in men at high risk of fracture and corticosteroid-induced osteoporosis. It is a portion of the full human PTH, consisting of only the amino acid sequence 1–34. Chronically elevated PTH will deplete bone stores through bone resorption; however, intermittent exposure to PTH **paradoxically activates osteoblasts more than osteoclasts**. Teriparatide works mainly on the periosteal surface of bone, but it also causes endosteal resorption, increasing the diameter of bone. Thus, once-daily subcutaneous injections of teriparatide have a net effect of stimulating new bone formation leading to increased bone mineral density. Treatment duration should last 18 months, after which no further course should be repeated. Minor adverse effects include gastrointestinal problems, leg cramps and dizziness.

Strontium ranelate

Strontium was originally detected in lead mines in the 1700s near Strontian in Scotland and is used in BMW car engines. It is a group 2, period 5 element in the periodic table, with atomic number 38. Strontium is similar to calcium, and thus dual-energy X-ray absorption (DEXA) scans following treatment with strontium look excellent. Its effects are **increased bone formation** (anabolic effect) and **decreased bone resorption** (anticatabolic effect). Strontium ranelate is licensed in the UK, as a once-daily tablet for the treatment of post-menopausal osteoporosis but restricted to those patients in whom bisphosphonates are contraindicated or not tolerated. Minor adverse effects include: nausea, diarrhoea and dermatitis. However, there have been reports of venous thromboembolism and severe allergic reactions.

Allopurinol

Allopurinol is a purine analogue and an inhibitor of the enzyme **xanthine oxidase**. Xanthine oxidase is responsible for the successive oxidation of hypoxanthine and xanthine, resulting in the production of uric acid, the product of human purine metabolism. Allopurinol is used for the long-term control of gout and should only be started 1–2 weeks after the acute attack has settled. Common adverse effects include diarrhoea and nausea.

Viva questions

1. What are the different methods of achieving pain relief after joint arthroplasty?

2. What thromboprophylaxis regimen would you use for total hip arthroplasty?

3. What are the indications for the use of bisphosphonates in orthopaedics?

4. What classes of drug can be used to treat osteoporosis?

5. How do local anaesthetics work?

Further reading

Bhattacharyya T, Smith RM. Cardiovascular risks of coxibs: the orthopaedic perspective. *J Bone Joint Surg Am* 2005;**87**:245–6.

Ekman EF, Koman LA. Acute pain following musculoskeletal injuries and orthopaedic surgery. Mechanisms and management. *J Bone Joint Surg Am* 2004;**86**:1316–27.

Parvizi J, Miller AG, Gandhi K. Multimodal pain management after total joint arthroplasty *J Bone Joint Surg Am* 2011;**93**(11):1075–84.

Morris CD, Einhorn TA. Bisphosphonates in orthopaedic surgery. *J Bone Joint Surg Am* 2005;**87**:1609–18.

Warwick D. New concepts in orthopaedicm thromboprophylaxis. *J Bone Joint Surg Br* 2004;**86**:788–92.

5 Inflammation and Infection

Vikas Khanduja, Sertazniel Singhkang and Manoj Ramachandran

Introduction

Inflammation and infection are large topics to cover in terms of the essentials required for day-to-day orthopaedic practice. Details of the virulence of microorganisms and the host response produced following an infection are beyond the scope of this chapter. However, a working knowledge of the common microorganisms causing infection in bones and joints, the common antibiotics used and the mechanisms of action of the latter is essential.

An in-depth knowledge of acute osteomyelitis and septic arthritis is invaluable and is thus covered in this chapter. Finally, a brief discussion on methicillin-resistant *Staphylococcus aureus* (MRSA) and tuberculosis (TB) is also required.

Overview of inflammation

The five cardinal features of acute inflammation are **rubor** (erythema), **calor** (heat), **dolor** (pain), **tumour** (swelling) and **functio laesa** (loss of function). Acute inflammation follows a specific sequence. The initial phase is **vasoconstriction**, followed immediately by **vasodilation** and increased **vascular permeability**. Further events include **leukocytic margination and emigration** (neutrophils, followed by monocytes) and **phagocytosis**, involving both intracellular degradation of ingested particles (oxygen-dependent and oxygen-independent mechanisms) and extracellular release of leukocyte products, e.g. lysosomal enzymes.

When bacteria invade the musculoskeletal system, the initial response is an acute inflammatory reaction. This results in polymorphonuclear cells attacking and phagocytosing bacteria.

There are three possible outcomes to acute inflammation: complete **resolution**, healing by **scarring**, and progression to **chronic inflammation**. Chronic inflammation can occur due to a variety of causes, including **persistent infection** by intracellular microbes (e.g. tubercle bacilli, viral infections) that are of low toxicity but evoke an immunological reaction, **prolonged exposure** to non-degradable but potentially toxic substances (e.g. lung silicosis, asbestosis), and **immune** (particularly autoimmune) **reactions**.

The key cells in chronic inflammation are:

- **Mononuclear cells** (principally macrophages, lymphocytes and plasma cells).
- **Fibroblasts**.
- **Eosinophils** (in immune reactions).

Macrophages are the central figures, their activation in inflammation being triggered by lymphokines (e.g. gamma-interferon) produced by immune-activated T-cells or non-immune factors such as exotoxin. The secretory products of macrophages induce characteristic chronic inflammatory changes, such as **tissue destruction** (proteases and oxygen-derived free radicals), **neovascularization** (growth factors), **fibroblast proliferation** (growth factors) and **connective tissue accumulation** (interleukin 1 [IL-1], tumour necrosis factor-alpha [TNF-α]).

Lymphocytes have a reciprocal relationship with macrophages in chronic inflammation. Activated lymphocytes produce lymphokines, and these (particularly gamma-interferon) are major stimulators of macrophages. Activated macrophages produce monokines, which in turn influence B- and T-cell function.

Systemic inflammatory response syndrome

In major traumatic events such as long bone fracture, pelvic and/or thoracic trauma or head injury, the post-injury inflammatory response, which in normal situations remains localized to the site of injury, may develop an imbalance in pro-inflammatory mediators. A generalized state of inflammation evolves, known as the **systemic inflammatory response syndrome** (SIRS).

The pathophysiology of SIRS is not fully understood. However, it appears that widespread **fibrin deposition**, **microvascular occlusion** and **tissue hypoxia** occur following an increased production of cytokines and inflammatory mediators.

Polymorphonucleocytes (PMNs) in the circulation bind to adhesion molecules on the surface of endothelial cells in organs distant from the initially injured tissue. Endothelial damage occurs due to PMNs releasing proteolytic enzymes and oxygen metabolites from cytoplasmic granules at their binding sites. This results in endothelial barrier impairment, with diffusely increased capillary permeability, and tissue infiltration. Widespread endothelial injury causes diffuse fluid infiltration and multiple organ failure (**Figure 5.1**).

In the management of polytrauma patients the second-hit concept acknowledges that post-injury surgical procedures have the potential to add further inflammatory insult in addition to the initial trauma. The timing of a surgical procedure before restoration of physiological balance may result in a hyperinflammatory state with the potential to cause systemic disease, including SIRS, acute respiratory distress syndrome (ARDS,) and multiple organ failure syndrome (MOFS.) This understanding has led to the development of Damage Control Orthopaedics (DCO) and a more cautious approach in the early care of polytrauma patients.

Bacteriology

Microorganisms that can cause infection include bacteria, viruses, parasites and fungi. Of these, bacteria are the most common source of infection in bones and joints. Bacteria are **prokaryotic cells,** as they do not have a nucleus (**Figure 5.2**).

The genetic material is aggregated in an area of the cytoplasm called the nucleoid. Bacteria do not possess a cytoplasmic compartment containing mitochondria and lysosomes. A consistent

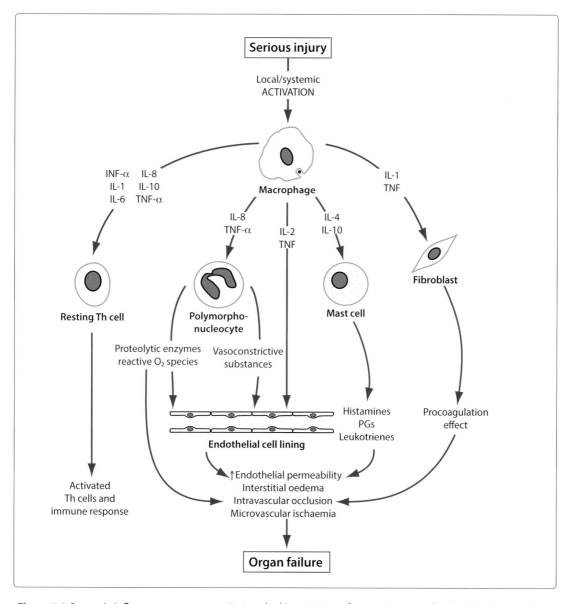

Figure 5.1 Systemic inflammatory response. IL: Interleukin; INF: interferon; PG: prostaglandin; Th: T-helper; TNF: tumour necrosis factor.

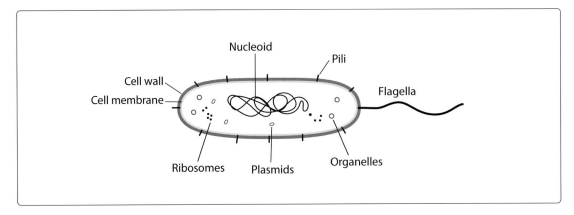

Figure 5.2 Structure of a bacterium.

feature of all prokaryotes but not eukaryotes is the presence of a **cell wall**, which allows bacteria to resist osmotic stress. This cell wall differs in complexity between species, and bacteria are usually divided into two major groups – **gram-positive and gram-negative** bacteria – which reflect their cell wall structure.

Bacteria are designated gram-positive or gram-negative depending on whether the cell membrane of the bacterium retains crystal violet indium dye after an alcohol rinse. Gram-positive bacteria retain the dye and, hence, appear bluish under a light microscope. Gram-negative bacteria do not retain the dye, but they do retain the safranin O counter-stain and, hence, appear pink under a light microscope.

Bacteria can be classified further into **cocci** and **bacilli** depending on their shape. Cocci are round and bacilli are small rods. Examples of the common bacteria and their classification are given in *Table 5.1*.

Table 5.1 Examples of common bacteria and their classification

Gram-positive cocci	Gram-negative cocci	Gram-positive bacilli	Gram-negative bacilli
Staphylococcus aureus S. epidermidis		Clostridium tetani C. perfringens	Pseudomonas aeruginosa
Enterococcus spp.	Neisseria gonorrhoea N. meningitides	Bacillus anthracis	Eikenella corrodens
Streptococcus spp.		Actinomyces spp.	Haemophilus influenzae Escherichia coli Salmonella typhi

Septic arthritis and osteomyelitis

Definition

Septic arthritis is a condition characterized by **infection of the synovium and the joint space**. The infection causes an intense inflammatory reaction and release of proteolytic enzymes, leading to rapid destruction of the articular cartilage.

Osteomyelitis is an **acute or chronic inflammatory process of the bone** and its structures secondary to infection.

Aetiology and pathogenesis

Septic arthritis and osteomyelitis are **common in children** but can also occur in adults, usually secondary to an immunocompromised state or an underlying medical condition such as diabetes. Septic arthritis and osteomyelitis can occur from **primary seeding of the synovial membrane**, secondarily from **infection in the adjacent metaphyseal bone** or directly from **infection in the adjoining epiphysis**. In the shoulder, elbow, hip and ankle joints, the capsule overlaps a portion of the adjoining metaphysis. If the focus of osteomyelitis breaks through the metaphyseal bone, it can directly infect the joint and lead to concurrent septic arthritis.

Destruction of the articular cartilage begins quickly and is secondary to proteolytic enzymes released from synovial cells. IL-1 triggers the release of proteases from chondrocytes and synoviocytes in response to polymorphonuclear leukocytes and bacteria. Degradation results in the **loss of proteoglycans** from the articular cartilage by 5 days and **loss of collagen** by 9 days.

Impairment of the intracapsular vascular supply secondary to elevation of the intracapsular pressure and thrombosis of the vessels also play a role in the destruction of articular cartilage. The common sites of involvement in children are the hip and knee, but in the adult about 85% of cases are monoarticular, the knee being the most common joint involved.

Clinical presentation

Typically, the disease has an **acute onset** and the child is irritable and febrile. If the infection involves the lower limb, the child usually has a **limp** and **refuses to bear weight**. Clinical examination of the involved joint reveals **resistance to passive motion** of the attempted joint and **severe pain on attempted motion**. In subcutaneous joints, increased **warmth**, **erythema**, **soft-tissue swelling** and **effusion** may be present. The joints are usually held in a position of maximal comfort; if the hip is involved, the child holds it in a position of flexion, abduction and external rotation.

Neonates with septic arthritis may exhibit only irritability, lethargy, difficulty in feeding and pseudo-paralysis of the affected limb. In osteomyelitis tenderness is most acute over the involved area of bone, which is usually metaphyseal.

Investigations

Initial laboratory tests include a full blood count, acute-phase reactants, including erythrocyte sedimentation rate (ESR) and C-reactive protein (CRP), and blood cultures. The **white cell count** is usually greater than 12,000/mm^3, with 40–60% polymorphonuclear leukocytes. **ESR** is usually elevated to more than 50 mm, and **blood cultures** are positive in about 30–50% of cases. **CRP** is elevated and returns to normal fairly quickly after treatment. A CRP less than 10 mg/ml in a limping child with a hip effusion would indicate that septic arthritis is unlikely.

Ultrasound of the affected joint, especially the hip, can detect an effusion, as well as periosteal elevation, and can be an aid in aspiration. **Radiographs** may show subluxation or dislocation of the joint and soft tissue swelling around the affected joint. Radiographs can also reveal subtle changes such as joint-space widening in septic arthritis and metaphyseal rarefaction in early osteomyelitis.

Bone scans may show a decreased-uptake 'cold scan' early in the disease process and an increased-uptake 'hot scan' later on.

Joint aspiration with immediate **Gram stain and microscopy** followed by **culture and sensitivity** remains the mainstay for diagnosis for septic arthritis. On direct examination, the aspirate may demonstrate **gross pus**. Gram stains are positive in only 30–50% of the cases, and cultures of the aspirate are positive in about 50–80% of cases.

The diagnosis of osteomyelitis is usually made by a combination of clinical findings, radiographs, bone scanning and magnetic resonance imaging (MRI) scans, along with the aspiration of pus from the involved area and positive blood cultures. In chronic osteomyelitis, radiographic signs of necrotic bone (**sequestrum**) and periosteal new bone formation (**involucrum**) are evident.

Management algorithms

These include clinical and serological parameters such as weight-bearing status, the presence of pyrexia, and raised white cell count, ESR and CRP. They are not necessarily applicable in all settings, and their validity must be tested locally. However, other than weight-bearing status, the currently published clinical algorithms do not include physical examination. Algorithms should supplement clinical decision-making in all cases as there is no substitute for the clinical acumen of experienced clinicians.

Treatment

Septic arthritis is an emergency, and treatment should be expedited to prevent any permanent damage to the articular cartilage. Appropriate management involves **prompt diagnosis** followed by **surgical drainage** and **irrigation of the involved joint** with appropriate constitutional support, including hydration and antibiotics. A drain can be left in place following irrigation until the volume of the drainage decreases. If surgery is not followed by rapid recovery, **re-exploration** should be considered.

Intravenous antibiotics should be commenced immediately after aspiration of the involved joints. **Broad-spectrum** antibiotics are commenced initially based on the organisms suspected and subsequently changed to **specific** antibiotics, depending upon culture and sensitivity. The organisms responsible in various age groups are summarized in *Table 5.2*. The traditional regimen of intravenous antibiotics being given for 2 weeks and then **converted to oral antibiotics** for a total of 4–6 weeks is being replaced by shorter duration treatments, depending on the clinical and serological response.

Table 5.2 Organisms responsible for septic arthritis and osteomyelitis by age

Age group	Organisms
Infants (<1 year)	Group B streptococci
	Staphylococcus aureus
	Escherichia coli
Children (1–16 years)	*S. aureus*
	Streptococcus pyogenes
	Kingella kingae
Adults (>16 years)	*Staphylococcus epidermidis*
	S. aureus
	Pseudomonas aeruginosa
	E. coli

The approach to management of acute osteomyelitis is similar but may involve open drainage of pus if, for example, a subperiosteal abscess forms. If osteomyelitis becomes **chronic**, the management principles involve **drainage and debridement** of all necrotic tissue, with **preservation of the involucrum**, **obliteration of dead spaces** (e.g. with vascularized bone graft or vacuum-assisted closure), **adequate soft-tissue coverage** (e.g. with local or free flaps) and **preservation of skeletal stability**.

Biofilm formation

A feature common to both osteomyelitis and prosthetic infections is the provision of a surface that facilitates bacterial attachment, subsequent biofilm formation and an established infection. **Strong bonds are formed between glycoproteins of host tissue and the biofilm**, which makes diagnosis and eradication of the bacteria from bone/implant difficult. The bacterial barrier created protects against antibiotics and the host's immune response. This virulence factor provides the basis for the principle of debridement of necrotic tissue or hardware exchange.

In the case of prosthetic infections, *Staphylococcus epidermidis* is the most common offending organism due to its ability to form biofilms. Treatment strategies to prevent biofilm formation include the local delivery of antibiotic impregnated cement and derivatization of implant surfaces with antibiotics.

Polymerase chain reaction (PCR) based amplification technology coupled with other molecular techniques such as ribonucleic acid (RNA) analysis could be used for more efficient diagnosis of prosthetic infections. *Propionibacterium acnes* has recently been isolated from more than one-third of infected shoulder arthroplasties, and this organism can take up to 2 weeks to culture, making this an excellent candidate for molecular detection.

Host response

The strongest determinant in the outcome following osteomyelitis is the effectiveness of the host response.

Antibiotics

Antibiotics are used for **prophylaxis**, to **eradicate infections** and for **initial care** in open fractures and wounds. A comprehensive list of the antibiotics commonly used for musculoskeletal infections along with their groups, subgroups and mechanism of action is shown in *Table 5.3*. *Table 5.4* summarizes the spectrum of activity and the common complications of these antibiotics.

Antibiotic delivery

Antibiotics can be delivered in a variety of ways:

- **Oral**.
- **Intramuscular**.
- **Intravenous and home intravenous therapy** (via Hickman line).
- **Antibiotic beads and spacers**:
  - aminoglycosides are impregnated in polymethylmethacrylate (PMMA) cement and used to treat infected total joint arthroplasty and osteomyelitis.
  - the antibiotic used in this form is stable during the process of PMMA polymerization.
  - elution of antibiotic from PMMA is for a maximum of 6–8 weeks.
  - this form delivers a very high local concentration of the antibiotic.
- **Osmotic pump**: delivers high concentration of antibiotic locally. Useful for osteomyelitis.

Antibiotic resistance

There are two types of microbiological resistance: innate (or intrinsic) and extrinsic.

Innate or intrinsic antibiotic resistance

This implies that the bacterial cell inherently has properties that do not allow the antibiotic to act on it. Examples of innate or intrinsic resistance include:

- Enzyme production that destroys the antibiotic.

Table 5.3. Antibiotics commonly used in orthopaedics

Antibiotic group	Examples and subgroups	Mechanism of action
Penicillins	**Natural** Penicillin G (IV) Penicillin V (oral) **Penicillinase-resistant** Flucloxacillin Cloxacillin Aminopenicillins Ampicillin Augmentin Amoxycillin **Antipseudomonal** Piperacillin Ticarcillin Mezlocillin	Penicillins are bactericidal and act by inhibition of bacterial peptidoglycan synthesis. This takes place by binding to the penicillin binding proteins present on bacterial cell membrane. Penicillins are also known as beta-lactam antibiotics.
Cephalosporins	**First-generation** Cephradine Cephalexin **Second-generation** Cefuroxime Cefaclor **Third-generation** Ceftriaxone Ceftazidime **Fourth-generation** Cefepime Cefpirome	Cephalosporins are also known as **beta-lactam antibiotics**, are **bactericidal** and act by **inhibition of bacterial cell wall synthesis.**
Carbapenems	Imipenem	Carbapenems are bactericidal and act by inhibition of cell wall synthesis.
Monobactams	Aztreonam	Monobactams are also bactericidal and act by inhibition of cell wall synthesis. They have a limited spectrum of activity, mainly against gram-negative anaerobes.
Aminoglycosides	Gentamicin Neomycin Tobramycin Amikacin	Aminoglycosides act by inhibition of bacterial protein synthesis by binding to cytoplasmic ribosomal RNA (to the 30S subunit). They are bactericidal.
Macrolides	Erythromycin Clarithromycin Azithromycin	Macrolides act by inhibiting dissociation of peptidyl transfer RNA from ribosomes during translocation (by binding to the 50S subunit).
Quinolones	Ciprofloxacin Ofloxacin Norfloxacin	Quinolones act by inhibiting DNA gyrase, an enzyme that compresses DNA into supercoils.
Glycopeptides	Vancomycin Teicoplanin	Glycopeptides act by inhibiting cell membrane synthesis by interference with insertion of glycan subunits in the cell wall.
Tetracyclines	Tetracycline Doxycycline Minocycline	Tetracyclines act by inhibition of bacterial protein synthesis by binding to cytoplasmic ribosomal RNA (to the 30S subunit). They are bacteriostatic.
Others	Rifampicin	Rifampicin acts by preventing RNA transcription by inhibiting DNA-dependent RNA polymerase. It is bactericidal.

DNA: deoxyribonucleic acid; IV: intravenous; RNA: ribonucleic acid.

Table 5.4. Antibiotic spectrum of activity and complications

Antibiotics	Spectrum of activity	Complications
Penicillins	Mainly against gram-positive cocci *Clostridium Bacillus anthracis* (cause of anthrax) Inactivated by bacterial beta-lactamases	Hypersensitivity reactions Haemolytic anaemia Central nervous system toxicity Colitis Same as for penicillin Cholestatic jaundice Hepatitis
Flucloxacillin	*Staphylococcus*	Same as for penicillin Cholestatic jaundice Hepatitis
Augmentin (Amoxycillin + beta lactamase inhibitor clavulanic acid)	*Staphylococcus aureus* *Escherichia coli* *Haemophilus influenzae* *Bacteroides* spp. *Klebsiella*	Hepatitis Cholestatic jaundice Skin reactions
Piperacillin	*Pseudomonas aeruginosa* Gram-negative bacilli	Same as for penicillin
Cephalosporins	The first-generation cephalosporins are very active against gram-positive-bacteria and the fourth-generation agents are active against gram-negative bacteria. The activity against gram-positive bacteria decreases from first to fourth generations.	Haemolytic anaemia Colitis Allergic skin reactions Disturbances in liver enzymes
Imipenem	Administered with cilastatin to prevent renal metabolism Active against aerobes and anaerobes and gram-positive and -gram-negative bacteria	Central nervous system toxicity – grand mal seizures Colitis
Gentamicin	Mainly against aerobic gram-negative bacteria *Pseudomonas aeruginosa* Enterobacteriaceae	Ototoxicity Nephrotoxicity Neuromuscular blockade
Erythromycin	Active against: *Streptococcus* *Listeria monocytogenes* *Moraxella catarrhalis* *Mycoplasma pneumoniae* *Legionella pneumophila* *Chlamydia pneumoniae*	Fairly safe but can cause gastrointestinal reactions – nausea, vomiting and abdominal cramps
Ciprofloxacin	Mainly against gram-negative bacteria	Gastrointestinal disturbances Tendonitis and increased risk of Achilles tendon rupture
Vancomycin	*Staphylococcus aureus* *Staphylococcus epidermidis* Enterococcus MRSA	'Red man syndrome' – flushing of head, neck and upper torso associated with hypotension Nephrotoxicity Ototoxicity Neutropenia and thrombocytopenia Colitis
Tetracycline	Mainly against gram-positive bacteria	Thrombocytopenia Colitis Staining of bone and teeth in children Hepatotoxicity in pregnancy

MRSA, methicillin-resistant *Staphlococcus aureus*; spp: species (plural).

- Changes in cell wall permeability.
- Alterations in structural target (e.g. 30S and 50S ribosomes).
- Mutations in efflux mechanisms.
- Bypass of metabolic pathway.
- Resistance via a combination of the above or multiple mechanisms.

Extrinsic antibiotic resistance

This implies that an organism acquires resistance to an antibiotic to which it was previously sensitive. This can take place due to a chance mutation in the genetic material of the cell or the acquisition of drug-resistant genes from other drug-resistant cells. This resistance is usually mediated via **plasmids**, small circles of double-stranded deoxyribonucleic acid (DNA). Plasmids carry genes for specialized functions and also carry one or more genes for antimicrobial resistance.

Methicillin-resistant *Staphylococcus aureus*

Definition and prevalence

MRSA is a gram-positive coccus and a **major nosocomial pathogen**. The prevalence of MRSA is reported to be around 1.6% within orthopaedic departments, compared with 0.3% within general hospital settings. MRSA is a cause for significant concern due to its associated high morbidity and mortality and the financial implications if total joint arthroplasties are infected.

Genetics

The staphylococci acquire their methicillin resistance due to the presence of an **acquired penicillin-binding protein**, PBP2a. This protein is encoded by the gene *mecA*, which is carried on the staphylococcal chromosome. The levels of resistance of the bacteria depend on the production of PBP2a.

Subclassification

Community- and healthcare-acquired (CA- and HA-) MRSA are different organisms. Each affects different patient populations, produces distinct infections and requires unique treatment. CA-MRSA has become more prevalent especially in the USA, and is defined as MRSA isolated as an out- or in-patient within 48 hours of admission. The importance of CA-MRSA is the presence of the **Panton-Valentine leukocidin** (PVL) locus whose gene product causes neutrophil lysis and subsequent severe soft tissue infection in healthy, often athletic patients. Fortunately, CA-MRSA has greater susceptibility to most beta-lactams, erythromycin and quinolones, whereas HA-MRSA has multiple drug resistance.

Colonization and risk factors

Most MRSA infections are acquired by proximity and contact with other colonized patients. It is postulated that up to 25% of hospital personnel are carriers of MRSA. Other important risk factors implicated in the acquisition of MRSA are:

- Old age.
- Previous hospitalization or surgery.
- Prolonged hospitalization.
- Open skin lesions.
- Chronic medical illness.
- Presence of invasive in-dwelling device.
- Prolonged antibiotic therapy.
- Exposure to another colonized or infected patient.

Prevention and prophylaxis

The main areas of focus for prevention are **effective screening** to pick up high-risk patients and staff and appropriate **isolation** and **treatment of carriers**. Once these patients have been identified, they should be treated with **nasal mupirocin**; bathing in **antiseptic detergent**, such as 4% chlorhexidine or 2% triclosan, should be encouraged.

Education of nursing and medical staff on hand hygiene is essential. Alcohol-based hand rubs have been shown to be effective against hospital-acquired MRSA infection. Ringfencing or segregation policies have been shown to clearly reduce the infection rate secondary to MRSA.

Management

Once infection is established, management involves administering **intravenous glycopeptides**, which have become the mainstay of treatment. Vancomycin and teicoplanin are the drugs of choice. The advantage of teicoplanin over vancomycin is that the former has better bone penetration, is better tolerated and can be administered as a bolus dose and, therefore, given on an outpatient basis. MRSA is adept at forming biofilms which makes it difficult to eradicate with antibiotic therapy alone. This provides the rationale for hardware removal in chronic infection.

Staphylococcal resistance to glycopeptides has been reported and is a cause for concern. There are also concerns about emergence of strains of *Staphylococcus aureus* with reduced sensitivity to vancomycin. Fortunately, the discovery of oxazolidinones, which inhibit an early step in protein synthesis, seems to have solved the problem of glycopeptide resistance.

Linezolid, which was the first in this class of antibiotics to be used, has excellent tissue penetration, has 100% bioavailability and can be given orally. Linezolid is recommended when conventional glycopeptides have failed or are not tolerated. The major adverse effect of linezolid is bone-marrow suppression with prolonged use.

Tuberculosis

TB is a **chronic granulomatous condition** commonly caused by *Mycobacterium tuberculosis*. The incidence in developed countries is much lower than in developing countries. However, TB is on the rise again, partly due to the human immunodeficiency virus (HIV) epidemic. In addition, multiple drug-resistant strains of *M. tuberculosis* appear regularly.

Pathogenesis

Mycobacteria are **obligate aerobic acid-fast rods**. The infection usually **begins in the lung** and the subpleural region along with the draining lymphatics. The mediastinal lymph nodes are also involved. This is known as the primary (Ghon) complex. This primary infection can undergo complete resolution and remain quiescent, or it can spread systemically. Local spread into the lung can lead to **bronchopneumonia**, and haematogenous spread can lead to **miliary TB**, which involves the lung, bones, joints and spine; this is known as **secondary TB**.

Clinical presentation

Patients with pulmonary TB present with low-grade fever, productive chronic cough, weight loss and generalized weakness. Although skeletal involvement usually follows pulmonary involvement, only half of the patients with skeletal involvement have pulmonary disease. Skeletal involvement commonly includes the spine (**tuberculous spondylitis**), the fingers (**tuberculous dactylitis**), the appendicular skeleton (where **metaphyseal lytic lesions** with little or no sclerosis are found) and, rarely, the hip and knee joints (presenting as **monoarthritis**). The important features of tuberculous monoarthritis include florid synovitis, preservation of joint space and periarticular osteopenia.

Diagnosis

The diagnosis is difficult to establish and requires a minimum of three large-volume **early-morning sputum samples**. The presence of **acid-fast bacteria under Ziehl–Neelsen stain** confirms the diagnosis. The bacteria appear as red acid-fast organisms under the stain. If microscopy is negative, the specimen is subjected to culture on **Lowenstein–Jensen medium** for a period of 6 weeks at 35–37°C; growth of bacteria in this medium confirms diagnosis.

If both microscopy and culture are negative, then the gold standard for diagnosis remains **biopsy**. Histological sections reveal a **classic granuloma with caseating central necrosis**. The development of DNA probes, PCR assays and liquid media has allowed more sensitive and rapid diagnosis, but these tests are not always specific.

Skin tests

The basis of skin tests is a **delayed hypersensitivity reaction**. The two commonly employed tests are the Heaf test and the Mantoux test. Both tests involve exposing the patient's skin to purified protein derivative. A positive response includes the formation of papules on the skin after a designated number of hours. A positive response implies an active infection or previous bacillus Calmette–Guèrin (BCG) vaccination.

Blood tests

There are several problems with skin tests, which has led to the development of selective immunological **interferon gamma tests** (IGTs). These IGTs identify three different tuberculosis antigens – early secretion antigen target 6 (ESAT 6), culture filtrate protein 10 (CFP-10) and tb7.7 – from whole blood samples.

IGT shows a stronger correlation with exposure than Mantoux tests, but NICE guidelines recommend a two-step approach of an initial Mantoux test followed by an IGT to confirm positivity.

Bone and joint treatment

A combination regime of **first-line chemotherapeutic agents** initially lasting for 12 months, comprising isoniazid, pyrazinamide, rifampicin and a fourth drug (for example, ethambutol) for the first 2 months, followed by isoniazid and rifampicin for the remaining treatment period is recommended by the latest NICE guidelines (2011).

TB is usually treated for an extensive time period, as the organism grows slowly and there is a possibility of it becoming dormant. By using two or more antibiotics, the chance of developing resistance during this extended time is minimized.

Multi-drug resistant TB

Multi-drug resistant (MDR) TB comprises approximately 0.8–0.9% of culture-confirmed TB cases in the UK. A risk assessment for drug resistance should be made for each patient with TB, based on the risk factors listed below:

- History of prior TB drug treatment.
- Prior TB treatment failure.
- Contact with a known case of drug-resistant TB.
- Birth in a foreign country, particularly high-incidence countries.
- HIV infection.
- Age profile, with highest rates between ages 25 and 44 years.
- Male gender.

In the absence of clinical improvement, or if cultures remain positive after the 4 months of treatment ('treatment failure'), drug resistance should be suspected and treatment reviewed with a clinician experienced in the treatment of MDR TB.

Viva questions

1. Classify bacteria. Give some examples of gram-positive bacteria.
2. How do penicillins act? What are the different classes of penicillins? How do the classes differ?
3. How do bacteria develop resistance?
4. Describe the pathogenesis of septic arthritis.
5. What is MRSA, and how is it acquired?
6. How is musculoskeletal TB diagnosed and treated?
7. Why are prosthetic infections difficult to diagnose and treat? What methods are available for diagnosis in such cases?

Further reading

Kang S-N, Sanghera T, Mangwani J, Paterson JMH, Ramachandran M. The management of septic arthritis in children: Systematic Review of the English Language Literature. *J Bone Joint Surg Br* 2009;**91**-B:1127–33.

Lazzarini L, Mader JT, Calhoun, JH. Osteomyelitis in long bones *J Bone Joint Surg Am* 2004;**86**:2305–18.

Mader JT, Wang J, Calhoun JH. Antibiotic therapy for musculoskeletal infections. *J Bone Joint Surg Am* 2001;**83**:1878–90.

NICE. Tuberculosis: Clinical diagnosis and management of tuberculosis, and measures for its prevention and control. NICE clinical guideline 117 March 2011.

Patel A, Calfee RP, Plante M, Fischer SA, Arcand N, Born C. Methicillin-resistant *Staphylococcus aureus* in orthopaedic surgery. *J Bone Joint Surg Br* 2008;**90**:1401–6.

Sears BW, Stover MD, Callaci J. Pathoanatomy and clinical correlates of the immunoinflammatory response following orthopaedic trauma. *J Am Acad Orthop Surg* 2009;**17**(4):255–65.

Tuli SM. General principles of osteoarticular tuberculosis. *Clin Orthop Relat Res* 2002;**398**:11–19.

Wong KC, Leung KS. Transmission and prevention of occupational infections in orthopaedic surgeons. *J Bone Joint Surg Am* 2004;**86**:1065–76.

6 Imaging Techniques

Manoj Ramachandran, Dennis Kosuge, Navin Ramachandran and Asif Saifuddin

Introduction

The orthopaedic surgeon should have a working knowledge of the various imaging modalities available as in addition to a detailed history and thorough examination, investigations in the form of imaging are often required to narrow down the differential or confirm the diagnosis. This chapter initially covers the effects of radiation exposure and then details the commonly encountered imaging modalities.

Risk of exposure

As clinicians who request a wide range of radiological investigations, it is important to understand the radiation doses associated with these investigations. In order to allow levels of exposures from different radiological modalities to be compared, the **effective dose** is described – this is the **estimated whole body radiation dose associated with a specific modality** (*Table 6.1*). To put things into perspective, the average person receives an effective dose of 2.4 mSv per annum from natural background radiation.

The risk of cancer is dependent on the dose of radiation exposure and the sensitivity of the tissues to radiation (thyroid and breast tissue are particularly sensitive). It is estimated that a 10 mSv effective dose leads to a lifetime risk of one radiation-induced cancer per 1000 patients. Bearing in mind the lifetime risk of developing cancer in the United Kingdom (UK) is 1 in 3, the risk from radiation exposure is relatively low. However, radiation doses are cumulative and this may be relevant in patients who undergo multiple radiological investigations. In the UK, the annual limit for radiation exposure for those who work with radiation is 20 mSv.

Table 6.1 Common radiological investigations and their effective radiation dose

Radiological modality	Average effective radiation dose to patient (mSv)	Equivalent number of radiographs
PA chest radiograph	0.02	1
Cervical spine	0.2	10
Shoulder radiograph	0.01	0.5
Pelvic radiograph	0.6	30
Hip radiograph	0.7	35
Knee radiograph	0.005	0.25
CT neck	3.0	150
CT abdomen	8.0	400
CT pelvis	6.0	300
CT spine	6.0	300
DEXA	Adult spine 0.013 Adult hip 0.009	0.65 0.45
Bone scan (99mTc-MDP)	6.3	315
Gallium-67 citrate scan	15	750
White cell scan (111In)	6.7	335
Pelvic vein embolization	60	3000
Fluoroscopy (C-arm)	12–40 per minute (lower for extremity and higher for pelvis)	600–2000
Fluoroscopy (mini C-arm)	1.2–4.0 per minute	60–200

CT: computed tomography; DEXA: dual energy X-ray absorptiometry; mSv: milliSieverts.

For orthopaedic surgeons who are regularly exposed to fluoroscopy, the effective dose varies according to screening time and it is important to keep screening to a minimum whilst ensuring protection of sensitive organs with protective gowns.

Ionizing Radiation (Medical Exposure) Regulations (IRMER) 2000

IRMER was introduced in the UK to protect patients against the dangers of ionizing radiation in relation to medical exposure. These regulations define four 'duty holders', namely the employer, referrer, practitioner and operator. Employers are responsible for providing a framework of procedures for medical exposures. Orthopaedic clinicians will commonly act as a 'referrer' but also to a lesser extent as an 'operator' – the referrer requests that the patient undergoes a radiological investigation or treatment and is required to provide sufficient clinical information to allow justification; the operator carries out any practical aspect of the radiological investigation or treatment, such as operating fluoroscopy. The practitioner is involved in justifying and authorizing each exposure undertaken. The practitioner may be radiologists or radiographers. These regulations also cover the justification and optimization of medical exposures. The recommendation is that doses arising from exposure for any radiological modality must be kept 'as low as reasonably practicable.' The other facets of IRMER include investigation of human errors that leads to an exposure 'much greater than intended', training and equipment.

Plain radiography

Wilhelm Roentgen discovered X-rays in 1895 and his work led to him receiving the first Nobel Prize in Physics in 1901. Another significant moment in radiography was the introduction of filmless digital radiography in the 1980s. In most developed countries, this has surpassed the use of conventional screen film radiography (SFR).

X-rays

X-rays are a form of **high-energy electromagnetic radiation that possess a shorter wavelength than visible light** (**Figure 6.1**). It is one of the most commonly used diagnostic tools in orthopaedics.

X-ray generation is achieved by heating a fine filament (the negative cathode, usually made of tungsten) to incandescence in a vacuum of around 2200°C. This results in the emission of electrons, a process known as **thermionic emission** (**Figure 6.2**).

These free negatively charged electrons leave the surface of their atoms and are drawn towards the positive anode, a smooth metal fragment usually made of tungsten. The electrons hit the anode at about half the speed of light on an area known as the focal spot. Here the free electrons may interact with:

- **Outer electrons of the target nucleus**, generating heat, which can lead to tube over heating. In order to reduce the generation of excess heat, the rotating anode disc was developed.

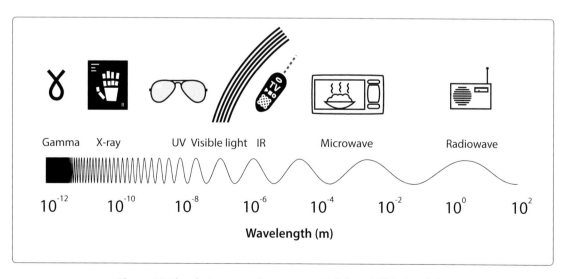

Figure 6.1 The electromagnetic spectrum. IR: infrared; UV: ultraviolet.

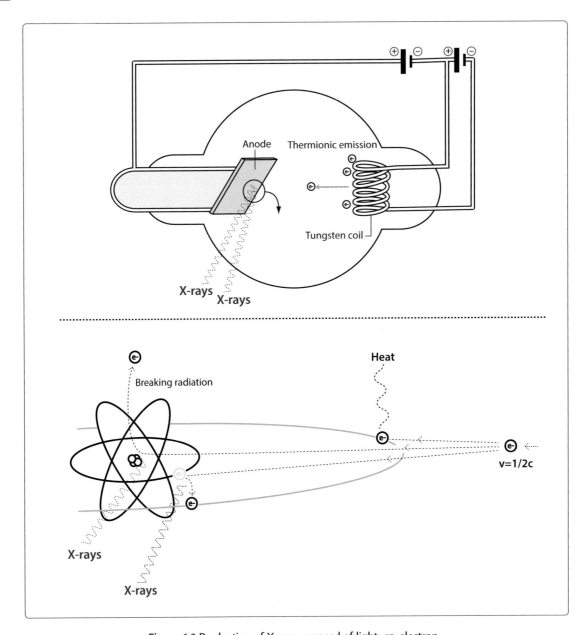

Figure 6.2 Production of X-rays. c: speed of light; e⁻: electron.

- **The inner electrons,** knocking them out of their orbit, with subsequent X-ray production.
- **The nucleus,** causing the free electrons to slow down and change direction, resulting in the emission of X-rays from braking radiation (bremsstrahlung). This constitutes 80% of the X-rays generated in the X-ray tube.

The vacuum tube is shielded throughout but has a narrow opening to allow escape of the X-ray beam in a concentrated fashion. The X-ray beam then passes through the body and is differentially absorbed by tissues, causing differential attenuation of the X-ray beam:

- **High beam attenuation** – absorbs high proportion of X-rays, therefore appearance on film is radio-dense e.g. bone, metalwork.
- **Low beam attenuation** – absorbs little or no X-rays, therefore appearance on film is radio-lucent e.g. air and fat.
- **Scattering** – the X-ray beam may deviate from the straight-line path between the source and image receptor, leading to image degradation. This is as a result of interactions between the X-ray beam and electrons of tissues/materials it comes into contact with.

The X-ray beam then passes through to the film detector with variations in quality (energy of electrons) and quantity (number of electrons flowing from cathode to anode). In addition, scattering will affect the quality of the final images.

There are **three basic types of X-ray receptors, namely conventional SFR, digital receptors and fluoroscopic receptors**.

Conventional screen film radiography

The basic components include a film sandwiched between two intensifying screens within a cassette:

- Intensifying screen – absorbs the X-ray and produces light (fluorescence). An ideal screen would have 100% absorption efficiency but this is never the case. Absorption efficiency is determined by screen material and thickness. However, increasing the latter leads to degradation of image quality. Materials used are phosphor compounds such as barium lead sulphate and gadolinium oxysulfide.
- Film – light produced by the intensifying screen exposes the film. Intensifying screens are used because film is much more sensitive to light than to X-ray. A significantly higher dose of X-rays is required to expose a film without use of intensifying screens.

Digital radiography

In digital radiography (DR), the basic components required include digital receptors, an image processing system (Digital Image Management System [DIMS], Patient Archiving and Communications System [PACS]), storage system, display system and a communication system. The advantages of DR over conventional SFR have led to its widespread use (*Table 6.2*).

Digital receptors substitute the cassettes used for SFR. There are two forms of receptors:

- Direct radiography – the receptor is made of up of numerous pixelated elements. Each pixel has the ability to absorb X-ray and produce an electrical signal. This signal is converted to a digital number and stored as one pixel in the final image.
- Computed radiography – similar to SFR with use of a phosphor receptor that absorbs X-rays and produces light. Unlike SFR, there is a delay between the absorption of X-ray and production of light. The production of light occurs when the cassette is fed into the processing unit within which a laser beam stimulates production of light based on the X-ray exposure. The data is then converted into digital values for each pixel and stored as a digital image.

Table 6.2 Comparison of screen film radiography (SFR) and digital radiography (DR)

	SFR	DR
Cost	Film is expensive	High set-up costs but savings in the long-term, e.g. reusable phosphor plates
Radiation exposure	Higher	Lower
Processing	Dark room/chemical processing of film	Environmentally friendly with elimination of chemical costs and disposal issues
Exposure time	Longer	Shorter (at same energy level)
Storage	Loss or deterioration of image with time	Physically less space required
Retrieval	Difficult	Multiple sites/user
PACS	Not compatible	Compatible
Spatial resolution	Higher	Lower
Image contrast	Not adjustable	Adjustable

PACS: Patient Archiving and Communications System.

Fluoroscopic receptors (FRs)

Image intensification is used for real time images and converts transmitted X-rays into a brightened, visible light image. The image intensifier houses the fluoroscopic receptors, amongst other components, within a vacuum setting.

Components

- Input window – often convex shaped (minimizes patient distance) and made from aluminium or titanium. It contains the vacuum and attenuates the X-ray beam only to a small extent.
- Input phosphor plate (caesium iodide) – fluorescent function by absorbing X-ray beam and producing light.
- Photocathode – conversion of light photons to electrons.
- Accelerating anode – a series of electrostatic focusing electrodes that accelerate electrons towards the output phosphor screen.
- Output phosphor screen (silver-activated zinc–cadmium sulphide) – conversion of electrons to light photons which are then captured by an imaging device. Approximately 2000 luminescence photons are generated for every accelerated electron, equating to a few thousand light photons produced for each X-ray photon reaching the input phosphor.

The radiation dose from fluoroscopically guided procedures depends on a number of factors including the procedure performed, fluoroscopy time and proximity of the image receptor, as well as the X-ray source and image quality setting of the machine.

The main methods that an orthopaedic surgeon may influence radiation exposure from scatter are:

- Fluoroscopy time – this is dependent on the procedure performed, the surgeon as well as the radiographer. The radiation exposure from fluoroscopy to the orthopaedic surgeon during

Table 6.3 Plain radiography as an imaging modality

Advantages	Disadvantages
Good for bony assessment	Radiation exposure
Readily available	Subtle bony pathology missed
Cheap	Two-dimensional – difficult to interpret in areas with overlapping tissues or complex anatomy

    various procedures has been investigated: e.g. intramedullary nailing, 1–1.3 mSv; dynamic hip screw, 5.7 mSv.
- Distance from the beam – doubling the distance reduces the amount of exposure by a factor of four.
- Shielding – more than 90% of radiation is attenuated by a lead gown with a thickness of 0.25 mm. This improves to 99% attenuation at a thickness of 0.5 mm but with the disadvantage of a doubling in its weight. Thyroid gland shields at 0.5 mm thickness attenuate 90% of radiation. Although not routinely worn, it should especially be considered in women due to their propensity to developing radiation-induced thyroid tumours, relative to men.

Other methods for reducing radiation exposure from scatter include:

- Equipment maintenance – fluoroscopy equipment and lead gowns should be checked on a regular basis for leakage from the X-ray generator and through the gowns.
- Fluoroscopy setting – increasing the current in the X-ray generator leads to increased photon production, hence more radiation. Conversely, increasing the voltage leads to increased rate of transmission of the X-ray beam, thereby reducing radiation exposure. The ideal setting is with a low current and high voltage but this may not lead to an optimal image. Collimation reduces the size of the beam, therefore reducing the amount of scatter.

The advantages and disadvantages of plain radiography are listed in *Table 6.3*.

Computed tomography

Sir Godfrey Hounsfield was an engineer who began development of the computed tomography (CT) scanner in 1967. The first clinical CT scanner was built in 1971.

CT scanning overcomes the three main limitations of plain radiography: (1) radiographs convey a two-dimensional image of a three-dimensional structure; (2) radiographs are limited in distinguishing tissues of differing densities; (3) radiographs record the mean absorption of all the tissues that the X-ray beam has penetrated and therefore do not provide data that separate the densities of individual tissues. In addition, due to the inefficient absorption of X-ray beams by the film/screen cassettes, wastage of the beam, and therefore information, is a problem.

The CT gantry contains a **collimated X-ray source** that projects a **fan-shaped beam**, along with a **collimated detector** that is rigidly linked to and sits opposite the X-ray source (**Figure 6.3**).

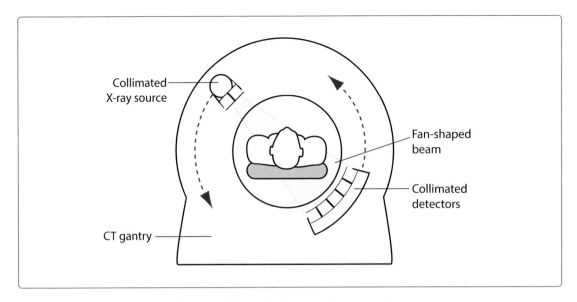

Figure 6.3 Schematic of computed tomography.

The source–detector combination measures parallel projections at that particular level in order to create a CT slice. Images are built as the gantry rotates to a new position to obtain another projection at that given level. The CT gantry then translates in a linear fashion to repeat the process at another level. Each CT slice may be visualized to compose of numerous three-dimensional rectangular boxes (voxels) of tissue (**Figure 6.4**).

The x and y axes are within the plane of the slice and the z axis corresponds to the thickness of the slice. This was how traditional CT scanning was performed but one of the main drawbacks was the time required to acquire a section, even on a low-resolution setting.

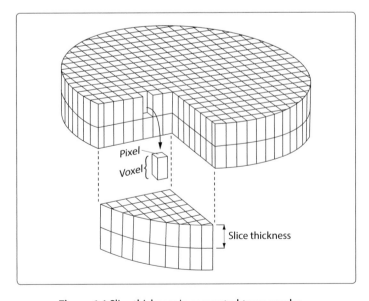

Figure 6.4 Slice thickness in computed tomography.

CT scanning has been revolutionized by the development of **helical scans** and **multi-detector technology**. The former involves activation of the X-ray tube throughout the duration of the scan whilst the patient table moves continuously during the exposure. The path of the X-ray beam traces a helix/spiral around the patient, hence the nomenclature. In order to reduce imaging time, multiple rows of detectors are stacked together to acquire multiple slices with each revolution of the X-ray tube. The combination of these developments have led to **reduced time required to acquire volumetric data, decrease in motion artefacts and generation of data to facilitate three-dimensional reconstruction images**. The major drawback of multi-detector technology is the **significantly increased radiation exposure** relative to conventional CT methods.

The CT image is based on tissue attenuation of the X-ray beam – the higher the tissue attenuation, the higher the density (whiteness) of the image. **The Hounsfield unit (HU) scale describes tissue attenuation coefficients and is a scale in which the radio-density of water is defined as zero at standard pressure and temperature** (*Table 6.4*). There is a much wider range of attenuation coefficients than the shades of grey that the eye can differentiate between and therefore the image has to be **manipulated by changing window levels and widths** to allow the whole range of CT attenuations to be displayed. This is of relevance to orthopaedics as settings are different for visualizing soft tissues and bone.

Contrast CT

Some of the limitations in soft tissue visualization with CT may be overcome by use of contrast media. **Single (iodine-based) or double (iodine-based and air)** contrast studies can be performed. Contrast may be injected intra-articularly (CT arthrography), intrathecally (CT myelography) or intradiscally (CT discography). By and large, these investigations have been superseded by magnetic resonance (MR) arthrography but CT is useful in cases where MR arthrography is contraindicated. The most common joints CT is reserved for are the shoulder and knee joints.

The advantages and disadvantages of CT are listed in *Table 6.5*.

Table 6.4 Tissues and their corresponding coefficient of attenuation

Tissue	Hounsfield Unit (HU)
Air (black)	-1000
Lung	-500
Fat	-100
Water	0
CSF	15
Blood	30
Muscle	10–40
Soft tissue	100–300
Cortical bone (white)	1000

CSF: cerebrospinal fluid.

Table 6.5 Computed tomography as an imaging modality

Advantages	Disadvantages
Three-dimensional imaging	Higher ionizing radiation doses relative to plain radiographs
Improved delineation of soft tissues relative to plain radiographs	Inferior soft tissue contrast resolution to MRI

MRI: magnetic resonance imaging.

Magnetic resonance imaging

Magnetic resonance imaging (MRI) is based on the use of **superconducting magnets** and **radiofrequency (RF) coils** to manipulate hydrogen protons, creating a detailed, high-contrast image. The stationary magnet leads to alignment of the protons within tissues parallel to the main magnetic field. When an RF pulse is applied, protons absorb energy and two things occur: **(1) protons change alignment and lose parallelism to magnetic field; (2) protons spin (precess) in a synchronized fashion (Figure 6.5).**

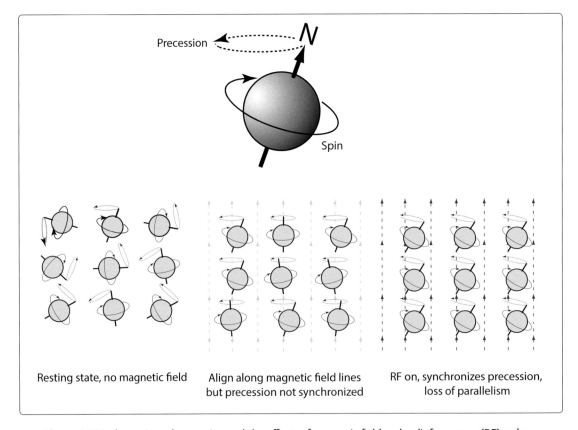

Figure 6.5 Nuclear spin and precession and the effects of magnetic field and radiofrequency (RF) pulse.

On terminating the RF pulse, the protons release the absorbed energy and realign themselves to the magnetic field (**T1** refers to the time this takes) as well as lose their synchronized spinning (**T2** refers to the time this takes) (*Table 6.6*). The RF coil detects the energy emitted (signal) from the protons whilst smaller magnets are used to acquire spatial information and images are formed based on this.

Tissues abundant in hydrogen atoms (e.g. fat and fluid) are responsible for most MRI signals and tissues devoid of hydrogen atoms (e.g. cortical bone and ligaments) give off very little signal. Different 'sequences' are utilized based on what the possible underlying diagnosis may be (*Tables 6.7, 6.8*).

Table 6.6 Useful definitions and terms in relation to magnetic resonance imaging

Definitions	
T1	Time for magnetization to return to the longitudinal axis after application of a radiofrequency pulse
T2	Time for loss of phase coherence of a group of spins and the resulting loss in the transverse magnetization signal
TR (Repetition time)	Time between successive excitations
TE (Echo time)	Time between the middle of the excitation pulse and the middle of the spin echo (see below)
T1-weighted image	Short TR and short TE which emphasizes differences in T1 between tissues
	Useful for demonstrating anatomy – as most tissues appear dark (low-intensity signal) and generally are surrounded by fat, which appears bright (high-signal intensity), T1 sequences demonstrate anatomic detail well Magic angle artefact
T2-weighted image	Long TR and long TE which emphasizes differences in T2 between tissues
	Best at demonstrating pathology associated with fluid and/or oedema as these appear bright (high-signal intensity) on T2 sequences
	However, if fluid and/or oedema within marrow or fat needs to be isolated, a fat suppression sequence should be utilized

Table 6.7 Common magnetic resonance imaging sequences

Sequences	
Spin echo (SE) sequence	One of the most commonly used sequences in which an echo is produced by a 90° radiofrequency pulse followed by one or more 180° radiofrequency pulse Both T1- and T2-weighted images can be obtained with the SE sequence
Short-tau inversion recovery (STIR) sequence	Fat suppression sequence Used to detect fluid or oedema within bone marrow or from tissues with high fat content
Metal artefact reduction sequence (MARS)	Used to reduce the size and intensity of susceptibility artefacts from magnetic field distortion

Table 6.8 Normal tissue specific signal intensity on various magnetic resonance imaging sequences

Tissue	T1-weighted	T2-weighted	STIR
Fat	High	Moderate	Low
Fluid	Low	High	High
Cancellous bone	Moderate/high	Moderate	
Cortical bone	Low	Low	Low
Synovium	Low	High	High
Articular cartilage	Moderate	High	High
Ligament	Low	Low	Low
Tendon	Low	Low*	Low
Muscle	Moderate	Moderate	Moderate
Spinal cord	Moderate	Low/moderate	Low/moderate
Cerebrospinal fluid	Low	High	High
Intervertebral disc	Low	High	High

NB: high signal (white); moderate signal/isointense (grey); low signal (black). *Larger tendons such as the Achilles or quadriceps tendons may have linear areas of high signal.

STIR: short-tau inversion recovery sequence.

As this technique involves creation of a magnetic field, patients should undergo screening prior to MRI. **Absolute contraindications** to MRI include cardiac pacemakers or implanted cardiac defibrillators, electromagnetic implants and cochlear implants. **Relative contraindications** include intracranial aneurysmal clips, vascular stents/clips, intraorbital metallic foreign body, retained shrapnel and any metallic prosthesis.

Gadolinium

This is a **para-magnetic agent** with a plasma half-life of 2 hours that is cleared from bloodstream within 24 hours of intravenous administration. It **strongly reduces the T1 times of tissues** to which it has access to, and therefore leads to an **increased signal on T1-weighted images**. It is often used to facilitate the differentiation of a solid soft tissue mass from a fluid filled cyst.

If intravenous contrast is to be given, patient allergy status and renal function must be known. Gadolinium has a dose-dependent nephrotoxicity effect, but of more concern is it is associated with nephrogenic systemic fibrosis (NSF) in patients with abnormal renal function. NSF is a rare but devastating disease that primarily involves the skin and subcutaneous tissues but has been associated with effects on internal organs.

The advantages and disadvantages of MRI are listed in *Table 6.9*. *Table 6.10* compares the features of plain radiography, CT and MRI.

Ultrasound

Ultrasound (US) is part of the acoustic spectrum, and may be defined as **sound of a frequency above the human audible range (>20 kHz)**. The frequency range for diagnostic US is generally between **2 and 18 MHz**. Ultrasonography is based on the principle that the sound wave will travel until it encounters a border between two tissues that conduct sound differently. The sound wave has two main fates – **reflection** back towards the transducer as an 'echo' sound wave and **transmission** through the tissues.

An US signal is generated by a transducer and the signal is in a waveform. There are two modes of signal generation in medical US:

- **Continuous wave** US – continuous excitation of the transducer with an electrical sine wave at constant amplitude.
- **Pulse wave** US – excitation of transducer with short electrical signals intermittently.

Ultrasonography requires the following components:

- **Transducer** – contains crystals that are **piezoelectric** in nature, such that when a voltage is applied the material contracts or expands, creating sound waves of a certain frequency. When the sound wave of a returning 'echo' hits the transducer, the piezoelectric crystal within converts this into an electrical signal.
- **Monitor** – the brightness on the monitor is determined by the magnitude of the electrical signal created by the returning 'echo' and therefore structures reflecting the ultrasonic waves appear bright (**hyperechoic**) and in contrast, structures that do not reflect waves appear dark (**hypoechoic or anechoic**).
- **Computer unit** – responsible for transmission of electrical signals to the transducer and processing of data to create an image.

Table 6.9 Magnetic resonance as an imaging modality

Advantages	Disadvantages
Excellent soft tissue imaging	Image artefact
No ionizing radiation	Claustrophobia

Table 6.10 Comparison of radiography, computed tomography (CT) and magnetic resonance imaging (MRI)

	Radiography	CT	MRI
Spatial resolution	Highest	High	Moderate
Soft tissue contrast	Poor	Moderate	High
Calcium measurement	Direct	Direct	Indirect
Metal artefact	None	Moderate	Moderate/severe

Doppler

Christian Doppler, an Austrian physicist, discovered the Doppler effect in 1842. It describes the **phenomenon of a change in the frequency of sound waves as a result of motion of either the source or the receiver of the waves**. An example of this would be the changing pitch of an ambulance siren as it drives past a stationary person.

This principle is used in assessment of blood flow in vessels. When the sound wave is reflected from a target that is moving, the 'echo' will have a different frequency to that of the transduced pulse – if the reflecting target is moving away from the transducer, the echo frequency will be lower than the transduced frequency and *vice versa*. This may be represented in the form of a colour flow map superimposed on a regular US image.

The advantages and disadvantages of US are listed in *Table 6.11*.

Table 6.11 Ultrasound as an imaging modality

Advantages	Disadvantages
Real-time dynamic assessment	Ultrasound waves do not reflect clearly from bone or air (hence the need for gel between transducer and skin)
Portable	Operator dependent
Non-invasive	
No ionizing radiation	

Bone scintigraphy

Bone scintigraphy is a form of nuclear medicine imaging that **detects distribution of injected radiolabelled tracer in tissues sensitive to gamma ray emissions** (**Figure 6.6**). The process involves **injection of a radiolabelled tracer** followed by **gamma camera recording of photoemissions**. It is indicated in metastatic or primary bone tumours, trauma (stress or occult fractures), loosening or infection of arthroplasty, arthritis and complex regional pain syndrome.

Radiolabelled tracers

- Technetium-99m – affinity for osteoblasts; $t_{1/2}$ 6 hours.
- Gallium-67 – affinity for inflammatory proteins; $t_{1/2}$ 3.2 days.
- Indium-111 – autologous leukocytes are obtained and labelled with indium-111 then reinjected; $t_{1/2}$ 2.8 days

Different tracers may be used depending on the pathology suspected. The tracers are excreted through the urinary tract and therefore exposure of radiation to the bladder must be minimized by instructions to frequently micturate post-examination.

Gamma camera

The camera detects radio-active decay and records images in three phases:

- **Flow phase** (nuclear angiogram) – images immediately post-injection; **demonstrates arterial flow and areas of hyperperfusion.**
- **Blood pool phase – images 5 minutes post-injection; demonstrates relative vascularity where areas of inflammation result in 'pooling' of blood due to stagnant flow in dilated capillaries (soft tissues and bone).**
- **Static phase – images 3 hours post-injection; demonstrates bone activity.**

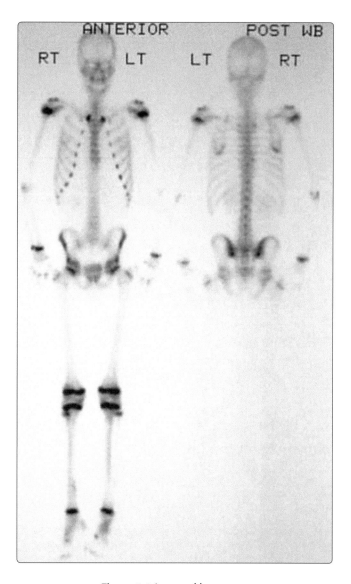

Figure 6.6 A normal bone scan.

Although the specificity of bone scintigraphy is low, abnormalities based on the three phases may point the investigator towards the possible diagnosis (*Table 6.12*). The advantages and disadvantages of bone scintigraphy are listed in *Table 6.13*.

Table 6.12 Bone scintigraphy findings in common conditions

Pathology	Flow phase	Blood pool phase	Static phase
Cellulitis	Increased	Increased	Normal
Osteomyelitis	Increased	Increased	Increased
Acute fracture (<4 weeks)	Increased	Increased	Increased
Chronic fracture (>12 weeks)	Normal	Normal	Increased

Table 6.13 Bone scintigraphy as an imaging modality

Advantages	Disadvantages
High sensitivity	Low specificity
Localization of bone lesions for subsequent investigations	Two dimensional image – poor localization of small lesions
	High radiation dose

Positron emission tomography

A positron emission tomography (PET) scan is a form of nuclear imaging that has distinctive advantages relative to other imaging modalities as it is **capable of measuring body function such as blood flow, oxygen consumption and glucose metabolism** (*Table 6.14*). It is predominantly used for investigation and surveillance of cancers, but its role in orthopaedics is developing.

Table 6.14 Positron emission tomography as an imaging modality.

Advantages	Disadvantages
High sensitivity	High radiation dose (especially when combines with CT)
Tomographic – three-dimensional image; precise location of tracer retention	Expensive
Information regarding metabolism/function	

CT: computed tomography.

Its basic components are:

- **Cyclotron** – machine that produces positron emitting isotopes e.g. nitrogen-13, oxygen-15, carbon-11, fluorine-18. The isotope is then tagged to a naturally occurring chemical such as glucose, water or ammonia depending on the indication for the scan. This radiotracer is then injected into the patient. For example, fluorodeoxyglucose (FDG) is a radiotracer used to analyse glucose utilization.
- **Camera** – as the radiotracer undergoes positron emission decay, positrons travel in tissues to interact with electrons within the tissues (**positron annihilation event**). This produces a back-to-back emission of two gamma rays that travel in opposite directions (180°) on the same axis. The gamma detectors used are sensitive only to such gamma rays.
- **Computer** – the data collected is then reconstructed to form an image.

Technologies combining PET with modalities such as CT and MRI are being developed with a view to combining metabolic data and anatomical data:

- **PET–CT** – the CT component is used to relate tracer signal with bony (and soft tissue) anatomical landmarks, e.g. assessment of bone formation/mineralization associated with uncemented hip arthroplasty components.
- **PET–MRI** – the MRI component is used to relate tracer signal with soft tissue anatomical landmarks, e.g. use in diabetic foot to distinguish uncomplicated diabetic foot, Charcot's neuroarthropathy and osteomyelitis.

Bone densitometry

Bone mineral density (BMD) may be measured using a number of bone densitometry techniques, the commonest of which is dual-energy X-ray absorptiometry (DEXA). These imaging modalities are most widely used for diagnosis and surveillance of osteoporosis.

Dual-energy X-ray absorptiometry (DEXA)

This modality makes use of **X-ray beams of two different energies that are absorbed in different proportions by bone and soft tissue**. A DEXA scan provides BMD measurements both **axially** (spine, proximal femur, forearm) and **peripherally** (calcaneum) in a matter of a few minutes. The routinely measured sites include the lumbar spine and proximal femur. Volumetric data are not collected; therefore, although it is a measurement of density, it is expressed as g/cm^2.

The World Health Organisation (WHO) definition of osteoporosis is based on BMD in the spine and proximal femur measured with DEXA:

- **Osteoporosis** – BMD 2.5 standard deviations (SD) below the mean value of a young reference sex and ethnically-matched population (T-score $\leq$-2.5)
- **Osteopenia** – BMD 1 to 2.5 SD below mean value of a young reference sex and ethnically-matched population (-2.5< T-score <-1.0)
- **Normal** – T-score $\geq$-1.0

T-score = $\dfrac{\text{(measured BMD } - \text{ young adult mean BMD)}}{\text{young adult population SD}}$

Z-score* = $\dfrac{\text{(measured BMD } - \text{ age-matched mean BMD)}}{\text{age-matched population SD}}$

*Z-score – comparison to age, sex and ethnically-matched population and therefore abnormal Z-scores are suggestive of aetiology independent of age.

It is important to understand that the WHO definitions refer only to BMD values obtained via DEXA and should not be extrapolated to include BMD values obtained from other modalities such as quantitative CT or US. The reason for this is because the curves of T-scores obtained from the various modalities plotted against age are quite different.

The advantages and disadvantages of bone densitometry are listed in *Table 6.15.*

Table 6.15 Dual energy X-ray absorptiometry as an imaging modality

Advantages	Disadvantages
High-resolution images – able to detect small changes in BMD	No differentiation between cortical and cancellous bone
Low radiation dose	Two-dimensional measurement of three-dimensional structures
Short acquisition time	False positives particularly in lumbar spine secondary to arthritis, trauma and surgery

BMD: bone mineral density.

Quantitative CT

This technique involves CT imaging of the area of interest in the presence of a mineral calibration phantom. The phantom (often hydroxyapatite) acts as a reference source used to calibrate bone density measurements, as its BMD is known. Quantitative CT overcomes the limitations of DEXA as it allows separate assessment of cortical and cancellous bone and also provides volumetric assessment of BMD (g/cm^3). The main drawbacks are the higher costs and radiation dose involved.

Quantitative US

The basis for quantitative US is that the velocity and attenuation of US waves varies as the biomechanical properties of bone varies. Accessible sites for quantitative US involve the periphery and include the calcaneum, patella and to a lesser extent the radius, tibia and phalanges. In addition to providing information regarding BMD, mechanical properties may also be measured. Quantitative US is not associated with radiation exposure and hence is an emerging modality for BMD.

Viva questions

1. What is the difference between how X-rays work in plain radiography versus fluoroscopy?
2. What are the advantages of digital radiography compared to conventional radiography?
3. What do you understand by the term 'scatter'? Name some of the ways in which you can reduce radiation exposure from scatter during fluoroscopy.
4. Here is a DEXA scan report. Talk me through it.
5. How does ultrasound work? Talk me through the principles behind Doppler scanning.

Further reading

Bansal GJ. Digital radiography. A comparison with modern conventional imaging. *Postgrad Med J* 2006;**82**:425–8.

Davies HE, Wathen CG, Gleeson FV. The risks of radiation exposure related to diagnostic imaging and how to minimise them. *BMJ* 2011;**342**:d947.

Hartley KG, Damon BM, Patterson GT, Long JH, Holt GE. MRI techniques: a review and update for the orthopaedic surgeon. *J Am Acad Orthop Surg* 2012;**20**:775–87.

Hounsfield GN. Computed medical imaging. *Science* 1980;**210**(4465):22–8.

Kanis JA, Joseph Melton III L, Christiansen C, Johnston CC, Khaltaev N. The diagnosis of osteoporosis. *J Bone Min Res* 1994;**9**(8):1137–41.

7 Orthopaedic Oncology

Nimalan Maruthainar, Rej Bhumbra and Steve Cannon

Introduction

A **tumour** (neoplasm) is a mass of tissue formed as a result of abnormal, excessive or inappropriate proliferation of cells. Growth continues independently of the normal mechanisms that determine cellular turnover, division or programmed cell death.

Traditionally tumours are categorized into **benign or malignant** lesions. Wholly benign tumours do not metastasize. They may cause symptoms by their pressure effect upon related structures or secondary to normal tissue loss, such as pathological fracture. Cells that take origin from malignant tumours may spread to distant sites via the vascular or lymphatic systems. The distant deposits of malignant tumours are termed metastases. Malignant neoplasms taking cellular origin from mesenchyme or its derivatives are termed **sarcomas**.

Tumours may present in a variety of ways to the orthopaedic surgeon in either bone or soft tissue or both. Although most malignant lesions in bone will be metastatic in an adult, it is important to consider a primary bone tumour in the differential diagnosis and refer to a bone tumour centre if any uncertainty exists. A soft-tissue tumour greater than the size of a golf ball that demonstrates rapid growth or is deeply located should also be referred to a specialist unit.

Sarcomas of bone and soft tissues have an approximate annual incidence of 1 and 3 per 100,000 respectively. Timely appropriate referral of these neoplasms is reliant on the treating healthcare professional maintaining a high index of suspicion.

Diagnosis

A critical aspect in the recognition of a tumour in bone and soft tissue is being aware of the possibility of its presence. Once the presence of a tumour is apparent, there is considerable available guidance on appropriate assessment and further management, including referral to specialist treatment centres.

Bone and soft-tissue tumours tend to present **incidentally** (either clinically or on imaging), with a **mass**, **pain**, as **sequelae of local or related pressure effects** or a **pathological fracture**. As we discuss in this chapter, appropriate management of these fractures is often different to that of their traumatic counterparts. On occasion, other symptoms at presentation include altered sensation or function from **neurological compression** or **lesions arising within neural elements.**

The presenting complaint of pain, whether persistent for more than 4 weeks and/or relapsing or remitting, particularly at night or at rest is a red flag symptom. The attribution of pain symptoms in children to 'growing pains' is a relative pitfall, leading to missed or late diagnoses.

A history of trauma may well be present and more likely to be the event that draws the patient's attention to the lesion rather than the precipitant of the lesion. Persisting pain for greater than 4 weeks or swelling after trauma should also raise a suspicion of possible neoplasia and subsequent imaging requested.

In establishing the likely diagnosis, the patient's age may provide some indication. Lesions of bone in the first three decades are most often primary or haemopoietic in origin. In older patients, metastases are more likely. Omnipresent **differential diagnoses at all ages include infection, haematological and metabolic conditions**.

A complete history must be taken, establishing the duration and timing of symptoms and any associated weight loss, lethargy or fever. Documentation of either the presence or absence of a **pre-existing malignancy** or **previous radiotherapy treatment** is essential. A history of smoking may also point to a possible primary cause. With a few exceptions (e.g. neurofibromatosis, Li–Fraumeni syndrome), family history does not appear to be a significant factor in bone and soft-tissue tumours.

Tumours that most commonly give rise to metastases in bone are carcinomas of the breast, prostate, lung, kidney and thyroid. These metastatic lesions can be both osteolytic and sclerotic on plain film imaging. The presence of a mono-ostotic metastasis, especially in the case of renal, thyroid or breast, yields the possibility of cure following resection and reconstruction as per a primary lesion of bone. The advances being made in oncology in overall survival, an increasingly aging population, as well as the improvement in management of other cardiovascular co-morbidities, are increasing the disease burden of bone metastases.

Investigations

The assessment of a case of suspected neoplasia includes the following:

- **Plain radiographs** are essential in suspected bone lesions (see below for interpretation).
- **Full (complete) blood count** and **inflammatory marker assays**.
- **Serum electrophoresis** in older patients to investigate possible myeloproliferative disorder and, if appropriate, **urine analysis** for Bence Jones proteins.
- **Urea and electrolytes** and **liver function assays** may establish baseline renal and liver function before potent cytotoxic therapy. In addition, alkaline phosphatase may provide an indication of prognosis in osteosarcoma.

- **Prostate specific antigen (PSA) assay** (and acid phosphatase).
- **Magnetic resonance (MR) imaging** of the lesion, whether bone or soft tissue, further characterizes the pathology and stages the lesion locally, demonstrating the extent of oedematous reaction and presence of skip lesions.
- **Computed tomography** (CT) of the lesion may be of value in tumours of bone. Additionally, CT of the chest is regularly employed in the distant staging of malignant lesions.
- **Tissue biopsy** and **histological analysis** is a critical part of diagnosis. If performed inappropriately, it may considerably compromise the outcome.
- **Bone scintigraphy** is also used in the assessment of the rest of the skeleton. Approximately 20% of cases of Ewing's sarcoma present with bone metastases. Multifocal osteosarcoma is rare but usually fatal. The role of bone scintigraphy is beginning to be replaced by whole body MR to exclude polyostotic disease in bone sarcomas.
- **CT–positron emission tomography (PET) scanning** represents a relatively recent advance into functional metabolic imaging that will become part of routine distant staging for particular tumours in the future.

Radiographs

Plain film radiography can determine whether or not a lesion is likely to be 'aggressive' or 'non-aggressive'. Without histology, it cannot describe a lesion as malignant or benign. Where a lesion arises in bone and, more importantly, the matrix it produces, may indicate the most likely cellular origin. The position within the bone may be considered in relation to the epiphysis, metaphysis and diaphysis and also to the medullary cavity and cortex (**Figure 7.1**).

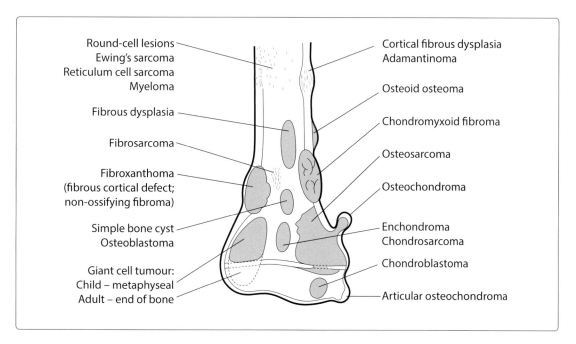

Figure 7.1 Common anatomical locations of bone tumours.

Generally speaking matrix types can be divided into cartilaginous, lytic, osteoid and fibrous (**Figure 7.2a–d**).

Concepts employed in the study of the radiographs are those of **the effect of the lesion on the bone and the effect of the bone on the lesion**. Lesions may precipitate a variable reaction of the adjoining bone. Slow-growing lesions tend to allow bone reaction at the margin, leading to a well-demarcated appearance with a **narrow zone of transition** (**Figure 7.3**). Rapidly enlarging aggressive lesions allow little bone-forming response to develop. These lesions yield a poorly-demarcated, **permeative** appearance with a **wide zone of transition** (**Figure 7.4**) as the tumour grows through the bone relatively rapidly.

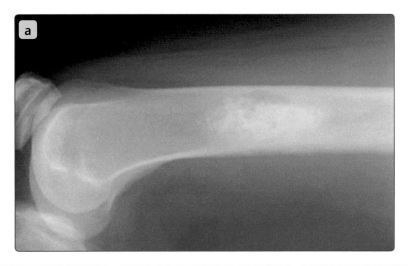

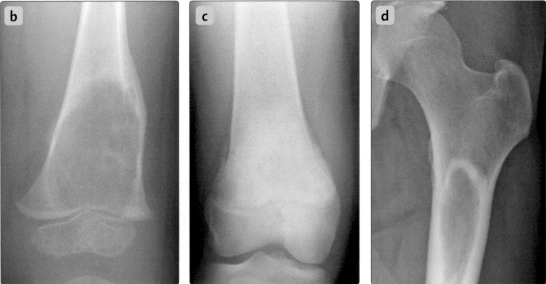

Figure 7.2a–d Radiographic examples (a) cartilaginous, (b) lytic, (c) osteoid and (d) fibrous types.

Rapidly growing subperiosteal lesions, such as some osteosarcomas, may elevate, destroy or simply just grow directly through the periosteum. In the axilla between the periosteal undersurface and the junction between the outer cortical bone and the tumour, bone deposition in response to rapid periosteal elevation produces the so-called **Codman triangle** appearance (**Figure 7.4**). Disorganized or radial osteoid production may result in streaks of calcification termed **sunray spiculation** (**Figure 7.4**).

Relatively slow-growing lesions within bone may result in bony expansion and the production of a neocortex. More aggressive lesions from within the medulla may result in cortical resorption (**endosteal scalloping/thumb printing**).

Characteristic radiographic features of some tumours are given in the tumour descriptions below. Note that for a lesion to become apparent as lytic on plain radiographs, there must be loss of at least 33% of the bone mass in comparison with the surrounding bone.

Biopsy

Tissue may be obtained for histological analysis by **percutaneous (fine-needle/core-needle)**, or **open (incisional/excisional)** biopsy techniques. The technique utilized is based on tumour location, size, depth, biology, clinical resources and histological expertise within the unit.

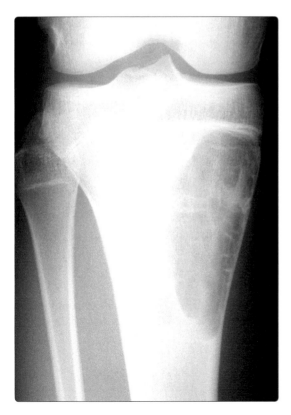

Figure 7.3 Narrow zone of transition in a benign tumour (non-ossifying fibroma).

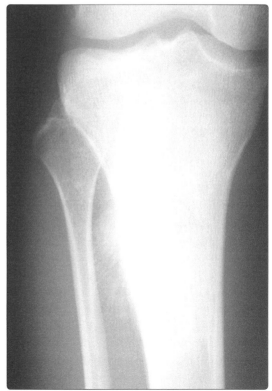

Figure 7.4 Wide zone of transition in osteosarcoma with Codman's triangle and sunray spiculation.

Instruments such as Trucut needles for soft tissue and Jamshidi needles for bone may be used to obtain core specimens. Tumours may have a necrotic core with viable tissue of histological use confined to the periphery. It is therefore vital that tissue from the appropriate zone of the lesion is obtained. Later excision of any tumorous lesion will need to include the biopsy tract. The potential for seeding of tumour tissue into joint cavities during biopsy needs to be recognized.

The selection of biopsy path and positioning of the biopsy needle within a lesion is a process best undertaken following consultation with the surgeon likely to undertake any later definitive resection and with specialist pathologists. The analysis of bone and soft-tissue tumour tissue requires knowledge and techniques not always available to the general pathologist. Initial processing of tissue in the laboratory differs from that of the specimens handled routinely in a general hospital environment. For example, tissue may be required fresh and without preservative in order to allow imprint and immunohistochemical analysis. Additional molecular studies and reverse ribonucleic acid (RNA) sequencing may also be conducted in modern tumour labs. Determining the precise origin and nature of bone and soft-tissue tumours often requires special expertise; bone tumour centres may request that any biopsy material and histological slides be forwarded for review. It is not unusual for tissue to be studied collectively by pathologists from more than one tumour centre.

Even in large tumours, the area from which the biopsy is obtained can greatly influence the ease of tissue diagnosis and accuracy of initial grading. The centre of large lesions may comprise necrotic non-specific tissue. It is common practice to obtain core-needle biopsies under ultrasound or CT guidance, allowing accurate targeting of the volume of tissue to be sampled. Multiple cores are obtained as both the cell appearances and stromal type are currently required to obtain an accurate diagnosis. A list of new molecular tumour-specific markers is being gathered to complete the diagnostic signature for different tumours. This will eventually lead to the production of new molecular targeted therapies.

Staging

To be useful, the surgical staging system for sarcomas should:

- Incorporate the most significant prognostic factors into a system that describes the patient's progressive degree of risk.
- Delineate progressive stages of disease that have specific implications for surgical management.
- Provide guidelines for the use of adjuvant therapies.

Based on these principles, Enneking (1986) proposed a staging system that considered **histological grade (G), local extent (T) and the presence or absence of distant metastases (M)**. Although strictly this system is based on the findings following surgical resection of the lesion, a representative pre-operative biopsy and appropriate imaging may yield an accurate approximation of the surgical stage.

Enneking staging system

Grade

- G1:
  - low-grade;
  - lower risk for metastases;
  - well differentiated;
  - few mitotic figures;
  - moderate cytological atypia.

- G2:
  - high-grade;
  - higher incidence of metastases;
  - poorly differentiated;
  - high mitotic rate;
  - high cell/matrix ratio;
  - necrosis;
  - microvascular invasion.

Site (local extent)

- Is lesion contained within a well-delineated anatomical compartment?
  - T1: intracompartmental;
  - T2: extracompartmental.

The definitions of compartments are debatable, but in principle the anatomical compartments are those natural barriers to tumour extension, such as cortical bone and the major fascial septae.

Metastases

Presence of regional or distant metastases:

- M0: no metastases.
- M1: metastases present.

This system has largely been replaced by the **TNM staging system**, which is used internationally. Pierre Denoix in France developed the TNM system between 1943 and 1952 for the classification of malignant tumours. TNM is a dual system that includes a clinical (pre-treatment – cTNM) and a pathological (post-surgical histopathological – pTNM) classification. Distinguishing between these classifications is important as they are based on different methods of examination and serve different purposes. Most sarcoma centres use cTNM as the basis for the choice of treatment and the pTNM for prognostic assessment.

For bone tumours, the TNM clinical classification is as follows (**Table 7.1**):

- T – primary tumour:
  - TX – primary tumour cannot be assessed;
  - T0 – no evidence of primary tumour;
  - T1 – tumour 8 cm or less in greatest dimension;
  - T2 – tumour greater than 8 cm in greatest dimension;
  - T3 – discontinuous tumours in the primary bone site.

- N – regional lymph nodes:
  - NX – regional lymph nodes cannot be assessed;
  - N0 – no regional lymph node metastasis;
  - N1 – regional lymph node metastasis.

- M – distant metastasis:
  - MX – distant metastasis cannot be assessed;
  - M0 – no distant metastasis;
  - M1 – distant metastasis;
  - M1a – lung;
  - M1b – other distant sites.

Table 7.1 TNM staging for bone tumours

Stage IA	T1	N0, NX	M0	Low grade
Stage IB	T2	N0, NX	M0	Low grade
Stage IIA	T1	N0, NX	M0	High grade
Stage IIB	T2	N0, NX	M0	High grade
Stage III	T3	N0, NX	M0	Any grade
Stage IVA	Any T	N0, NX	M1a	Any grade
Stage IVB	Any T	N1	Any M	Any grade
	Any T	Any N	M1b	Any grade

For soft-tissue sarcomas, TNM clinical classification (**Table 7.2**):

- T – primary tumour:
  - TX – primary tumour cannot be assessed;
  - T0 – no evidence of primary tumour;
  - T1 – tumour 5 cm or less in greatest dimension;
    - – T1a – superficial tumour;
    - – T1b – deep tumour;
  - T2 – tumour greater than 5 cm in greatest dimension;
    - – T2a – superficial tumour;
    - – T2b – deep tumour.

- N – regional lymph nodes:
  - NX – regional lymph nodes cannot be assessed;
  - N0 – no regional lymph node metastasis;
  - N1 – regional lymph node metastasis.

- M – distant metastasis:
  - MX – distant metastasis cannot be assessed;
  - M0 – no distant metastasis;
  - M1 – distant metastasis.

Table 7.2 TNM status of soft tissue

Stage IA	T1a	N0, NX	M0	Low grade
	T1b	N0, NX	M0	Low grade
Stage IB	T2a	N0, NX	M0	Low grade
	T2b	N0, NX	M0	Low grade
Stage IIA	T1a	N0, NX	M0	High grade
	T1b	N0, NX	M0	High grade
Stage IIB	T2a	N0, NX	M0	High grade
Stage III	T2b	N0, NX	M0	High grade
Stage IV	Any T	N1	M0	Any grade
	Any T	Any N	M1	Any grade

Treatment

Referral to a specialist centre

The complexity of the management of bone tumours, diagnosis, staging and treatment dictates referral to specialist centres. These units often have specialist radiologists, pathologists, oncologists, support professionals and surgeons experienced in the management of these rare lesions. Optimum management of a potential tumour must entail an **appropriate selection of biopsy tract**, such that prognosis and any future reconstructive surgery are not compromised. The most important factor in determining patient survival is the involvement of a specialized multi-disciplinary team.

Tumour excision

The methodology for tumour resection is determined by the biology, the appropriateness and planned margin status of the resected lesion.

Intralesional

The path of excision passes **through the pseudo-capsule (reactive zone) and directly into the lesion**. The entire operative field is to be considered as potentially contaminated. All incisional biopsies are intralesional procedures. An intralesional definitive procedure may be appropriate where the tumour is of a **benign nature** or as short-term **palliation** to overcome a mass effect. Indications for 'tumour debulking' are now very rare in modern sarcoma units.

Marginal

The **entire lesion is resected**, with the plane of dissection in the pseudo-capsule around certain points around the lesion. This is represented as oedema on T2-weighted images. Resections in the marginal category are performed to preserve critical structures such as nerve, vessel or bone. Sampling of tissues in the pseudo-capsule contains malignant cells in the case of some bone and soft-tissue sarcomas, especially those that grow with a more infiltrative pattern following fascial planes, such as myxofibrosarcomas.

Wide (intracompartmental)

The lesion is removed together with its **pseudo-capsule** and a **cuff of normal tissue** outside the field of oedema.

Radical (extracompartmental)

The **entire lesion and the plane of dissection is outside the limiting fascia or bone**. A true compartectomy is rarely performed and in reality, a radical resection is an amputation.

Although categorized into these four groups, modern surgical and pathological descriptions include a quantitative and qualitative margin status. For example, 1 mm of fascia or periosteum is a 'better' margin than 1 mm of muscle.

Amputation versus limb salvage

Malignant tumour management is a sequential process of life saving, limb-salvage and restoration of function treatments. This sequence is followed in this order and the treatment of a tumour should not **compromise its prognosis**. Treatment should aim **to preserve or maintain function** as best as possible, without compromising the 'oncological' aspects of the procedure. It should be noted that amputation does not equate to an equal or better prognosis than limb-salvage surgery *per se*, but may be a surrogate marker for an aggressive tumour. Indications for amputation include **primarily unresectable tumours that would compromise the oncological margin status and/or distal limb viability or function, secondary unresectability in a tumour that was initially resectable,** as seen with progression of tumour growth whilst on chemotherapy, and a **resectable tumour that post-resection would yield an unacceptable functional result,** as most commonly seen with distal lower limb sarcomas with extensive soft tissue involvement.

An amputation where the level is planned inadequately or where its execution is suboptimal will yield a guarded prognosis. Planning of an amputation must consider the possibility of skip lesions proximally in a bone, and the proximal anatomy of any affected compartment, hence imaging is mandatory.

Reconstruction in limb-salvage surgery

The reconstruction options for bony resection with limb-salvage surgery include **massive endoprosthesis**, **autograft** and **allograft**. Local recurrence of malignant tumours after limb-salvage surgery may be addressed by amputation without compromise of the overall prognosis depending on the staging.

Massive endoprosthetic replacement

The most commonly used method of reconstruction for bony resection is that of massive endoprosthetic replacement. This may be by **custom-made implants** (often with computer-aided design and manufacture) or by **modular systems**. These implants serve to replace the significant bulk of bone resected and often also an adjacent joint (**Figure 7.5**).

Early complications include **vascular injury, unpredicted neurological injury, thrombo-embolism, infection** and, if the implant has a subcutaneous location, **necrosis of overlying tissues**. Late complications include **implant loosening and failure, infection, pathological or implant fracture** as well as **local or systemic relapse**.

As the bony resection for tumour usually requires excision of juxta-articular bone, the endoprosthetic replacement includes a joint reconstruction. As an extensive amount of bone and ligaments is sacrificed, these endoprosthetic joints are usually fully constrained. Wear of bearing surfaces may require procedures to 'rebush' or renew their components.

Endoprosthetic replacements to the lower limbs in the immature skeleton require extending mechanisms to minimize final limb-length discrepancies. Extending prostheses have evolved from requiring repeated major surgery in order to insert lengthening sleeves, to needing smaller incisions in order to allow manual turning of in-built extending rack-and-pinion mechanisms (**Figure 7.6**). More recent systems employ externally applied pulsed magnetic fields in order to turn in-built motors within the prosthesis that enable non-invasive limb lengthening.

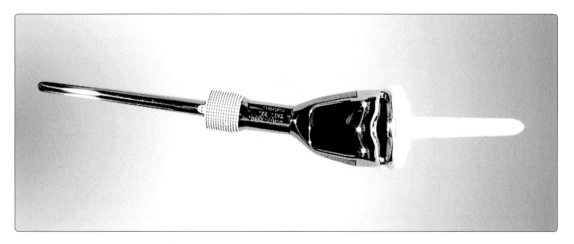

Figure 7.5 Custom-made distal femoral endoprosthetic replacement. Image courtesy of Stanmore Implants, Royal National Orthopaedic Hospital Trust, Stanmore, UK. www.stanmoreimplants.com.

Autograft

Reconstruction using the patient's own bone may be considered, particularly where **only resection of diaphyseal bone** is required. Here, a **strut graft**, typically from the **fibula**, may be interposed. This technique has been of use in **tibial tumours**, where the grafted fibulae have been shown to subsequently enlarge in response to loading. The fibula has also been employed in osteoarticular reconstruction for excision of **tumours of the distal radius**.

Autograft reconstruction may also be achieved by **resection of the pathological bone, irradiation and reimplantation**. This bone is **non-viable** when implanted and therefore has **reduced mechanical properties**. There are, however, limited indications for this technique, e.g. where a **resection of a large segment of the pelvic ring** is required.

Allograft

As in autograft reconstruction, a large bulk of the bone may be **non-viable**. In addition, there are risks of **disease transmission** from the donor and problems of the availability of cadaveric bone of the appropriate size. Bulk allograft reconstruction is used widely internationally, but less so in the UK.

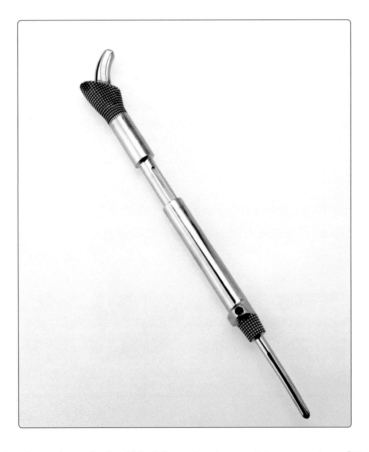

Figure 7.6 Growing endoprosthetic midshaft femoral replacement. Image courtesy of Stanmore Implants, Royal National Orthopaedic Hospital Trust, Stanmore, UK. www.stanmoreimplants.com.

Chemotherapy (adjuvant and neo-adjuvant)

The improved survival of patients with osteosarcoma in the past few decades has been through the development of multi-agent adjuvant chemotherapy treatment protocols. Further significant increase in survival has resulted from the use of neo-adjuvant chemotherapy. In this, the patient has a number of cycles of chemotherapy before surgery. After neo-adjuvant therapy, restaging is undertaken. These may even demonstrate shrinkage of the tumour and its reactive zone where the response has been good. This is particularly demonstrated in the soft-tissue mass of Ewing's sarcoma.

Radiotherapy

Radiotherapy may be considered as adjuvant treatment for primary bone and soft-tissue tumour resection where a **histological marginal resection** is demonstrated or where **patient factors** limit the surgical resection that can be achieved. Radiotherapy is also indicated in the management of **bone metastases** or **pathological fracture** after surgical stabilization. The effectiveness of radiotherapy is limited in osteosarcoma and chondrosarcoma, but is particularly effective in shrinking the tumour volume of myxoid liposarcomas. Radiation given preoperatively reduces the dose and field size, but doubles the subsequent wound complication rates, relative to post-operative radiation. The long-term problems with the greater doses and field size of post-operative radiation include a greater extent of limb fibrosis, oedema and joint stiffness. A balance needs to be achieved in selecting the appropriate sequencing of radiotherapy.

Treatment of benign bone tumours

Where a lesion can be confidently diagnosed as benign, more conservative treatments may be considered. The lesion may be **observed for further growth** or **spontaneous reossification**. Surgical intervention should be considered if there is pain. This may be reflected in radiographically-proven **thinning of the cortex by at least 50%** (associated with significantly increased risk of pathological fracture) or if there is a **mass effect** on adjacent structures due to the size and location of the lesion. The surgical strategies for benign bone tumours include **intralesional resection or curettage**. This may be augmented by local **cytotoxic therapies**, such as **phenolization, cryotherapy, phototherapy** or **cement in-filling**. Recurrence or particular large benign tumours may be addressed by **endoprosthetic replacement** or indeed **amputation**.

Key features of selected benign bone tumours

Benign epiphyseal tumours

Chondroblastoma

- Usually arises in the immature skeleton.
- Aggressive benign condition that very rarely has been known to metastasize.
- Local recurrence may be reduced by meticulous curettage with good technique including the use of high speed burrs, avoiding the need for joint resection and reconstruction.

Giant-cell tumour (GCT)

- Occurs after skeletal maturity (80%).
- Arises on the metaphyseal side of the physis, expanding into the epiphysis as a juxta-articular eccentrically placed lytic lesion with internal septation.
- Classically low signal intensity on both T1- and T2-imaging, but can undergo cystic degeneration, which changes the signal characteristics.
- Aggressive, locally recurrent tumour.
- Rarely malignant from outset (giant-cell sarcoma); malignant transformation may occur and is seen particularly after local recurrence and treatment with radiotherapy.
- Radiological grading system: cortex intact, expanded, broken (Campanacci).
- Treatment: essential to check calcium and phosphate to exclude brown tumour (primary hyperparathyroidism) prior to considering curettage and augmentation by bone graft/cement or cryosurgery. Consider resection or even amputation for recurrence or lesions demonstrating malignant features histologically.

Benign metaphyseal and diaphyseal tumours

Simple (unicameral) bone cysts

- Arises in the growing skeleton.
- Most common in the proximal humerus (67%) and proximal femur (15%).
- Usually asymptomatic until they fracture.
- Well-demarcated lytic lesions, expanding bone; 'fallen-fragment' sign.
- Diagnosis is usually made reliably on radiological features and the site of the lesion. If uncertain, consider bone scintigraphy, which should demonstrate a cold spot corresponding to the radiographic lesion.
- If diagnosis can be made confidently and the lesion is detected on incidental X-ray, the lesion may be monitored for spontaneous ossification. May consider invasive techniques if lesion fails to resolve or pathological fracture is impending. In case of pathological fracture, initiate supportive measures for fracture and observe healing. If ossification is not triggered, consider invasive techniques.
- Invasive treatment options include aspiration with instillation of steroid/bone marrow, or primary currettage.
- Intramedullary nails may also be used.

Osteochondroma (exostosis)

- Most common benign bone tumour.
- Usually solitary, except in patients with hereditary multiple osteochondromastoses.
- Pedunculated or sessile lesions arising from juxtaphyseal location and growing away from the joint.
- May cause local irritation and pain. Growth of lesion or new pain in adulthood may signify malignant change.
- Radiological appearance of the lesion may appear smaller than the clinically palpable mass due to the presence of a cartilaginous cap.
- Malignant change occurs in approximately 1% of lesions.
- Malignant transformation occurs in the cartilaginous cap to chondrosarcoma. If cap thickness exceeds 2 cm in an adult on MRI, consider resection.

Enchondroma

- May be solitary or multiple (Ollier's disease). If multiple and found in association with soft-tissue mineralized phleboliths, then this is Maffucci's disease, with a correspondingly increased risk of malignant change.
- Often an incidental finding.
- Those occurring in hands or feet are usually benign.
- Lesions in pelvis or shoulders should prompt a higher suspicion of malignancy (chondrosarcoma).

Osteoid osteoma

- Characteristic symptoms of localized pain, worse at night and relieved by salicylates.
- Can affect any bone, although femur, tibia and spine are most often involved.
- May affect any part of bone, although usually intracortical.
- Lesion itself is radiolucent but gives rise to surrounding sclerotic reaction.
- Fine-cut CT may be necessary to demonstrate the lesion.
- Bone scintigraphy demonstrates markedly increased uptake.
- Treatment is by percutaneous thermal ablation under CT guidance, or surgical excision for larger or recurrent lesions.

Key features of selected malignant bone tumours

Osteosarcoma

- Bimodal age distribution of incidence. First peak in childhood and adolescence, and further peak in later years. Second peak may be associated with Paget's disease, irradiation or polyostotic fibrous dysplasia.
- Most often affects bones about the knee (50%) or humerus (25%); rarely affects the axial skeleton.
- Radiological features of increased intramedullary sclerosis with permeative destruction. Elevation of periosteum gives rise to the appearance of Codman's triangle (**see Figure 7.4**). Extraosseous component gives rise to ossification in the soft tissues.
- Histologically a high-grade spindle-cell tumour.
- Variants of classical osteosarcoma described may occur. There may be a predominantly lytic appearance to the lesion. Lesions may also arise in cortex giving rise to parosteal or periosteal osteosarcomas.
- Neo-adjuvant chemotherapy is required.

Chondrosarcoma

- Malignancy of cartilaginous tissues.
- Peak incidence in middle life.
- Radiologically may demonstrate patchy calcification, giving rise to a 'popcorn' appearance. Where central (intramedullary) in site, may give rise to endosteal scalloping. Narrow zone of transition may lead to misdiagnosis as benign.
- Variable histological grade.
- Treatment is by surgical resection, with little effective adjuvant chemotherapy or radiotherapy.

Ewing's/primitive neuroectodermal tumour (PNET)

- These are small round-cell tumours believed to be of the same aetiology.
- The tissue type of origin is uncertain, although the condition is associated with the gene translocation (11:22).
- Occur in children and adolescents (80% of cases in first two decades), with median age 13 years.
- Most frequently affects the femoral diaphysis.
- Male-to-female ratio 3:2.
- Radiological studies may demonstrate pathognomonic onion skin appearance due to episodes of periosteal reaction and new bone formation. Often have a large soft-tissue element.
- Neo-adjuvant chemotherapy is highly effective in reducing tumour mass.

Haemopoietic tumours

These tumours (multiple myeloma, plasmacytoma) may present to the orthopaedic surgeon as incidental findings, with pain or after pathological fracture. Diagnosis should follow the principles outlined above, with appropriate referral for further management, such as surgical stabilization of pathological fractures.

Secondary tumours of bone

- Metastatic disease affecting bone is common and may be increasing in incidence with improved overall tumour survivorship.
- Long-established tumours with a predilection for spread to bone are those of the lung, breast, prostate, kidney and thyroid.
- Initial management of tumours presenting as bony metastases should follow the principles outlined above.
- In treating the osseous element, the key is avoidance of pathological fracture. Assessment of risk of fracture may be performed (Mirels, 1989) and prophylactic stabilization undertaken if appropriate.
- Where fracture through the lesion is already present, segmental reconstruction by a load-bearing prosthesis may be required, as union of the fracture may not occur. Mechanical and fatigue properties of the implant selected should preferably exceed the patient's predicted survival.

Conclusion

Orthopaedic surgeons are likely to encounter bone malignancy (primary or secondary) infrequently in their practice. A detailed knowledge of individual tumours is not expected of the general orthopaedic surgeon, and only a brief summary of the more common neoplasms is given in this chapter. The management, including diagnosis, should follow the simple principles outlined, i.e. suspect the diagnosis, refer early and avoid compromise of the prognosis by inappropriate intervention.

Viva questions

1. Describe this tumour (when showing an image).
2. How would you investigate a patient who presents with a possible malignant bone tumour?
3. How are bone tumours staged?
4. What are the principles of treatment of bone tumours?
5. What surgical options are available in the treatment of bone tumours?

Further reading

D'Adamo D. Is adjuvant chemotherapy useful for soft-tissue sarcomas? *Lancet Oncol* 2012;**13**(10):968–70.

Demicco EG. Sarcoma diagnosis in the age of molecular pathology. *Adv Anat Pathol* 2013;**20**(4):264–74.

Grimer R, Athanasou N, Gerrand C, *et al*. UK Guidelines for the Management of Bone Sarcomas. *Sarcoma* 2010;**2010**:317462. doi: 10.1155/2010/317462. Epub 2010 Dec 29.

Grimer R, Judson I, Peake D, Seddon B. Guidelines for the management of soft tissue sarcomas. *Sarcoma* 2010;**2010**:506182. doi: 10.1155/2010/506182. Epub 2010 May 31.

Grimer RJ, Briggs TW. Earlier diagnosis of bone and soft-tissue tumours. *J Bone Joint Surg Br* 2010;**92**(11): 1489–92.

Mirels H. Metastatic disease in long bones. A proposed scoring system for diagnosing impending pathologic fractures. *Clin Orthop Relat Res* 1989;**249**:256–64.

8 Ligaments and Tendons

Cheh Chin Tai, James Hui and Andy Williams

Introduction

Tendons and ligaments are dense connective tissues that contain a large amount of collagen. They play essential roles in joint motion.

Structure

Ligaments and tendons are similar in that **extracellular matrix** accounts for 80% of the total tissue volume, with **cells** (fibroblasts) occupying only 20% of this volume. Approximately 30% cent of the matrix is solid, comprising mainly collagen but also ground substance (including proteoglycans, which are critical for function) and a small amount of elastin.

There are important differences in the function, structure, and composition of ligaments and tendons.

Functional differences

Ligaments connect bone with bone and function:

- To augment the static mechanical stability of joints.
- To prevent excessive or abnormal motion.
- As a sensory source for protective reflexes and to provide proprioceptive feedback about movement and posture, thereby contributing to the neuromuscular dynamic control of stability.

Tendons attach muscle to bone and function:

- To transmit tensile loads from muscle to bone.
- To enable the muscle belly to be at an optimal distance from the joint without an extended length of muscle between origin and insertion.
- As a store of energy (analogous to a spring).

Structural differences

In tendons, the collagen fibers are arranged in an almost parallel fashion reflecting its function to transmit tensile loads. In ligaments, the fibres are less parallel in the different layers (see details below). Some tendons in the hand and feet have a synovial sheath covering.

Composition differences

The **collagen content is high** (over 70%) and **is greater in tendons than in ligaments.** In extremity tendons, the solid material may consist almost entirely of collagen (up to 99% of dry weight). There are two notable exceptions: the ligamentum nuchae and the ligamentum flava along the spinal column, which contain large amounts of elastic fibres (almost 75% of dry weight). There is generally **more elastin in ligaments than tendons.**

Collagen

Collagen is synthesized as a precursor, procollagen, by fibroblasts. Procollagen is secreted and cleaved extracellularly to form collagen fibres (**Figure 8.1**).

More than 90% of collagen in tendons and ligaments is type I, and less than 10% is type III. Type IV is present in small quantities. Type I collagen consists of **three polypeptide chains**: two (alpha 1) are identical and one differs slightly (alpha 2). The three alpha chains are combined to form a **right-handed triple helix**, which gives the collagen molecule a rod-like shape. The intra- and interchain bonding (**cross-linking**), which aggregates the chains into a triple helix, are due mainly to hydrogen bonds and provide stability to the molecule. Several collagen molecules aggregate in a **quarter-staggered array** to form microfibrils (each 0.02–0.2 μm in diameter) (**Figure 8.2**).

Further aggregation of the microfibrils results in the formation of collagen **fibres** (each 1–20 μm in diameter) and **bundles**. Fibroblasts are aligned between these bundles in the direction of ligament or tendon function. The arrangement of the collagen fibres is nearly **parallel in tendons**, allowing them to handle high unidirectional (uniaxial) tensile loads (**Figure 8.3**).

The **less parallel arrangement of the collagen fibres in ligaments** and the **layered arrangement** allows these structures to sustain predominantly tensile stresses in one direction but also smaller stresses in other directions for any applied external force. In any single layer the fibres lie parallel to each other, but in subsequent layers they lie in different directions. As a result of this arrangement, a ligament can resist applied forces from many directions. In addition, the fibres in ligaments are arranged in a **wavy pattern (crimp)**, increasing their capacity to absorb tension.

Ground substance

Ground substance consists of **proteoglycans** (PGs), **glycoproteins, plasma proteins** and a variety of **small molecules**. PGs are composed of sulphated polysaccharide chains (glycosaminoglycans) bound to a core protein, which in turn is bound via a link protein to a hyaluronic acid chain to form an extremely high-molecular weight PG aggregate. These PG aggregates bind most of the extracellular water of the ligaments and tendons, making the

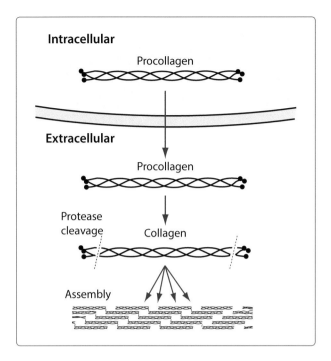

Figure 8.1 Collagen synthesis in fibroblasts.

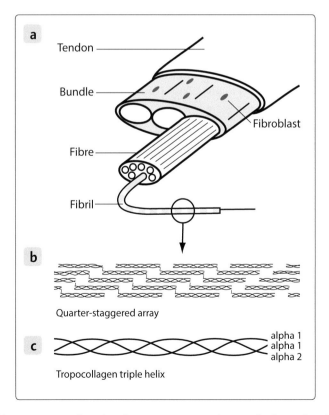

Figure 8.2 a: Macrostructure of tendon; b: quarter-staggered array of collagen forming microfibrils; c: type I collagen (three polypeptide chains).

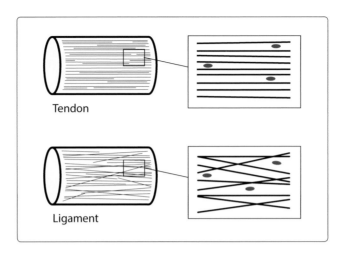

Figure 8.3 Arrangement of collagen fibres in a tendon and ligament.

matrix a highly structured gel-like material. By acting as a cement-like substance between the collagen microfibrils, they help to **stabilize the collagenous skeleton** of tendons and ligaments and contribute to the **overall strength** of these composite structures. However, only a small number of these molecules exist in tendons.

Elastin

Elastin consists of **hydrophobic non-glycosylated proteins** secreted by fibroblasts into the extracellular matrix. These proteins form an **extensive network** with highly **cross-linked filaments** and **sheets**, which allows the network to **stretch and coil** (up to 200% of their unloaded length at relatively low loads). Elastic fibres are of great importance to the recovery of tissues after loading. Their function, however, diminishes towards maximal loading levels because their maximum strength is about five times lower than that of collagen.

Surrounding connective tissue

Tendons and ligaments are surrounded by **loose areolar connective tissues,** known as the **paratenon** in tendons (no specific name in ligaments). These form a sheath, which can either run the entire length of the tendon or exist only at the point where the tendon bends in concert with a joint. The paratenon protects the tendon and facilitates gliding. It is also the major source for remodelling and healing responses, as it contains abundant cells and blood vessels (**vascular tendons**). In some tendons, a true synovial sheath replaces the paratenon (**avascular tendons**).

A synovium-like membrane, called the **epitenon**, is found just beneath the paratenon in tendons that are subjected to particularly high friction forces (e.g. in the palm and wrist). The epitenon enhances gliding of the tendon by producing synovial fluid from its synovial cells. The epitenon surrounds the endotenon, which in turn binds together the fascicles (groups of collagen bundles).

The flexor tendons in the hand and feet are in part surrounded by synovial sheaths. These sheaths enhance tendon gliding and produce synovial fluid, which is important for tendon nutrition. This double-walled synovial sheath consists of an inner visceral sheath and an outer parietal sheath. The two walls are linked by a **mesotenon**, which connects blood vessels, lymphatics and nerves to the tendon.

Insertion site

Tendons and ligaments are **highly resistant to lengthening**. Tendons in particular are also relatively flexible and can therefore be angulated around bone surfaces or deflected beneath retinacula to alter the direction of muscular pull. In ligaments, due to the organization of the fibres in layers, not all fibres are stretched when loaded along the main fibre axis. Consequently, **ligaments are less strong than tendons**.

The structure of the insertion into bone is similar in ligaments and tendons and consists of **four zones of indirect insertion**:

- **Zone 1: parallel collagen fibres at the end of the tendon or ligament.**
- **Zone 2: collagen fibres intermesh with unmineralized fibrocartilage.**
- **Zone 3: fibrocartilage gradually becomes mineralized.**
- **Zone 4: mineralized fibrocartilage merges into cortical bone.**

The **perforating fibres of Sharpey** cross all four zones. The gradual change in structural properties results in increased stiffness and decreased stress concentration, minimizing injuries at insertion sites. In addition, the collagen fibres of ligaments can also insert directly into bone by blending with the periosteum at an oblique or orthogonal angle.

In tendons, the musculotendinous junction is of equal importance, since high local stresses can occur here, predisposing to injury. Frequently, tendons have an internal portion within the muscle fascia known as the **aponeurosis**. The aponeurosis provides a large surface area for load transfer from muscle to tendon; the orientation of this junction enhances its strength.

Nutrition and blood supply

Compared with other connective tissues such as bone and skin, ligaments and tendons are poorly vascularized and have a lower metabolic rate. The blood supply of ligaments **originates mainly at the insertion sites, runs longitudinally** through the ligament and is **uniform**. Blood vessels come through tendon and ligament insertion sites, and through the myotendinous junction of tendons. The blood supply of paratenon-covered tendons is provided by a relatively **sparse array of small arterioles** that run longitudinally from the adjacent muscular tissues and surrounding areolar connective tissue. In sheathed avascular tendons such as digital flexor tendons, a **vinculum (mesotenon)** carries a vessel to supply one tendon segment; adjacent avascular areas receive nutrition via diffusion. 90% of flexor tendon nutrition in the digits is provided for via synovial diffusion, with the rest from blood vessels. Digital motion promotes the delivery of nutrients via synovial fluid. As a result of these differences, **paratenon-covered tendons heal better** than other tendons.

Nerve supply

The nerve supply is mainly afferent, with specialized **afferent** receptors. When these receptors are activated (during rapid increase in tension), myotactic reflexes are initiated, which inhibit the development of excessive tension during muscular contraction. Hence, tendons and ligaments play an important proprioceptive role in overall neuromuscular control of the limb.

Function

Load–elongation curves

The biomechanical properties can be measured in tensile loading experiments using isolated cadaveric tendon or ligament-bone complexes of human or animal origin. The tissue is elongated until it ruptures and the load–elongation curve plotted (**Figure 8.4**).

The first region of the load–elongation curve is concave and is usually called the **non-linear toe region**. The reasons for this behaviour are multifactorial. During the stretching of ligament or tendon, an increasing number of fibres are recruited under tension and **crimped fibres begin to straighten**. Initially, there is little resistance to tension as the fibres lengthen, but as elongation progresses an increasing number of fibrils become taut and carry load. Some studies suggest that sliding and shear of the interfibrillar ground substance may cause this elongation.

As elongation continues at higher loads, the stiffness of the tissue increases, and progressively greater force is required to produce equivalent amounts of elongation. This is known as the **linear region**, as the deformation of the tissue has a more or less linear relationship with load. At the end of this region, the load value is designated as **Plin**, the yield point for the tissue. The energy to Plin is represented by the area under the curve up to the end of the linear region.

Small force reduction (**dips**) can sometimes be observed at the end of the linear region in the loading curves for tendons and ligaments. These dips are caused by the **early sequential failure** of a few greatly stretched fibre bundles. Ultimately, as elongation exceeds the capacity of the

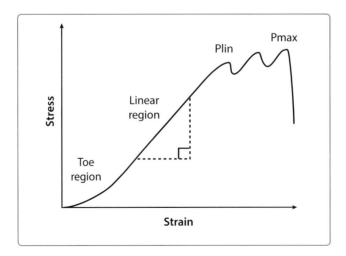

Figure 8.4 Stress–strain curve for ligaments and tendons. Plin:, linear yield point; Pmax: maximum load (ultimate tensile strength).

fibres, yield and failure of the tissue result from **progressive fibril failure**. This is when the curve begins to bend toward the strain axis and reaches a point of ultimate stress. With attainment of the maximum load, **Pmax**, which reflects the ultimate tensile strength of the specimen, complete failure occurs rapidly. The strain to failure is usually only a few percentage points of total length. However, in real life, ligaments and tendons are rarely stretched significantly, as muscular reflexes initiated by proprioceptive feedback provide protection.

The modulus of elasticity for tendons and ligaments is based on a linear relationship between load and deformation (structural property), or stress and strain (mechanical property). The stress (force or load divided by the cross-sectional area) is proportional to the strain (change in length or deformation divided by the original length):

$$E = \delta/\varepsilon$$

where E is the modulus of elasticity (slope of the stress–strain curve), δ is stress and ε is strain.

In the toe region of the graph, the modulus is not constant but increases gradually. The modulus stabilizes in the fairly linear region of the curve.

Not all ligaments and tendons are identical. The curve for ligamentum flavum, with its high proportion of elastic fibres, is different. When tensile testing human ligamentum flavum, elongation of the specimen reaches 50% before the stiffness increases appreciably. At 70% elongation, the stiffness increases greatly with additional loading, and the ligament fails abruptly with little further deformation. This is very uncommon, as most tendons and ligaments fail after a length increase of only a few percentage points of the original.

Viscoelasticity

Viscoelastic materials exhibit stress–strain behaviour that is **time-** and **rate-dependent**, i.e. the material deformation depends on the load and its rate and duration of application. In a tissue that is viscous (fluid-like), constant loading results in a progressive deformation over an extended period of time, known as **creep**. In contrast, a more elastic (solid-like) tissue returns to its original shape or length after load is removed and its stress–strain behaviour remains unchanged with cycled loads. Tendons and ligaments maintain the capacity for both viscous and elastic responses: at **low loads**, **viscous behaviour** dominates; at **higher loads**, **elastic behaviour** dominates. This balance allows normal ligaments and tendons to function within a fairly wide range of loads without damaging their fibres.

When ligaments and tendons are repetitively loaded, the stress–strain curve shifts to the right, indicating that the tissues have become less stiff and more compliant. However, when subjected to increased strain rates, the linear portion of the stress–strain curve becomes steeper, indicating greater stiffness of the tissue and more energy storage, thus requiring more force to rupture.

The three main features of viscoelastic behaviour are:

- **Hysteresis**: the load–elongation curve differs during loading and unloading, resulting in net internal energy loss, usually as heat (**Figure 8.5**).

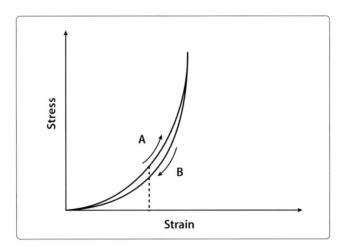

Figure 8.5 Hysteresis is the difference in stress between the loading curve (A) and unloading curve (B) for a given strain. The difference is energy lost.

- **Stress relaxation**: this is a decrease in stress in the tendon or ligament subjected to constant strain over an extended period (**Figure 8.6**). However, when the stress–relaxation test is repeated cyclically, the decrease in stress gradually becomes less pronounced. This is used as an argument for cyclic loading of hamstring grafts before fixation in cruciate ligament reconstruction.
- **Creep**: this is an increase in deformation or strain that occurs when a constant load is applied over an extended period (**Figure 8.7**). When this test is repeated cyclically, the increase in strain gradually becomes less pronounced. Clinically, this behaviour is applied in the application of plaster casts for deformity correction, e.g. the Ponseti method for treatment of congenital talipes equinovarus.

Under normal physiological conditions *in vivo*, ligaments and tendons are subjected to a stress magnitude that is only about one-quarter to one-third of the ultimate tensile load. The upper limit for physiological strain in tendons and ligaments (e.g. during running and jumping) is 2–5%.

Factors affecting the biomechanical properties of ligaments and tendons include the following:

- **Aging effect**: during maturation (up to age 20 years), the number and quality of cross-links increases, resulting in increased tensile strength of tendons and ligaments. After maturation, as aging occurs, the mean collagen diameter and content decrease, resulting in the gradual decline of mechanical properties. Before puberty, the weakest link in the ligament bone complex is the developing bone, but once skeletal maturity is reached, mid-substance failure of the ligament usually occurs. Similarly, in the growing skeleton tendon avulsion may occur, but in adolescent and older age groups failure tends to occur at the musculotendinous junction due to stress concentration and the relatively weak muscular tissue.
- **Endocrine effect**: increased laxity and decreased stiffness of the tendon and ligaments are noted in the pelvic region during the latter stages of pregnancy and in the post-partum period. It is also thought that the incidence of anterior cruciate ligament ruptures in females varies according to the phase of the menstrual cycle.

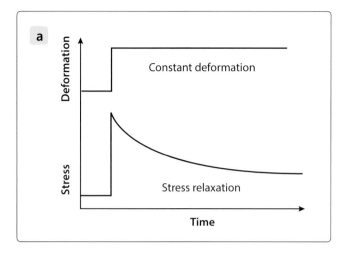

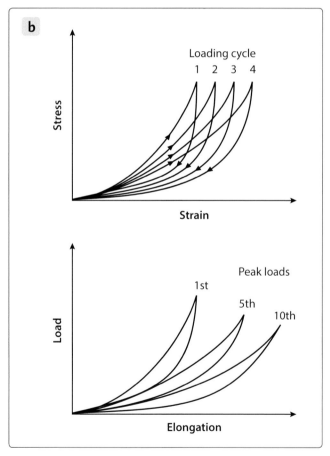

Figure 8.6 a: Graph showing stress relaxation being exhibited in a tendon. When the deformation is constant, the stress drops over time; b: when the tendon is loaded and unloaded repeatedly, the curve shifts to the right. This decrease in stress becomes less with repeated loading until the curve becomes repeatable, in about 10 cycles.

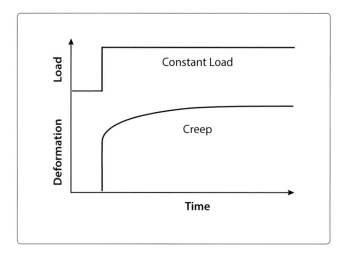

Figure 8.7 Graph showing creep being exhibited by a tendon. Under a constant load, the deformation increases over time.

- **Pharmacological effect**: some studies have shown that short-term treatment with indomethacin increases the tensile strength of tendons, probably due to an increased cross-linkage of collagen molecules. Other studies have shown that the rate and strength of tissue healing decreases as a result of such treatment. Corticosteroid injections have been shown to weaken the biomechanical qualities of both normal and healing tissues. The association of Achilles and patellar tendon ruptures with local steroid injections is well known. There are also many case reports of tendon ruptures associated with the abuse of anabolic steroids.
- **Mobilization and immobilization** effect: see Healing below.

Injury

The degree of injury is related to the rate of loading and the amount of load. There are **two main mechanisms of injury**:

- **Repetitive micro-trauma**: fatigue failure occurs due to repetitive loading well below the normal ultimate tensile strength. These injuries result in **micro-tears** followed by an **inflammatory reaction** (in an attempt to heal) and sometimes **calcification**, which alters the biomechanical properties of the tissues. This type of injury is common and is more likely to occur in tendons, since these structures tend to carry higher loads *in vivo* than ligaments.
- **Macro-trauma**: acute failure due to forces (excluding laceration) above the ultimate tensile strength results in partial or complete rupture. These injuries tend to have well-documented mechanisms of injury and are associated with forces resisted by specific tendons or ligaments, e.g. injury to the lateral collateral knee ligament by a varus force. In ligaments, ruptures of sequential series of collagen fibre bundles tend to be distributed throughout the ligament rather than being localized to one specific area.

Factors contributing to ligament injury include:

- **Loading rate of the the ligament or tendon:** the failure of a ligament or tendon – either an acute rupture or micro-tears – can occur at insertion sites (avulsion), with or without a bony fragment, within the substance itself or a combination of both. At a **low loading rate** the **bony insertion is the weakest component** of the tendon/ligament–bone complex, but at a **high loading rate the tendon or ligament is the weakest link.** This suggests that with increasing strain rate, the increase in tissue strength is higher at the tendon/ligament–bone complex junction than in the tendon or ligament itself. However, some studies have shown that failure modes are independent of strain rate and merely depend on the maturation of the loaded tendon/ligament–bone complex and so may be age-specific. Note that ligament avulsions typically occur between the mineralized and unmineralized fibrocartilage layers.
- **Cross-sectional area of the tendon in relation to its muscle:** the strength of both the muscle and the tendon depends on their physiological cross-sectional areas. The larger the cross-sectional area of the muscle, the stronger the force produced by the contraction, and therefore the greater the tensile loads transmitted through the tendon. Similarly, the larger the cross-sectional area of the tendon, the greater the load it can bear. If the tensile strength of a tendon is greater than that of its muscle, then muscle ruptures are more likely to occur.
- **Amount of force produced by the contraction of the muscle to which the tendon is attached:** when the muscle is maximally contracted, the tensile stress on the tendon is at its highest. This stress can be increased if eccentric contraction of the muscle rather than concentric contraction takes place. As a result, the load imposed on the tendon may exceed the yield point, causing tendon rupture.

Clinically, injuries to tendons and ligaments can be categorized according to their degree of severity:

- **Grade I** (mild): some pain is felt, but no joint laxity can be detected clinically, even though micro-failure of collagen fibres may have occurred.
- **Grade II** (moderate): severe pain and some joint laxity can be detected clinically. Progressive failure of the collagen has taken place, resulting in partial rupture. The joint laxity is often masked by muscle activity, and hence the clinical test for joint laxity is often positive only if performed with the patient under anaesthesia.
- **Grade III** (severe): severe pain occurs at the time of trauma, with less pain after injury. Clinically, the joint is found to be completely unstable. Most collagen fibres have ruptured, but a few may still be intact. However, the tissue can still be in continuity, even though it has undergone extensive macro- and micro-failure and elongation.

Healing

The response to injury of different tendons and ligaments differs significantly. This could be due to differences in intrinsic fibroblastic response to injury, the mechanical environment, intra-articular versus extra-articular environment (inhibitory effect of synovial fluid), blood supply and the degree of inflammatory response.

Unlike skin and bone, ligaments and tendons are believed to have a slower and more limited healing response (ligaments and tendons are not as well vascularized or innervated as skin and bone). **Healing can be divided into three phases** (analogous to healing in other connective tissues):

- **Phase one – haemorrhagic/inflammatory phase**: this phase is characterized by the formation of a haematoma within the damaged region and the initiation of a rapid **inflammatory response**. This results in invasion by polymorphonuclear cells and monocytes/macrophages, with the release of a complex cascade of cytokines and growth factors. The monocytes remove debris and **fibroblastic cells** begin to appear. This phase of ligament healing lasts for **hours to a few days**.
- **Phase two – proliferative phase**: in this phase, **new blood vessels** are formed and fibroblasts are recruited from the local environment or circulation to produce **new matrix material**, mainly collagen (type III is predominant initially). This is **extrinsic healing**. The native fibroblasts in the ligament and tendon also contribute to this healing process, termed **intrinsic healing**. The new matrix then increases in mass and becomes less viscous and more elastic as the inflammation decreases over the next few weeks of healing.
- **Phase three – remodelling phase**: this phase starts within weeks after the injury and can last up to several years. It is characterized by **progressive maturation** and **conversion of collagen fibres (to type I)**, alignment in a more physiological orientation (in response to loads) and reorganization of the matrix. Surgical tendon repairs are at their weakest in the first week, regaining most of their original strength by 3–4 weeks and achieving **maximum strength at 6 months**.

Ideally, healing should lead to complete restoration of the original tissue with identical morphological and functional characteristics. Unfortunately, even after years of remodelling, healed matrix remains different from normal tissue biochemically, mechanically and histologically (collagen is more disorganized and less orientated, more defects exist between collagen fibres, and the number of collagen fibres of larger diameter is reduced).

Factors affecting healing include the following:

- **Mobilization**: ligaments and tendons appear to remodel in response to the mechanical demands placed upon them. Controlled movement of a joint appears to have a beneficial effect on healing, increasing the tensile strength of tendons and of the ligament–bone interface by stimulating synthesis of collagen and PG, and by promoting proper collagen fibre orientation. In animal studies on healing of ligament injury, immobilization results in decreased strength and stiffness of tendons and ligaments; the tissue metabolism also increases, leading to proportionally more immature collagen, with a decrease in the amount and quality of the cross-links between collagen molecules. This decline in structural properties is reversible, but the process is slow.
- **Surgery**: the calibre of suture, the number of suture strands, the suture technique and the use of peripheral epitendinous or sheath repair can all affect the strength of the healing process. Suturing of mop-end tears with extensive overlapping of tissue ends and minimal gapping confers little benefit.

- **Biological and biochemical manipulation**: the use of growth factors, e.g. epidermal growth factor (EGF) and platelet-derived growth factor (PDGF), increases fibroblast proliferation *in vitro*. Other agents such as steroids and hyaluronate have been shown to decrease adhesion formation in the healing process. However, the latter also decrease the rate and strength of tendon healing and increase the rate of infection.
- **Joint instability**: in an unstable joint, the healing of ligament is inferior, especially if instability is due to multiple ligament injury.

Viva questions

1. What is the structure of collagen?
2. Describe the blood supply of tendons and ligaments.
3. How do tendons and ligaments heal after injury?
4. Draw the stress–strain curve of a ligament/tendon and explain its various parts.
5. Discuss injuries to tendons and mechanisms of fatigue failure.

Further reading

Benjamin M, Ralphs JR. Tendons and ligaments – an overview. *Histol Histopathol* 1987;**12**:1135–44.

Buckwalter, JA, Hunziker, EB. Orthopaedics: healing of bones, cartilages, tendons, and ligaments – a new era. *Lancet* 1996;**348**:sll18.

Butler, DL, Grood, ES, Noyes, FR, Zernicke, RF. Biomechanics of ligaments and tendons. *Exerc Sport Sci Rev* 1978;**6**:125–81.

Fleming, BC, Beynnon, BD. In vivo measurement of ligament/tendon strains and forces: a review. *Ann Biomed Eng* 2004;**32**:318–28.

Noyes, FR, DeLucas, JL, Torvik, PJ. Biomechanics of anterior cruciate ligament failure: an analysis of strain-rate sensitivity and mechanisms of failure in primates. *J Bone Joint Surg Am* 1974;**56**:236–53.

Sharma, P, Maffulli, N. Tendon injury and tendinopathy: healing and repair. *J Bone Joint Surg Am* 2005;**87**:187–202.

Strickland JW. Flexor tendon injuries: I. Foundations of treatment. *J Am Acad Orthop Surg* 1995;**3**:44–54.

9 Meniscus

Vijai Ranawat, Patrick C Schottel, Anil Ranawat and John Skinner

Introduction

The meniscus is a **fibrocartilaginous** structure that deepens the articular surface of the knee. Although first perceived as a vestigial structure, subsequent investigation has elucidated its importance in such functions as load transmission and joint stability. This chapter will concentrate on the anatomy, function and pathology of the meniscus.

Anatomy

The knee contains a medial and lateral meniscus interposed between the femoral condyles and tibial plateau. The medial meniscus (MM) and lateral meniscus (LM) cover approximately 60% and 80% of the peripheral corresponding tibial articular surface, respectively (**Figure 9.1**). They are typically described as containing three segments: the anterior horn, body and posterior horn. In **cross-section**, the menisci are **triangular shaped** with a **thick peripheral border attached to the capsule of the joint** and an **inner border tapering to a thin free edge**. The femoral surface of the meniscus is concave whereas its tibial surface is flat or slightly convex.

The **MM** has an **asymmetric C-shape** with a **considerably wider posterior than anterior horn**. The **peripheral border** is continuously attached to the joint capsule via the **coronary ligament** with a **capsular condensation at its midportion**, known as the **deep medial collateral ligament**. The anterior horn attachment of the MM is geographically the largest (61.4 mm^2) compared to the other meniscal insertions. Additionally, it has the greatest amount of variability with four differently identified attachment locations. However, the majority attach **anterior to the anterior cruciate ligament (ACL) insertion. Posteriorly**, the MM inserts onto the **posterior intercondylar fossa directly anterior to the insertion of the posterior cruciate ligament** (PCL).

The **LM is semicircular in shape** with the anterior and posterior horns attaching closer to each other than those of the MM. The **anterior horn inserts adjacent to the ACL** and is commonly used as a landmark during ACL reconstruction. The **posterior horn attaches anterior to the PCL and posterior horn of the MM insertion**, but **posterior to the lateral intercondylar**

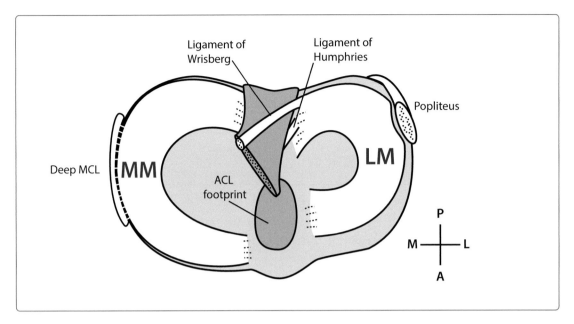

Figure 9.1 The superior aspect of the tibial plateau. ACL: anterior cruciate ligament; LM: lateral meniscus; MCL: medial collateral ligament; MM: medial meniscus.

eminence. Additionally, there are **two ligaments attaching the posterior horn of the LM to the medial femoral condyle** that are distinguished by their relationship to the PCL. The **anterior meniscofemoral ligament of Humphry** is located anterior to the PCL and the **posterior meniscofemoral ligament of Wrisberg** runs posteriorly. Additionally, unlike the MM, the LM is **not continuously attached to the joint capsule as a result of the popliteal hiatus** – a separation between the posterolateral LM and the joint capsule to allow passage of the popliteal tendon.

The MM and LM are perfused by an arborizing network of vessels arising predominately from the **inferior and superior branches of the lateral, medial and middle genicular arteries**. Branches of these vessels give rise to a **peri-meniscal capillary plexus** (PCP) within the synovial and capsular tissues of the knee that supplies the attached peripheral border of the menisci (**Figure 9.2**).

Understanding the vascular supply to the menisci is clinically important as more peripheral tears have greater perfusion and therefore increased healing potential.

Embryology and anatomical abnormalities

The menisci appear by developmental day 45. They are formed from the **middle of the three layers of fibroblastic tissue** present in a developing synovial joint. This central layer not only gives rise to the menisci but also to the synovium and other enclosed ligaments of the knee joint.

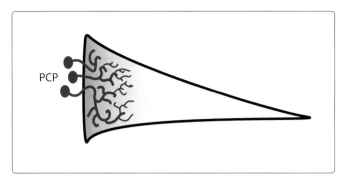

Figure 9.2 Cross section of meniscus showing blood supply. PCP: peri-meniscal capillary plexus.

At birth, the menisci are **completely vascularized**. However, regression of the vascularized zone occurs so that by age **9 months an avascular central third** of the meniscus is present. This devascularization continues until approximately **age 10 years** when the vascularity of the meniscus closely resembles that of the adult. In the adult, only the peripheral **10–25% of the LM** and **10–30% of the MM** demonstrate vascular penetration.

Three notable meniscal variants include a discoid meniscus, congenital hypoplasia or absence and meniscal cysts.

Discoid menisci

A discoid meniscus is a congenital anomaly that presents morphologically as a block-shaped meniscus instead of the typical crescentic shape. Thus, a discoid meniscus covers a larger area of the underlying tibial plateau. Although previously believed to be a failure of degeneration of the inner portion of the meniscus, it is now known that discoid menisci represent an **anatomic variant**.

A discoid LM is the most common, with a reported incidence of 4–15.5%. It usually presents in childhood with the classic complaint of 'snapping' and pain. Magnetic resonance imaging (MRI) scans are diagnostic. Arthroscopic partial meniscectomy gives good short-term results. A discoid MM is rare, with a reported incidence of 0.06–0.3%.

Hypoplasia and congenital absence

The incidences of hypoplasia and congenital absence of either or both menisci are unknown but invariably occur in association with ipsilateral knee abnormalities. This association is likely due to the common mesenchymal origin of these structures.

Meniscal and ganglion cysts

Ganglion cysts associated with the menisci are common and are related to cystic degeneration of the tissue. Meniscal cysts are a subgroup that occurs in association with trauma.

Histology and ultrastructure

The meniscus is a fibrocartilaginous structure whose **extracellular matrix** is predominately composed of **water** (70%). Of its dry weight, **collagen** comprises 60–70% with a majority being **type I** (90%) with types II, III, V and VI present in smaller quantities. Other components of the dry weight include **non-collagenous proteins** (8–13%), **elastin** (0.6%) and **proteoglycans** (<1%).

The cellular component of the meniscus consists of **fibrochondrocytes**. These cells are anaerobic with abundant endoplasimic reticula and Golgi complexes and few mitochondria. They are responsible for synthesizing and maintaining the extracellular matrix. Microscopically, there are two types of fibrochondrocytes: **fusiform cells (found in the superficial layer) and ovoid cells (found in surface and middle meniscal layers)**.

Studies have shown that the menisci are innervated and contain abundant axons, nerve bundles, free nerve endings and specialized receptors such as complex end-bulbs and Golgi-type type III endings. Additionally, mechanoreceptors present predominantly in the anterior and posterior horns are hypothesized to play an important role in knee proprioception.

Ultrastructure studies demonstrate three layers of collagen fibers: **superficial, surface and deep. Circumferentially-orientated** fibres following the C-shape of the meniscus can be found in all three layers but are most predominant in the **deep** layer. In addition to circumferential fibres, the **surface and superficial layers** contain fibres that are orientated **radially**. The radial fibres act as ties, thus providing structural rigidity against compressive forces and preventing longitudinal splitting (**Figure 9.3**). The orientation of the collagen fibres is clinically relevant such as in meniscal repairs when vertical sutures have been found to be stronger than horizontal sutures due to the circumferential nature of the majority of fibres.

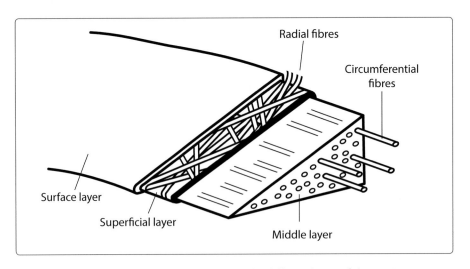

Figure 9.3 Collagen fibre arrangement in the different layers of the meniscus.

Function

The menisci perform several functions:

- Load transmission across the knee.
- Role in anteroposterior (AP) stabilization of the knee.
- Enhancement of articular conformity.
- Distribution of synovial fluid across the articular surface.
- Proprioception.

Meniscal function was first clinically inferred by Fairbanks in 1948 after noting the severe radiographic signs of degenerative joint change that developed following total meniscectomy. It is this role of load transmission that is the most important. Presently, the meniscus is believed to contribute to the following:

Load transmission

The meniscus has been shown to play a vital role in load transmission across the knee joint. Biomechanical studies have shown that at least 50–70% of the compressive load is transmitted through the menisci when the knee is in extension with an increase to 85% at 90° of flexion. In the **meniscectomized knee**, the contact area of the articular surfaces is **reduced by 50–70% medially and by 40–50% laterally** thus drastically increasing the load per unit area resulting in accelerated articular cartilage degeneration (**Figure 9.4**). **Partial meniscectomy** also significantly decreases articular contact area, especially as more of the meniscus is removed. The medial contact area decreases by **20% with a 50% meniscectomy and by 35% with a 75% meniscectomy**. Additionally, tears of the posterior horn attachment of the medial meniscus – known as a **posterior meniscal root tear** – have been shown to **increase contact pressures in the medial compartment by 25%** which is comparable to a subtotal meniscectomy. All of these studies quantitatively demonstrate the importance of the meniscus in load transmission and the decrease in contact area and subsequent increase in contact pressures when it is compromised.

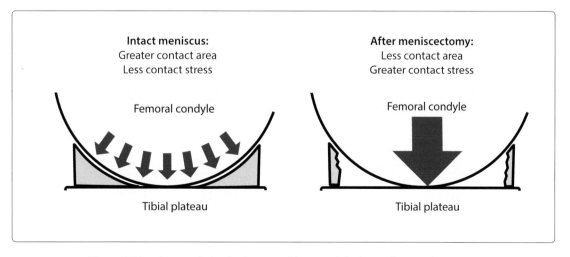

Figure 9.4 Load transmission in the normal knee and the knee after meniscectomy.

Joint stability

The MM plays a role in AP stability in ligamentously compromised knees. Studies have shown that at 90° of knee flexion, there is a **58% increase in AP tibial translation in ACL-deficient knees with medial meniscectomy** compared with ACL-deficient knees with the MM intact. Medial meniscectomy alone has no effect on AP laxity.

Articular conformity

As the knee passes through its range of motion, the menisci move with respect to the tibial articular surface. During **flexion**, both **menisci displace in an AP direction along the tibial plateau** with the **LM displacing more than the MM** (11.2 mm *vs.* 5.1 mm). In addition to the AP translation, the menisci **deform to remain in constant congruity to the tibial and femoral articular surfaces**. This deformable property of the meniscal tissue not only aids load transmission but also is thought to play a role in shock absorption. This is accomplished by the frictional drag exerted by the interstitial fluid as it is forced through the porous permeable solid matrix of the meniscus.

Joint lubrication

When meniscal compression and unloading occur, interstitial fluid is pushed out of and back into the meniscus. This **sponge phenomenon** not only contributes to load transmission and shock absorption as described above, but also it is responsible for the circulation of synovial fluid around the joint accomplishing joint lubrication and distribution of nutrients.

Proprioception

The menisci may serve a proprioceptive role as demonstrated by the presence of **type I and II nerve endings** concentrated in the anterior and posterior horns. In addition to similar structures seen on and within the adjacent cruciate ligaments, neural structures may be part of a complex proprioceptive reflex arc that contributes to the functional stability of the knee. As they are concentrated anteriorly and posteriorly, they may contribute to afferent feedback at the extremes of knee flexion and extension.

Meniscal tears

Presentation

Patients with an acute meniscus tear complain of knee pain and can present with swelling and tenderness to knee palpation along the joint line of the affected side. Patients typically describe a twisting or hyperflexion movement that initiated the symptoms. In addition to pain, they may complain of catching, locking or loss of motion secondary to a mechanical block to extension. Meniscal tears are often present in patients presenting with a popliteal cyst. Popliteal cysts, also known as Baker's cysts when associated with underlying joint pathology such as osteoarthritis, are masses present in the posteromedial aspect of the knee that arise from a pathologic one-way valve communication of synovial fluid between the knee joint and semimembranosus bursa. The accumulation of synovial fluid in this bursa results in distention and eventual formation of a popliteal cyst. Up to 82% of popliteal cysts are associated with a meniscal tear.

Classification

Two methods of classification exist:

- Based on location with reference to blood supply.
- Based on tear pattern.

Location: as mentioned previously, the menisci of the knee are relatively avascular structures. With vascular penetration accounting for only 10–30% of meniscal width (**red zone**) the remaining portion of the inner meniscus lies in a gradient (**red–white zone**) that extends into the entirely avascular free edge (**white zone**) (**Figure 9.5**).

The clinical importance of the blood supply is that **peripheral tears**, particularly those in the **red zone**, are **suitable for repair** whereas **central tears** are **less likely to heal** due to a relative lack of healing potential. The cell responsible for meniscal healing is the **fibrochondrocyte**. **A fibrin clot** forms in response to peripheral vascular zone injury that is rich in inflammatory cells. This inflammation leads to localized vessel and undifferentiated mesenchymal cell proliferation, eventually creating a **fibrovascular cellular scar**. This process is less likely to occur in the avascular inner zones.

Tear pattern: tears can be subdivided into the following:

- Vertical longitudinal – commonly peripheral; bucket-handle tears are extensive longitudinal tears with subluxation of the free edge between the articular surfaces.
- Radial – occur in the vertical plane; commonly at the lateral aspect of the LM; asymptomatic when small.
- Root – variant of a radial tear that occurs at the meniscal horn insertion.
- Horizontal – cleavage tear starting at inner margin that extends in a horizontal plane.
- Complex – combination of the above patterns; normally associated with degenerative meniscal tissue.

Management

Meniscus tears are treated either non-surgically or surgically. Non-surgical treatment can consist of oral anti-inflammatory medication, intra-articular corticosteroid injections, physiotherapy and/or activity modification. Surgical management includes partial or complete removal of the torn meniscus (meniscectomy), meniscus repair or allograft transplantation.

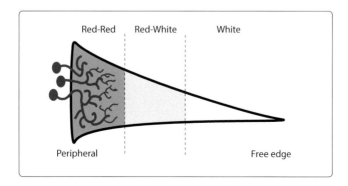

Figure 9.5 Diagram of the zones of vasculature of the meniscus.

Meniscectomy

Partial or complete removal of a meniscus occurs when there is an irreparable tear. Meniscectomy can occur by either an open or arthroscopic method. The choice of either removing the entire meniscus or restricting resection to just the affected portion is situation dependent; however, there is a general consensus that as much of the meniscus should be saved as is possible. Therefore, although open total meniscectomy was once the treatment of choice for meniscus tears, it has fallen out of favour and has largely replaced been with arthroscopic partial meniscectomy.

Meniscal repair

Surgical repair is performed by either an open or arthroscopic method. The location, type of tear and surgeon preference dictate the appropriate suture technique and whether to employ an open or arthroscopic approach. Additionally, augmentation of the surgical repair with injection of exogenous fibrin clot or, more recently, platelet-rich plasma (PRP) into the repaired tissue, is growing in popularity although longer-term results are awaited.

When to repair

Suggested criteria for repair are:

- Presentation: patients with significant pain and/or mechanical symptoms such as knee locking or catching.
- Location: large tears >1cm located in the red–red zone (0–3 mm from periphery) and some tears in the red–white zone (3–5 mm from periphery).
- Tear pattern: vertical longitudinal tears longer than 1 cm and radial tears extending into red zone.
- Tissue quality: repairable meniscal tissue that is neither macerated nor severely degenerate.
- Concomitant injury: if surgical repair or reconstruction is planned for an ipsilateral knee injury, such as an ACL reconstruction, meniscal repair may also be performed at the time of surgery.

Meniscal allograft transplantation

Transplantation of a cadaveric LM or MM can be undertaken in selected patients who have failed non-surgical management of a meniscal-deficient knee. Operative candidates are typically <40 years of age, have normal mechanical knee alignment and have no evidence of advanced degenerative joint disease. Initial clinical outcomes demonstrate improved knee pain and function; however, further long-term clinical data are needed.

Viva questions

1. Can you describe the anatomy of a meniscus?
2. What are the three vascular zones of the meniscus?
3. What are the functions of the meniscus?
4. Is a vertically or horizontally orientated suture more biomechanically advantageous? Why?
5. What is the usual mechanism of injury for a meniscal tear?
6. What are the indications for surgical repair of a meniscal tear?

Further reading

Arnoczky SP, Warren RF. Microvasculature of the human meniscus. *Am J Sports Med* 1982;**10**(2):90–5.

Greis PE, Bardana DD, Holmstrom MC, Burks RT. Meniscal injury: I. Basic science and evaluation. *J Am Acad Orthop Surg* 2002;**10**(3):168–76.

Fairbank TJ. Knee joint changes after meniscectomy. *J Bone Joint Surg Br* 1948;**30B**(4):664–70.

Kocher MS, Klingele K, Rassman SO. Meniscal disorders: normal, discoid, and cysts. *Orthop Clin North Am* 2003;**34**(3):329–40.

Krause WR, Pope MH, Johnson RJ, Wilder DG. Mechanical changes in the knee after meniscectomy. *J Bone Joint Surg Am* 1976;**58**(5):599–604.

McDevitt CA, Webber RJ. The ultrastructure and biochemistry of meniscal cartilage. *Clin Orthop Relat Res* 1990;**252**:8–18.

Wojtys EM, Chan DB. Meniscus structure and function. *Instr Course Lect* 2005;**54**:323–30.

10 Articular Cartilage

Tim S Waters, Nima Heidari and George Bentley

Introduction

Hyaline (literally, 'glass-like') cartilage coats the articular surfaces of synovial joints. It is composed of individual chondrocytes bound together by an extracellular matrix. The function of hyaline cartilage is to distribute weight-bearing forces and reduce friction. It is **avascular, aneural, alymphatic** and almost **non-immunogenic**. It is nourished entirely via diffusion from the synovial fluid.

The major constituent of the extracellular matrix is **water** (75% wet weight of articular cartilage), which is held in place by the negative charge of the **proteoglycans** (10–15% wet weight). **Collagen** fibres (almost exclusively **type II**) constitute around 10–20% wet weight (40–70% dry weight), forming a meshwork with high tensile strength. **Chondrocytes** (5% wet weight) manufacture and maintain the extracellular matrix.

Constituents of articular cartilage

- Cells (chondrocytes).
- Extracellular matrix:
  - water;
  - fibres:
    - collagen – type II, IX, XI
    - type VI, X;
    - elastin.
  - proteoglycans and glycosaminoglycans:
    - aggrecan;
    - hyaluronan;
    - decorin, byglycan, fibromodulin, syndecan, lumican, superficial zone protein.
  - glycoproteins:
    - cartilage oligomeric protein (COMP), laminin, lubricin, chondro-adherin;
    - cartilage matrix protein (CMP), cartilage matrix glycoprotein (CMGP), chondronectin, fibronectin, anchorin CII.
- Degradative enzymes (matrix metalloproteinases).
- Extracellular ions.

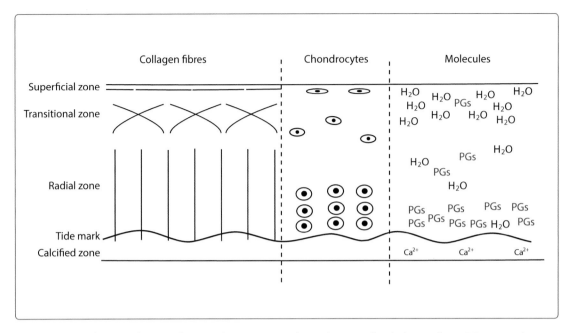

Figure 10.1 Schematic diagram showing the structure and constituents of articular cartilage. PG: proteoglycan.

Proteoglycan aggrecan, type II collagen and hyalronan account for 90% of the dry mass of articular cartilage.

Structure

Layers

The structure of articular cartilage can be divided into layers as seen on histological examination (**Figure 10.1**). The uppermost superficial layer is almost entirely collagen, with a few elongated cells. The **collagen concentration decreases** through the deeper layers, as does the **water concentration**, from 80% in the superficial layer to 65% in the deep zone. Conversely, the **proteoglycan concentration increases** with depth.

Zone 1: the **superficial /gliding zone**. This separates the cartilage from the surrounding tissue and fluid. This zone consists of a **lamina splendens**, a clear film of small collagen fibrils and a cellular layer of flattened chondrocytes one to three cells thick. The chondrocytes produce their own specific proteins and exhibit macrophage-like features, including phagocytosis and inflammatory characteristics. The superficial zone is **the thinnest layer**. It has the **highest water and collagen content** and the **lowest level of proteoglycan synthesis**. The superficial zone may also function as a barrier to the passage of large molecules from the synovial fluid. The **collagen fibres** lie parallel to the articular surface, and this tangential orientation allows the articular surface to resist shear stresses. In osteoarthritis, this zone is the first to show degenerative changes.

Zone II: the **transitional zone**. Here the fibres are arranged obliquely and the proteoglycan concentration is higher. This zone forms the transition between the shearing forces of the surface layer to compression forces in the deeper layers.

Zone III: the **radial/deep zone**. This is the largest part of the articular cartilage. The perpendicularly arranged collagen fibres distribute loads and resist compression.

The chondrocytes in zones II and III produce all the components of the extracellular matrix. The chondrocytes are spherical in shape. Although there are no intercellular junctions between chondrocytes, communities of two or more cells form chondrons. These share the same peri-cellular matrix, which differs in its composition and has a higher rate of turnover compared with the interterritorial extracellular matrix between the chondrons.

The **tidemark** is the boundary between the calcified and uncalcified cartilage made visible by histological staining. It is cell-free and represents a **calcification front** that tends to migrate towards the surface with age.

In the **calcified zone**, hydroxyapatite crystals anchor the cartilage to the subchondral bone. It forms a barrier to diffusion from blood vessels supplying the subchondral bone. **Type X collagen** is present mainly in the calcified cartilage layer.

Collagen

Collagen synthesis takes place in stages both within and outside the chondrocyte (see Chapter 8). Polypeptide chains are formed and modified following messenger ribonucleic acid (mRNA) translation within the rough endoplasmic reticulum. The signal peptide is cleaved, lysine and proline residues are hydroxylated and hydroxylysine residues are glycosylated. N-linked sugars are added to the terminal portion, and the modified polypeptide chains form **triple-helical molecules**. Disulphide bonds between and within the chains define the shape of the molecule. In the Golgi apparatus, the resultant **procollagen** is packed into secretory granules and released into the extracellular matrix via microtubules. Outside the cell, the terminal ends of procollagen uncoil and are cleaved to form **tropocollagen fibrils**. These molecules combine via the cross-linkage of lysine and hydroxylysine residues. The resulting fibrils aggregate to form **collagen fibres**. See Chapter 8 for further structural detail on collagen.

Approximately 90% of the collagen in articular cartilage is type II. The collagen fibres comprise a core of types XI and II collagen surrounded by multiple layers of type II collagen. **Type XI collagen** is thought to regulate the diameter of the fibres, which is greater in the deeper zones.

Type IX collagen is found on the surface of the fibre. It has a chondroitin sulphate side chain and may act as a link to form collagen–proteoglycan complexes and regulate type II fibril formation. The collagens in articular cartilage form a cross-linked network. These inter- and intramolecular cross-links add to the three-dimensional stability and tensile properties of the tissue. One of the functions of type IX collagen is thought to be the stabilization of the collagen II network by forming these cross-links.

Type VI collagen does not from fibres but is found in the peri-cellular region in a three-dimensional meshwork. It may help to carry some of the shear stresses and is probably involved in cell–matrix interactions. Its levels increase significantly in early osteoarthritis.

Type X collagen similarly forms a meshwork and is present in the calcified cartilage layer. It is associated with **cartilage calcification** and is produced by hypertrophied chondrocytes during endochondral ossification. It is therefore found in the physis, fracture callus, heterotopic ossification, calcifying cartilaginous tumours and osteoarthritis.

Type I collagen is not found in normal articular cartilage but is present following injury in the subsequently formed fibrocartilage.

Proteoglycans and glycosaminoglycans

Proteoglycans are responsible for most of the water content of cartilage and also provide compressive strength to cartilage. They are large **hydrophilic** molecules containing chains of **glycosaminoglycans** (GAG) (chondroitin sulphate, keratan sulphate) bound by **covalent bonds** to a **linear core of protein**. GAGs have high negative charges from attached carboxyl and sulphate groups, which attract cations and water, thus increasing the osmotic pressure in the tissue. **Aggrecan** is the predominant proteoglycan in articular cartilage. Lesser proteoglycans present include decorin, byglycan, fibromodulin, syndecan, lumican and superficial zone protein.

Aggrecan is heavily glycosylated with GAG components such as chondroitin sulphate and keratan sulphate. Aggrecan interacts with hyaluronic acid, stabilized via a link protein, to form a large (up to 50–106 molecular weight [MW]) proteoglycan aggregate (**Figure 10.2**). Influx of water is limited to approximately 40% of maximum hydration by the collagen meshwork, which physically prevents further expansion. These properties provide the compressive strength of the tissue to mechanical loading.

Degradative enzymes

The matrix metalloproteinases are classified into **collagenases, stromelysins, gelatinases and membrane-associated metalloproteinases**. These degrade collagen and proteoglycan aggregates as part of the normal turnover of the matrix constituents. Balancing this action are the proteinase inhibitors. **Tissue inhibitors of matrix metalloproteinase** (**TIMPs**) are acidic polypeptides that prevent degradation by the metalloproteinases by binding to the matrix proteins. The avascular nature of articular cartilage is maintained by TIMPs that inhibit the proteases produced by migrating vascular endothelium. TIMPs may form the basis of future drugs that inhibit the excessive expression of matrix metalloproteinases, as this may be responsible for the progression and severity of osteoarthritis.

Ions

Cartilage typically has a high **sodium** and **potassium** ion content. The sulphate residues on proteoglycans attract these cations. Extracellular calcium tends to be highly concentrated in the calcified zone. In the deep and superficial zones, calcium ions are in lower concentrations than in the plasma and are buffered by the sulphate residues.

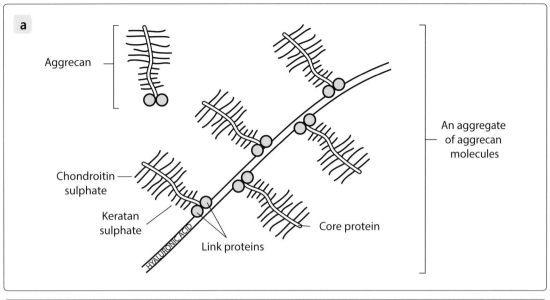

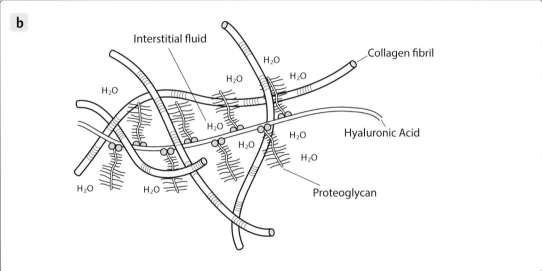

Figure 10.2 a: The aggrecan molecule is a complex of proteoglycans that all are connected to a central long chain of hyaluronic acid via link proteins. The proteoglycans in the large aggrecan complex are feather-like structures composed of a number of regularly spaced glycosaminoglycan chains, such as keratan sulphate and chondroitin sulphate, which are covalently linked to a protein core; b: molecular organization of the solid matrix of articular cartilage as a fibre reinforced composite solid matrix. The swelling pressure exerted by the proteoglycan keeps the collagen network inflated.

Glycoproteins

Sparsely distributed through the extracellular matrix, these macromolecules act as 'tissue glue', binding to various constituents of the matrix and the chondrocyte surface. Glycoproteins include **COMP**, which binds to various matrix proteins, **chondrocalcin**, a calcium-binding glycoprotein, and **laminin**, which is found in the peri-cellular matrix of chondrocytes. **Lubricin**, found in synovial fluid, is thought to act as a joint lubricant. Other glycoproteins involved with the anchorage of chondrocytes include chondroadherin, CMP, CMGP and chondronectin.

Chondrocytes

The articular chondrocyte is **derived from uncommitted mesenchymal stem cells** (MSCs). Chondroblasts proliferate during fetal development, and the majority of cartilage transforms into bone through endochondral ossification, with the growth plate and cartilaginous epiphyses persisting after birth. At skeletal maturity, the articular surface is the only remaining cartilaginous part. Articular chondrocytes and growth plate chondrocytes represent different pathways of terminal differentiation. The matrix and synovial fluid environment play extremely important roles in the maintenance of the phenotype of articular chondrocytes. Once committed to one of these pathways, the cell phenotype is not usually reversible, although if growth plate chondrocytes are positioned in an articular defect the surface layers take on the appearance of articular cartilage.

Being avascular, cell nutrition takes place via diffusion from the synovial fluid. Although the exact mechanism is poorly understood, a simple explanation is that when the joint is not under load, the cartilage (being highly hydrophilic) absorbs synovial fluid. Under load, fluid is squeezed out, and with it metabolic waste. Absence of joint loading fails to maintain adequate nutrition and therefore predisposes to degeneration.

The metabolic rate of chondrocytes is generally very low. Deeper cartilage zones contain chondrocytes with decreased rough endoplasmic reticulum and increased degenerative products (increased intraplasmic filaments). The half-life of proteoglycans is weeks to months; that of collagen is several years or possibly even longer. The extracellular matrix in the immediate vicinity of the chondrocytes or chondron may, however, have a relatively high turnover. A large proportion of chondrocyte energy utilization is via the lactic-acid pathway, even in the presence of high oxygen and glucose concentrations.

Various hormones, growth factors and cytokines influence chondrocytes. Fibroblast growth factor (FGF) stimulates adult chondrocyte deoxyribonucleic acid (DNA) synthesis. Insulin-like growth factor I (IGF-I) stimulates adult chondrocyte DNA and matrix synthesis. Parathyroid hormone (PTH) and thyroxine stimulate matrix synthesis. Abnormal production of some of these factors has been implicated in the pathogenesis of rheumatoid arthritis and osteoarthritis.

Function

The main functions of articular cartilage are **joint lubrication** (allowing movement between opposing surfaces with the minimum of friction and wear) and **shock absorption** (distributing joint loads and therefore reducing the stresses experienced). Articular cartilage has a very low coefficient of friction (0.002), 30 times smoother than most modern joint replacements. This coefficient of friction can be lowered further by fluid-film formation, elastic deformation of articular cartilage, synovial fluid and efflux of fluid from cartilage. The coefficient of friction can be increased by fibrillation of articular cartilage.

Biomechanical properties

Cartilage is ten times more effective a shock absorber than bone. Cartilage protects bone by diffusing the load. Cartilage is a **biphasic** material that is **viscoelastic** (like a water-soaked sponge). With respect to its viscoelasticity, cartilage undergoes **creep** (under constant load, it initially deforms rapidly, increasing the surface area through which to dissipate the force, followed by slow deformation until a steady state is reached) and **stress relaxation** (under constant deformation, high initial stress is followed by progressively decreasing stress to the level required to maintain the deformation). These properties occur through **macromolecular** and **water movement**. Seventy per cent of the water present is intermolecular and can move when a load or pressure gradient is applied.

Cartilage is freely **permeable to water**, but under high compressive loads water movement is hindered by the frictional drag of the macromolecules. This decreases the flow and stiffens cartilage, allowing greater resistance to higher loads. Cartilage is also **anisotropic**, having different mechanical properties depending on the direction in which it is loaded. This is due to the collagen fibre arrangements, cross-links and collagen–proteoglycan interactions.

In tension, the molecular structure of articular cartilage, the organization of collagen fibres, and the collagen fibre cross-links are altered. Cartilage is pulled apart, which increases water permeability. This in turn decreases compressive stiffness.

Lubrication (see Chapter 25)

In classical engineering terms, there are two types of lubrication: **boundary** and **fluid-film**. The ideas behind joint lubrication have been extrapolated from these, although the exact mechanisms have not been elucidated fully in humans. Each type of lubrication probably comes into play at a different point in the movement of the joint.

Boundary lubrication involves a monolayer of lubricant molecule (probably the glycoprotein lubricin) adsorbed on each surface (boundary) of the joint. This prevents direct articular contact and is most important at rest or under load. In **fluid-film lubrication**, a thin layer of fluid increases the separation of the two surfaces. The following methods are described:

- **Hydrodynamic lubrication:** the two surfaces are at an angle to each other. The viscosity in the resulting wedge of fluid separates the two surfaces.
- **Squeeze-film lubrication:** the two surfaces are parallel and move perpendicularly to each other. The viscosity of the incompressible fluid maintains the lubrication. High loads can be carried for short lengths of time. As the layer of fluid lubricant is forced out, it becomes thinner and the joint surfaces come into contact, but they are still protected by the lubricin.
- **Elastohydrodynamic lubrication:** this occurs as speed increases and is similar to squeeze film, but the yielding articular surface creates a larger surface area when compressed by the fluid. There is less dissipation of the fluid-film, and therefore the load is sustained for a longer period. This is the **predominant lubrication mechanism in synovial joints during dynamic joint function.**

Synovial joints, being non-rigid structures, exhibit modified forms of boundary and fluid-film lubrication. When movement begins, boundary lubrication is exhibited at points of close contact of the two surfaces and fluid-film elsewhere.

Two other forms of lubrication are also thought to occur between the static state with boundary lubrication and the elastohydrodynamic lubrication seen at speed:

- **Weeping or self-lubrication**: articular cartilage is variably permeable to fluid, depending on whether it is loaded. As the articular cartilage of the joint slides under compression, fluid is exuded under and in front of the leading edge of the load, enhancing lubrication. As the load decreases after maximum compression, water is once again imbibed and the articular cartilage reforms its shape.
- **Boosted lubrication**: the solvent part of the lubricant enters the articular cartilage, which leaves behind the concentrated hyaluronic acid complexes as a lubricant in 'trapped pools' of concentrated synovial fluid.

Injury and healing

Superficial injuries

Superficial lacerations (**above the tidemark**) **do not heal**. This region is completely avascular. Although peripheral chondrocytes may increase matrix synthesis and proliferate, they do not migrate actively enough into the defect to effect repair.

Deep injuries

Lacerations that extend **below the tidemark** to subchondral bone result in haematoma, fibrin clot and **activation of the inflammatory response**. This acts as a scaffold for the formation of **fibrocartilage**, produced by the **undifferentiated mesenchymal cells** that have migrated into the defect. This differs from hyaline cartilage in that it consists of disorganized bundles of type I collagen and is therefore not really suitable for repetitive load-bearing.

Infection and inflammation

Infection can be devastating to the articular surface. This can be as a direct result of the organism itself, such as the chondrocyte proteases of *Staphylococcus aureus,* or due to the host's inflammatory response. Polymorphs stimulate production of cytokines and other inflammatory products, which cause hydrolysis of collagen and proteoglycans. Destruction of cells and the release of lysosomal enzymes (e.g. collagenases, proteases, galactosidases) further injures the joint.

Osteoarthritis and cartilage

Changes to cartilage in osteoarthritis are covered in detail in Chapter 30.

Treatment

Non-operative treatment options for injured cartilage

Physiotherapy

The maintenance of motion is vital to nutrition and healing of the damaged joint. As detailed above, loading of the joint is essential in order to allow diffusion of synovial fluid and thus metabolic turnover of the cartilage. Hence, immobilization leads to cartilage atrophy, whereas physical therapy is therapeutic. Salter (1989) has shown that continuous passive movement may be beneficial in the healing of full-thickness articular defects in rabbits, although this has yet to be demonstrated in humans.

Oral visco-supplementation

Nutritional supplements, especially those advertised as being beneficial to joints, constitute a multi-million-pound industry. **Glucosamine** is an amino-monosaccharide sugar and is a naturally occurring component of the glycosaminoglycans keratan sulphate and hyaluronate. **Chondroitin** is another glycosaminoglycan. Of these, glucosamine is the only substance to have been evaluated in clinical trials and to have shown some benefit. Produced either synthetically or from shells, glucosamine is sold as glucosamine sulphate and glucosamine hydrochloride. *In vitro* studies have demonstrated the effect of glucosamine in reversing the inhibition of proteoglycan synthesis by interleukin-1 (IL-1) and suppressing the inflammatory response of neutrophils. Several randomized studies have shown the efficacy of glucosamine in knee osteoarthritis, but the methodology and outcome measures used have been criticized widely in the literature. Nonetheless, it is likely that some benefit is obtained from glucosamine comparable to analgesic therapy, and in view of the very low risk of side-effects (shellfish allergy, occasional gastrointestinal symptoms) and the low cost of glucosamine, it is worth trying. Most trials used a dose of 1500 mg/day, but there is variety in the consistency of available formulations. Currently, glucosamine and chondroitin are not NICE-recommended (see Chapter 30).

Intra-articular visco-supplementation

This aims to replace lost hyaluronan and improve the viscoelastic properties of the articular cartilage. Several products have been produced. Preparations are of relatively low MW (e.g. Hyalgan™), intermediate MW but lower than that of normal healthy synovial fluid (e.g. Orthovisc™), or cross-linked hyaluronan of high MW (e.g. Synvisc™). As with oral supplements, many of the studies showing efficacy have an element of publication bias, with poor numbers and outcome measures. Currently, intra-articular visco-supplementation is not NICE-recommended (see Chapter 30).

Operative treatment options for injured cartilage

Abrasion arthroplasty

This is essentially **cartilage repair from subchondral bone**. By turning the cartilage defect into a 'deep injury', undifferentiated MSCs proliferate in the defect when the subchondral bone plate is penetrated. They subsequently differentiate into fibrocartilage. This repair tissue initially has a moderately high proportion of proteoglycan and some type II collagen, but, as mentioned above, the proteoglycan content decreases and the disorganized collagen reverts to predominantly type I collagen. Moreover, there is usually incomplete integration of the fibrocartilaginous tissue with the adjacent normal articular cartilage, and the resultant tissue therefore is not very resistant to shear stress. However, this crude repair may still alleviate symptoms for several years.

Autograft/mosaicplasty

Full-thickness osteochondral grafts from the least weight-bearing periphery of the articular surface (superomedial margin of the femoral notch) are transplanted into the cartilage defect. This method has been found to be of most benefit in the medial compartment of the knee and of less value for patellar lesions. However, modern tissue engineering therapies appear to be superseding this form of treatment. The use of other autografts, such as a portion of the patella in the recreation of the tibial articular surface, has generally had poor results.

Allograft

Cadaveric osteochondral allografts have been used most extensively for reconstruction after resection of malignant tumours. The cartilage is usually **frozen with a cryoprotectant such as glycerol,** which prevents rupture of the cell membranes during the freezing process. Some of the chondrocytes will therefore remain viable when the tissue is thawed. The bony part of the graft acts as a scaffold for the allograft cartilage surface, which can integrate into the adjacent host bone. It is this integration that is crucial for the graft's survival, and therefore it is important to size it correctly. Any mismatch increases degradation due to excessive contact forces. Since the collagen and proteoglycan matrix makes the cells inaccessible to antibodies and T-cells, cartilage is considered an immunogenically privileged tissue. However, several reports of infection with spore-forming organisms following transplant have been published, and there is concern regarding the possibility of viral or prion transmission.

Periosteal/perichondrial mesenchymal stem cells

Periosteum and perichondrium both contain significant numbers of stem cells, which can be used to differentiate into hyaline cartilage. Rib perichondrium or periosteum can be used. The cambium layer contains the greatest number of MSCs and is positioned towards the synovial side of the defect. In the case of deep defects, the periosteum is sutured into place on top of the bone graft. The periosteum or perichondrium may differentiate into hyaline cartilage under these circumstances. Unlike abrasion arthroplasty, type II collagen and high levels of proteoglycan are seen in the repair tissue. There are no convincing reports of the efficacy of this method in clinical practice.

Chondrocytes from mesenchymal stem cells

MSCs are isolated from bone marrow using tissue culture plates. The stromal cells, including the MSCs, adhere and can then be cultured. Using periosteum, the MSCs are released from the cambium layer using an enzymatic treatment. By placing the MSCs in a three-dimensional matrix (e.g. collagen or alginate), the MSCs will differentiate into chondrocytes. These continue to proliferate when introduced into a collagen gel, which is inserted into the defect and forms hyaline cartilage. The deep part undergoes endochondral ossification, leading to a normal bone–cartilage interface. This technique is not routinely used in clinical practice.

Autologous chondrocyte implantation

Brittberg *et al.* (1994) first reported the autologous chondrocyte implantation (ACI) technique. A small amount of cartilage from a non-weight-bearing articular surface can be harvested and the cells isolated. Although the rate of chondrocyte proliferation is extremely low *in vivo*, chondrocytes can undergo many cell divisions in tissue culture, expanding the population considerably. After 4–5 weeks, the cells are suspended in a collagen gel carrier and reimplanted at a subsequent operation. A periosteal or collagen flap is sutured over the articular cartilage defect, and the cultured chondrocytes are injected beneath it. Needle biopsies have demonstrated histologically normal hyaline cartilage grown in the defect after 1–2 years. More recent techniques involve growing the cells on a collagen membrane before implantation – matrix-induced autologous chondrocyte implantation (MACI) – and suspending the cells in a three-dimensional polymer fleece or hyaluron-based scaffold, which is implanted into the defect without the need for a covering flap.

Role of growth factors

A variety of growth factors are produced by chondrocytes, including FGF, IGF-1, transforming growth factor (TGF), platelet-derived growth factor (PDGF) and bone morphogenetic proteins (BMPs). There have been limited studies into the effect of these factors on articular cartilage repair. Although promising, none of these studies has shown any overall efficacy in human trials.

TGF, IGF-1 and FGF stimulate chondrocyte proliferation. IGF-1 appears to stimulate collagen and proteoglycan production; TGF stimulates proteoglycan synthesis while suppressing type II collagen synthesis. TGF, when injected subperiosteally, leads to chondrocyte differentiation from the periosteum; unfortunately, when administered intra-articularly, TFG causes a synovitis that masks any therapeutic effect on the articular cartilage.

Intra-articular FGF has been shown to increase the amount of articular cartilage, but it enhances proteoglycan degradation and essentially weakens the overall cartilage. However, FGF injected into partial-thickness defects has been shown to stimulate filling of the defect with fibroblasts from MSCs recruited from the synovium. No differentiation to hyaline cartilage occurred.

Some success in reconstituting relatively normal-appearing hyaline cartilage has been shown with defects implanted with BMPs and also filled with a collagen gel containing liposomes of encapsulated TGF.

Viva questions

1. What is the composition of articular cartilage?
2. Draw the structure of articular cartilage.
3. What are the functions of articular cartilage? How is structure related to function?
4. What pathological processes are involved when cartilage is injured?
5. What are the different options available for treating cartilage defects?

Further reading

Bentley, G, Biant, LC, Carrington, RW, *et al*. A prospective, randomised comparison of autologous chondrocyte implantation versus mosaicplasty for osteochondral defects in the knee. *J Bone Joint Surg Br* 2003;**85**:223–30.

Brittberg, M, Lindahl, A, Nilsson, A, *et al*. Treatment of deep cartilage defects in the knee with autologous chondrocyte transplantation. *N Engl J Med* 1994;**331**:889–95.

Heinegård D, Saxne T. The role of the cartilage matrix in osteoarthritis. *Nat Rev Rheumatol* 2011;**7**(1):50–6.

Salter, RB. The biologic concept of continuous passive motion of synovial joints: the first 18 years of basic research and its clinical application. *Clin Orthop* 1989;**242**:12–25.

Ulrich-Vinther M, Maloney MD, Schwarz EM, Rosier R, O'Keefe RJ. Articular cartilage biology. *J Am Acad Orthop Surg* 2003;**11**:421–30.

11 Nerve

Mike Fox, Caroline Hing, Sam Heaton and Rolfe Birch

Introduction

The nervous system enables the body to react to environmental and physical changes. A nerve's structure and mechanism of action relate to its function and also determine how well it can recover from injury.

Structure of a nerve

Components of the nervous system

- **Central nervous system**: brain and spinal cord.
- **Peripheral nervous system**: cranial, spinal and peripheral nerves.
- **Autonomic nervous system**: sympathetic, parasympathetic and enteric systems.

The **central nervous system** (CNS) sends and processes information. The **peripheral nervous system** (PNS) relays information from the CNS to the periphery and vice versa. **Afferent** (sensory) nerve fibres transmit somatic (voluntary) and visceral information from the periphery to the brain. **Efferent** (motor) nerve fibres transmit somatic and autonomic information from the brain to the periphery.

Cells of the nervous system

The nervous system comprises two main cell types: **neurons** and **glial cells** (cells that support neurons).

Neurons specialize in sending and receiving chemically-mediated electrical signals. The functional unit of a nerve is the neuron; it has a **cell body** (perikaryon) and an **axon**. The **axolemma** (cell membrane) encloses the **axoplasm** (cytoplasm). The cell body contains all the subcellular organelles found in a typical cell but is specialized to provide high levels of protein synthesis, by having densely packed ribosomes on the rough endoplasmic reticulum. **Dendrites** are extensions of the cell body and receive signals from other neurons. Each neuron

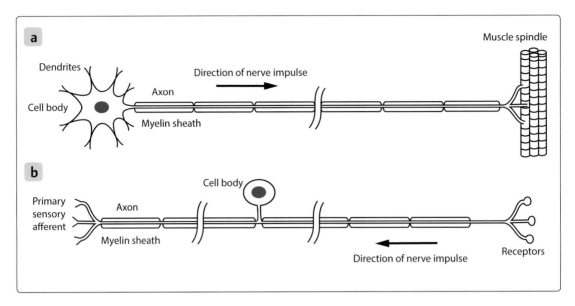

Figure 11.1 Motor (a) and sensory (b) units.

generally has a single axon arising from the cell body that typically conducts impulses away from the cell body. This may be encapsulated in a myelin sheath (**Figure 11.1**).

Glial cells fill the extracellular space that supports the neurons. They comprise **oligodendrocytes (CNS)/Schwann cells (PNS), astrocytes and microglia**. In the CNS, the myelin sheath is formed by oligodendrocytes; unlike the myelin sheaths of the PNS, the CNS myelin sheath does not possess a neurilemma. Astrocytes regulate extracellular potassium concentration, the synthesis of neurotransmitters, the removal of neurotransmitters from the synaptic cleft and the storage and transfer of metabolites from blood vessels to the neurons. Microglia are immune cells derived from monocytes and play a phagocytic role, defending the CNS from noxious stimuli while being involved in the inflammatory processes that accompany nerve repair.

Schwann cells are the glial cells that arise from the neuroectoderm and are responsible for myelination of peripheral nerves. The size of the axon determines whether it will be myelinated. Larger axons are invaginated into by a series of Schwann cells that lay down a myelin sheath in spiral layers and form a neurilemma on the outside, with each Schwann cell contributing myelin to one segment (internode) of the axon. The myelin sheath has a multilaminar structure that is high in lipids and proteins and is traversed by cytoplasmic channels that facilitate conduction. The smaller axons are arranged in bundles enveloped by Schwann cell cytoplasm with no myelin sheath.

Nodes of Ranvier are gaps between adjacent Schwann cell internodes along myelinated axons. The nodes are important in **saltatory conduction**, where the action potential jumps electrically from one node to the next. In this region, the axon diameter is reduced slightly, the diameter of the axon being inversely proportional to the length of the node of Ranvier. The concentration of sodium channels is increased in this region to facilitate saltatory conduction.

Axonal transport occurs in both an antegrade and a retrograde fashion along the axon. Axonal transport is important in maintaining the structure of nerves and the supply of neurotransmitters. Transport can occur in a fast or slow fashion and is adenosine triphosphate (ATP) energy-dependent, making it vulnerable to injury, anoxia and ischaemia. Microtubule and microfilament components are transported slowly in an antegrade direction. Neurotransmitters are also transported in an antegrade direction, but by a faster mechanism. Once the neurotransmitters have been released at the synapse, the neurotransmitter vesicles are transported in a retrograde direction for recycling by the cell body.

Nerve macrostructure

A nerve is composed of **fascicles** or **bundles** of nerve fibres (axon sheathed in myelin). The endoneurium is the connective tissue covering each nerve fibre (consisting of longitudinally arranged collagen fibres, fibroblasts and blood vessels). These are bundled together to form a fascicle that is enveloped by the **perineurium** (made of alternating layers of collagen and cell processes acting as a diffusion barrier). Finally, the **epineurium**, consisting of collagen and fibroblasts, acts as a supporting structure for the nerve fascicles grouped into a nerve trunk (**Figure 11.2**).

The proximal parts of most nerves tend to be monofascicular (containing both motor and sensory fibres) whereas more distally, they are polyfascicular (branching into individual motor and sensory subunits).

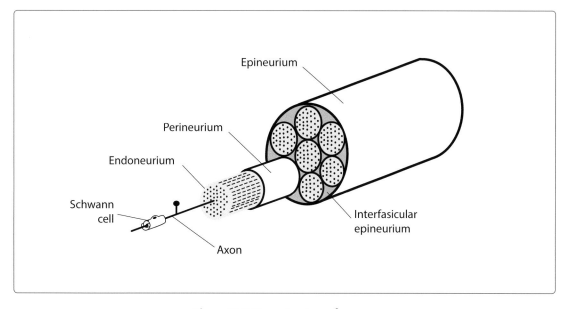

Figure 11.2 Macrostructure of a nerve.

Nerves can be classified according to their degree of myelination, diameter and speed of conduction (*Table 11.1*). Conduction is faster when axonal diameter increases and when they are myelinated.

The blood supply to nerves consists of **extrinsic** and **intrinsic plexuses**. The extrinsic vessels are arteries that enter the epineurium at sections along the nerve and form the **vasa nervorum**. They divide into epineural arterioles and form an anastomotic network found in the **paraneurium**, a layer external to the perineurium. The **intrinsic vessels** are distributed in a longitudinal fashion within the **endoneurium**. They form orientated capillaries whose endothelial cells are connected by tight junctions: the blood–nerve barrier. There are extensive connections between the extrinsic and intrinsic systems; following surgical mobilization, nerves are more dependent on the intrinsic supply although excessive tension further compromises this supply. Venules return blood to the venous system. Lymphatic drainage only occurs in the epineurium.

Action potentials

Neurons are bound by a lipoprotein cell membrane and possess a **resting membrane potential of -70 mV** due to difference in the ions inside and outside of the cell. This voltage difference is due to the **high concentration of potassium ions [K⁺]** and low concentration of sodium ions [Na⁺] and chloride ions [Cl⁻] **within the cell**. In the **extracellular space**, there is a low concentration of [K⁺] and a **high concentration of [Na⁺] and [Cl⁻]**. The different ionic concentrations in the intracellular and extracellular spaces are maintained by:

- A **lipid membrane**, which prevents the passage of water soluble ions.
- **Selectively permeable** ion channels.
- A metabolically active **Na+/K+ exchange pump**.
- **Donnan equilibrium** (irregular distribution of permeant ions across an impermeant membrane when a large impermeable organic ion is present on one side).

Table 11.1. Classification of nerves by Erlanger and Gasser

Axon Type	Myelination	Diameter (μm)	Conduction velocity (m/s)	Function
Aα	Myelinated	20	100	Efferent to skeletal muscle Afferent from muscle spindles and tendon stretch organelles
Aβ	Myelinated	10	50	Organised sensory receptors, e.g. Merkel, Pacinian, Ruffini, hair follicles
Aγ	Myelinated	5	20	Efferent to muscle spindles
Aδ	Myelinated	5	20	Fast pain (e.g. knife), crude touch, cold sensation
B	Myelinated	3	10	Pre-ganglionic autonomic
C	Unmyelinated	1	2	Post-ganglionic autonomic, slow pain (e.g. nettles), thermoreceptors, reflex responses

Cl⁻ ions diffuse out of the cell through the lipid membrane. The Na⁺/K⁺ exchange pump maintains a high concentration of K⁺ in the cell and a high concentration of Na⁺ in the extracellular space. Voltage-dependent ion channels exist for both K⁺ and Na⁺. The voltage-gated Na⁺ channel can be in a resting closed state, or an active open state following membrane depolarization, or an inactivated closed state. The voltage-gated K⁺ channels can be open when the membrane is depolarized or closed during the resting potential.

The **threshold stimulus** is the minimum stimulus intensity needed to produce an action potential. A smaller stimulus (**subthreshold**) will not produce a stimulus. However, **summation** of a number of subthreshold stimuli may be sufficient to incite a response.

Neurons are stimulated by synaptic inputs into their dendrites or by receptor potentials from sensory organs. This stimulation results in the opening of Na⁺ channels and an in rush of Na⁺ ions into the cell. The channels are dependent on oxygen and ATP. This results in **depolarization** of the membrane from its initial resting state of -70 mV due to **ionic conductance**, and the polarity across the cell membrane becomes **positive**. This also triggers the opening of more Na⁺ channels and the propagation of an action potential (nerve impulse). The Na⁺ channels remain open for 1 ms before closing. For a few milliseconds after closing, they cannot reopen (the **refractory period**), thus limiting the number of stimuli to which a nerve can respond.

Repolarization of the membrane results from the passage of K⁺ ions out of the cell through K⁺ channels. The **electrical potential falls** to below the original -70 mV resting potential due to the delay in closure of the K⁺ channels and the time taken for the Na⁺ channels to convert from an inactive to a resting state. The Na⁺/K⁺ exchange pump then restores the cell to its original resting potential (**Figure 11.3**).

The local change in potential of an area of the nerve fibre membrane compared with an adjacent area at resting potential generates a current, resulting in the **propagation** of the action potential. In myelinated fibres, the action potential cannot propagate across the myelin and instead 'jumps' (**saltatory conduction**) across the nodes of Ranvier. This increases the efficiency of the cell, resulting in fast conduction with minimum metabolic activity. Saltatory conduction is analogous to the electrical conduction of a capacitor, in contrast to the wave of chemical depolarization present in non-myelinated fibres.

Neurons communicate with each other via a **synapse**, which can be chemical or electrical. In humans, chemical synapses predominate. Synapses occur between the terminal branch of one axon and the cell body dendrites of another axon. An action potential causes the release of **neurotransmitters** from synaptic vesicles. The neurotransmitter diffuses across the synaptic cleft to the post-synaptic membrane, which it either excites (**excitatory post-synaptic potentials**) or inhibits (**inhibitory post-synaptic potentials**). Examples of neurotransmitters include **acetylcholine** (pre-ganglionic synapses, parasympathetic post-ganglionic synapses, sympathetic efferent to sweat glands, somatic efferent synapses), **adrenaline** (sympathetic post-ganglionic synapses), **noradrenaline** (sympathetic post-ganglionic synapses), **serotonin** and **histamine**.

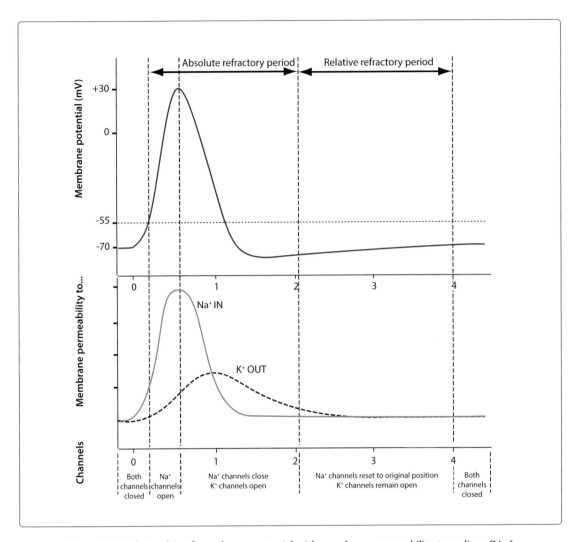

Figure 11.3 Relationship of membrane potential with membrane permeability to sodium (Na⁺) and potassium (K⁺).

Function of nerves

The CNS consists of the brain and spinal cord, which terminates at the level of the first lumbar vertebra. The PNS consists of **12 pairs** of **cranial** nerves and **31 pairs** of **spinal** nerves.

Peripheral nervous system

The spinal nerves divide close to the spinal cord, forming a **sensory dorsal root** and a **motor ventral root**. The cell body of the sensory nerve is situated in the dorsal root ganglion. The motor nerve's cell body is situated in the spinal cord (**Figure 11.4**).

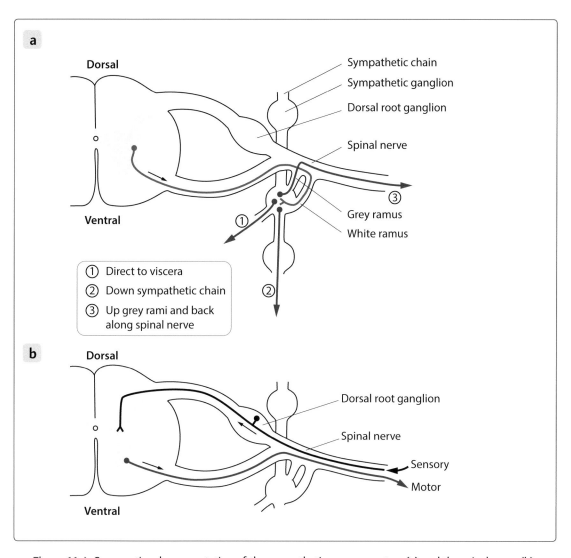

Figure 11.4 Cross sectional representation of the sympathetic nervous system (a) and the spinal nerve (b).

The **sensory** (afferent) nervous system relays impulses from superficial and deep sensory receptors. There is a functional specificity of nerve fibres and their organelles. Superficial sensory receptors can be divided further into **mechanoreceptors, thermoreceptors and nociceptors**.

Mechanoreceptors in and below human skin are fast myelinated Aβ fibres and include Merkel cells (slowly adapting), Meissner's corpuscles (rapidly adapting mechanical sensitivity), Ruffini's corpuscles (deep lying and important in skin creases), Pacinian corpuscles (rapidly adapting deep receptors) and hair follicle receptors.

Thermoreceptors are of two types – **cooling receptors** and **warming receptors**. Warming receptors are unmyelinated C fibres (low velocity) and are stimulated by a rise in temperature, which increases their action potential discharge rate. Cooling receptors include both C and Aδ (faster velocity) fibres and their firing increases during cold and decreases during warmth.

Nociceptors (pain receptors) are found in virtually every organ (except the brain). Their activity leads to the perception of pain and tissue injury. They have a high threshold for activation and often respond to more than one energy form (e.g. mechanical, thermal, mechanothermal) so are termed **polymodal** receptors. Myelinated fast Aδ and unmyelinated slow C fibres innervate these receptors.

Deep sensation from muscles, ligaments, tendons and joints occurs via free nerve endings and receptors, such as the following:

- **Muscle spindles**: consist of intrafusal nuclear bag fibres and nuclear chain fibres within the muscle itself. Innervated by myelinated afferent sensory Aα fibres and efferent motor Aγ fibres.
- **Golgi tendon organs:** activated by stretch and important in proprioception. They sense maintained tension in muscle and send impulses to the cerebellum and the cortex. Located at musculocutaneous junctions, they consist of small bundles of tendon fibres enclosed in a capsule of concentric cytoplasmic sheets. The capsule is pierced by Aα nerve fibres that divide and wrap around the tendon fasciculi. They are slowly adapting and the firing rate is proportionate to tension. They play a crucial part in the inverse stretch reflex during the application of acute traction in fracture reduction, whereby a prolonged constant stretch leads to relaxation of muscle contraction, allowing manipulation of the displaced fracture fragments.
- **Paciniform receptors**: lamellated receptors. Smaller than Pacinian corpuscles. Rapidly adapting low-threshold mechanoreceptors found in joint capsules. Supplied by myelinated Aα afferent fibres.

In the **motor system**, transmission of impulses to the muscle is via the **neuromuscular junction/motor end plate**. The two components making up the end plate are neural and muscular, separated by about 30 nm. There are two types of neural ending – the **extrafusal Aα (en plaque)** ending, which transmits to all parts of the muscle fibre, and the **intrafusal Aδ (plate)** ending, which excites the fibre at several specific points.

Autonomic nervous system

The autonomic nervous system can be divided into the **sympathetic** and **parasympathetic** systems. It comprises both central and peripheral components and forms the visceral part of the nervous system. The visceral and somatic afferent pathways are similar, with neurons from the periphery passing without interruption through autonomic ganglia or plexuses before accompanying somatic afferents in the dorsal spinal roots to the CNS. Unlike the somatic counterpart, the visceral efferent pathways comprise multiple pre-ganglionic and post-ganglionic neurons with corresponding synapses. This facilitates the relay of many autonomic effects.

The **sympathetic system** controls sweating, vasoconstriction, contraction of erector pilae, sphincteric contraction, bronchial dilation, papillary dilation, reduction of gut motility and cardiac stimulation. The sympathetic nervous system consists of **pre-ganglionic myelinated efferent axons** from the grey matter of the first thoracic to second lumbar levels of the spinal cord. The axons emerge from the spinal cord through the ventral spinal roots, before passing via the **white rami communicantes** to synapse in the para-vertebral or axial ganglia. The ganglia function as relay stations, where axons traverse or synapse with other axons, allowing amplification and dissemination of signals. The ganglia consist of a connective tissue capsule surrounding groups of neurons, fibroblasts, satellite cells and capillaries. Post-ganglionic neurons leave the ganglia and reach their target in one of several ways:

- Pass direct to the viscera.
- Pass direct to adjacent blood vessels.
- Pass via the grey rami communicantes, the axons return to their originating spinal nerve and on to blood vessels, erector pilae and sweat glands.
- Pass along the sympathetic trunk to another level.

The functional difference between white and grey rami communicantes is illustrated by **Horner's syndrome**. Interruption of the white rami communicans of the cervicothoracic ganglion interrupts the pre-ganglionic fibre pathways to the superior cervical ganglion, which supplies post-ganglionic fibres to muscles of the eyelid, dilator pupillae and secretory glands. Hence, injury to the white ramus causes ptosis, meiosis, enophthalmos and loss of sweating – Horner's syndrome. Interruption of the grey rami communicans at this level sympathectomizes the limb alone and does not cause Horner syndrome, as the axons have already synapsed in the cervicothoracic ganglion.

The **parasympathetic** nervous system consists of efferent myelinated pre-ganglionic fibres from nuclei in the brain (via the **oculomotor, facial, glossopharyngeal, vagus** and **accessory nerves**) and **second to fourth sacral spinal nerves.** The peripheral ganglia of the parasympathetic system include the cranial ganglia (**ciliary, pterygopalatine, submandibular** and **otic**), which are efferent. Afferent and post-ganglionic parasympathetic fibres also pass through these ganglia but do not synapse within them. The post-ganglionic parasympathetic non-myelinated axons synapse close to their target organs. The parasympathetic nervous system has an inhibitory effect on the heart (as well as causing dilation of blood vessels), bladder and bowel.

Nerve injury and repair

Aetiology of nerve injury
- Physical: traction, trauma, injection, thermal.
- Inflammation.
- Infection.
- Ischaemia.
- Pharmacological.
- Tumour.
- Systemic disease.
- Iatrogenic.

The mechanism of nerve injury includes:

- Open/closed injuries.
- Acute/chronic injuries.
- Single/continuing/repeated injuries.
- Whole/part of a nerve.
- Depth of the lesion.
- Nerve state (healthy/diseased).

Nerve injury has been classified by **Seddon** (1943), **Sunderland** (1951) and **Thomas and Ochoa** (1964) (*Table 11.2*). Sunderland's classification is based on an anatomical description of the lesion, rendering it a retrospective diagnosis with less clinical relevance than Seddon's or Thomas and Ochoa's classification systems. Thomas and Ochoa's classification system divides injuries into those resulting in neuronal degeneration and those that do not. This has been expanded further by **Birch and Bonney** (1998) into **injuries with no block to conduction** and **those leading to a conduction block**. Birch and Bonney's classification has the most direct relevance to clinical practice and prognosis.

Table 11.2. Classification of nerve injuries

Classification system Seddon	↓Amplitude proximal,	Classification system Thomas and Ochao, Birch and Bonney	Pathology	Potential for recovery
Neurapraxia	Normal	Transient conduction block (non-degenerative)	Anoxia with recoverable disturbance of membrane potentials at molecular level	Complete
Neurapraxia	I	Prolonged conduction block (non-degenerative)	Distortion of myelin sheath	Complete
Axonotmesis	II	Degenerative (favourable prognosis)	Axonal disruption; basal lamina, endoneurium and perineurium intact	Regeneration restores full function
Axonotmesis	III	Degenerative (intermediate)	Axonal disruption; basal lamina and endoneurium damaged	Dependent on degree of endoneurial scarring
Axonotmesis	IV	Degenerative (unfavourable prognosis)	Axonal disruption; endoneurium and perineurium damaged; epineurium intact	None without surgical intervention
Neuronotmesis	V	Degenerative (unfavourable prognosis)	Nerve completely transected	None without surgical intervention

The degree of nerve injury affects the outcome. A **neurapraxia** comprises a **transient concussion or crushing of the nerve**. There is **no Wallerian degeneration** (see below), but instead there is a block to flow of nerve impulses, with consequent interruption of physical function. A neurapraxia has a favourable outcome, provided the source of the injury is removed. **Axonotmesis** and **neuronotmesis** have less favourable outcomes as they are degenerative lesions.

Distinguishing between degenerative and non-degenerative lesions on clinical grounds is therefore possible. A **degenerative lesion** manifests as a **progressive loss of all peripheral function**. This includes peripheral autonomic function (sudomotor and vasomotor) due to interruption of post-ganglionic sympathetic fibres. A **non-degenerative lesion** comprises a **block of nerve transmission preserving some elements of peripheral function**, such as the sympathetic fibres and deep-pressure sensation.

The duration of injury also affects the type of nerve lesion sustained and its outcome. With the example of the radial nerve trapped within a fracture of the humeral shaft, if the nerve is not freed, the lesion to the radial nerve progresses rapidly from one of simple conduction block to prolonged conduction block and ultimately to what is effectively neuronotmesis.

Nerve fibres react differently to injury. A clinical example is the effect of a tourniquet left on a limb, with the severity of symptoms and potential recovery related to the duration of the tourniquet. A transient ischaemia (causing neurapraxia) results in a loss of superficial sensibility, followed by pain and finally a loss of motor power. This is due to the initial effect on large myelinated fibres followed by C fibres, with little effect on autonomic fibres, reflected in the preservation of pilomotor and vasomotor function.

Neurapraxia involves a local conduction block. The nerve and axon are in continuity, and segmental demyelination is the only histological finding. Full recovery is likely with this degree of nerve injury, which is a non-degenerative non-progressive lesion resulting in a conduction block only. Pure neurapraxia is rare in clinical practice and should not be diagnosed in the presence of complete palsy, Tinel sign, neuropathic pain, sympathetic paralysis or progressive symptoms when an open wound lies over the course of a nerve. In such cases, a working diagnosis of neuronotmesis or axonotmesis (degenerative lesions) should be made. However, distinguishing between a degenerative lesion capable of recovery with a favourable prognosis (axonotmesis) from a degenerative lesion of unfavourable prognosis (neuronotmesis) is not possible on clinical grounds alone.

More severe injuries with axonal damage or interruption cause a degenerative type of lesion, first described by Waller (1850) as **Wallerian degeneration**. Waller's work on the hypoglossal nerve of the frog after transection showed that distal degeneration of the nerve axon occurred, with later regeneration of neural tissue from the proximal stump.

Degenerative lesions correspond to axonotmesis or neuronotmesis (Sunderland second-, third-, fourth- and fifth-degree injury). With a **second-degree Sunderland injury** (axonotmesis), the axon is disrupted, but the endoneurium and perineurium remain intact. Wallerian degeneration occurs distal to the site of injury, but the Schwann cells around the distal segment of the injured axon remain intact and the regenerating axon follows its normal course to its normal target. Regeneration occurs at a rate of 1 mm/day and complete recovery is possible.

In **neuronotmesis**, the connective tissue envelopes of the nerve are interrupted and above all the basal lamina is transected or ruptured. Recovery, if any, is poor. Only repair of the nerve offers any chance of useful recovery. The Sunderland third, fourth and fifth degrees indicate deepening injury to the connective tissue envelope. Third- and fourth-degree lesions are seen in long traction injuries without complete rupture. Fifth degree represents complete loss of continuity in all elements of the nerve and is the most severe lesion.

Proximal to the sectioned nerve, the axon atrophies proximally, the cell body dendrites retract and the axon distal to the site of injury degenerates. The cell body's role changes from that of neurotransmission to the production of components for nerve regeneration. The cell nucleus migrates to the periphery of the cell body and chromatolysis occurs. The cell volume increases and production of ribonucleic acid (RNA) and regenerative enzymes also increase.

Distal to the site of injury, the myelin sheath degenerates, a haematoma forms and macrophages are stimulated to remove the axonal debris. Although the endoneurium and basement membrane may be intact, the neural tube will collapse once the myelin and axonal debris have been phagocytosed. Schwann cells and macrophages eventually replace the neural tube. Next, Schwann cells start to proliferate and migrate, forming columns (bands of Bungner). The mitotic activity of the Schwann cell increases, and the cell starts to produce growth factors as its phenotype changes and it becomes non-myelinating. Myelination occurs at a later stage in the regeneration process.

The axon proximal to the site of injury forms multiple axon sprouts with a **growth cone** situated at the tip of each sprout. **Filopodia** in the growth cone use **contact guidance** for **fibronectin** and **laminin** in the Schwann cell basement lamina to facilitate regeneration. Regeneration of axons can be followed by the presence of an **advancing Tinel sign**.

If the axon does not regenerate, permanent changes occur to the target organs. This is a time-dependent phenomenon, with the motor end plates the first to disappear after 3 months, followed by the muscle spindles and cutaneous sensory organs.

Factors determining prognosis following nerve injury include the following:

- **Violence of injury**: high-energy injuries have worse prognosis. A cleanly divided nerve repaired accurately has a better prognosis than a repaired nerve following a violent traction injury because of the extensive damage to nerve, connective tissue and bone.
- **Delay between injury and repair**: there is strong evidence that very early surgery (grafting or repair) promotes target reinnervation, nerve regeneration and neuromuscular function following axonotomy.
- **Age**: there is generally a better prognosis in younger patients due to the plasticity of the developing nervous system, although the immature nervous system is also more vulnerable to injury.
- **Gap between nerve ends**: the larger the gap, the worse the prognosis.
- **Level of injury**: repairs of nerve injuries at a distal level (e.g. posterior interosseous nerve) have a better prognosis than those at a more proximal level (e.g. radial nerve in the axilla).
- **Condition of nerve ends**: a tidy knife wound has a better prognosis than an untidy crush injury.

- **Association with arterial/bony injury**: nerve injuries associated with injury to bone or major vessels at the same level have a worse prognosis.
- **Type of nerve**: nerves that innervate one or two muscles (e.g. accessory and musculocutaneous nerves) have a better prognosis than those with mixed cutaneous and muscle innervation (e.g. median nerve). Some nerves (e.g. superficial radial nerve) have a poor prognosis following injury because of poor sensory recovery, often complicated by pain.

The **type of neuropathic pain following nerve injury** can aid in the diagnosis of nerve injury and can be divided into the following (*Table 11.3*):

- **Post-traumatic neuralgia**: pain after nerve injury with no sympathetic involvement. Pain is spontaneous but may be worsened by physical stimulus. Pain is expressed within the territory of the nerve. Treatment is to repair the nerve but outcome may be poor, e.g. following repair of the superficial radial nerve.
- **Neurostenalgia**: pain caused by persistent nerve compression/distortion/ischaemia of a nerve that is anatomically intact. Pain is severe and usually confined to the territory of the nerve. It indicates that the nerve is still subject to a damaging lesion. Examples include compression of the sciatic nerve from expanding haematoma and entrapment of the radial nerve within a humeral shaft fracture. Treatment of the cause carries a good prognosis, with early relief from pain and full recovery of the nerve.
- **Causalgia/chronic regional pain syndrome (type 2)**: burning pain with allodynia, hyperpathia, disturbance of skin colour, altered temperature and sweating. This is a rare but severe injury, often seen with partial division of a nerve. The pain is intense and extends beyond the territory of the damaged nerve. Sympathetic involvement is characteristic. Examples include penetrating missile injury to the root of the upper or lower limb. Repair of the nerve carries a good prognosis, as does repair of the commonly associated vascular injury such as false aneurysm or arteriovenous fistula.
- **Central pain**: caused by root avulsions. Two types of pain are described: a constant crushing or burning pain felt within the anaesthetic part, and a sharp shooting pain within the dermatome of the affected nerve.

Table 11.3. Terms used to describe patient symptoms with nerve injuries

Paraesthesia	Spontaneous abnormal sensation
Dysaesthesia	Unpleasant spontaneous normal sensation
Allodynia	Pain from stimulation that does not normally cause pain
Hyperalgesia	Increased response to a stimulus that is normally painful
Hypersensitivity	Over-reaction sensitivity of regeneration
Hyperpathia	Deep-seated, poorly localized, fiery pain radiating throughout the limb that is induced by palpation of the muscles

Nerve conduction studies

Diagnosis of nerve injury relies primarily on clinical examination but can be supplemented by **nerve conduction studies** (NCS) and **electromyography** (EMG) to document focal or continuous abnormalities in the length of the mixed, motor or sensory nerve and also to help determine the pathological processes responsible.

NCS involve the application of depolarizing electrical pulses to the skin over a peripheral nerve producing a propagated **nerve action potential** (NAP) at different points in the same nerve and a **compound muscle action potential** (CMAP) in the muscle fibres supplied by that nerve. These action potentials can then be recorded with **surface or needle electrodes**. **Surface electrodes** use stimulators placed on the skin to give information about the whole of the muscle, while **needle electrodes** are placed close to the nerve or its root and are useful for deep lying muscles and when severe wasting has occurred.

Measurements of **latency, amplitude** and **conduction velocity** are made:

- **Latency**: the time between onset of the stimulus and the response in milliseconds (ms).
- **Amplitude**: the size of the response in microvolts (μV) or millivolts (mV).
- **Velocity**: distance between the stimulating and recording electrodes divided by the time, measured in metres per second (m/s).

The amplitude of the response indicates the **quantity** of axons contributing to the action potential. The latency and velocity indicate the **quality** of conduction along the axons.

Motor nerve conduction studies. These are performed by electrical stimulation of a nerve and recording the **motor unit action potential** (MUAP) from the muscle supplied by that nerve. Hence, the **amplitude** of the MUAP indicates the number of functioning motor units. The **latency** of the MUAP records the time taken from motor nerve stimulation to muscle response and includes synaptic transmission and muscle depolarization. The **conduction velocity** is calculated by stimulating the motor nerve at two different sites. The distance between the distal stimulation site and the recording electrode is subtracted from the distance between the proximal stimulation site and the recording electrode. This distance is then divided by the distal latency subtracted from the proximal latency to give velocity for the motor nerve. CMAP is a sum of the MUAPS of all the motor units in the muscle and reproducible values are only possible when supramaximal levels of stimulating current or voltage are used.

Sensory nerve conduction studies. Sensory nerve action potentials (SNAP) are measured by electrically stimulating sensory fibres and recording the NAP at a separate point further along that nerve. The stimulus must again be supramaximal. The recording electrode can be proximal to the stimulation (**orthodromic**/normal direction) or distal to the stimulation (**antidromic**/reverse of normal direction). Different laboratories prefer different directions for different nerves. Amplitude (μV) and latency (ms) can be measured directly, and velocity (m/s) is calculated by dividing the distance between the electrodes by the latency (**Figure 11.5**).

CNAPs are usually measured antidromically (distal to proximal) from mixed sensory and motor nerves, with the recording electrode situated proximal to the stimulating electrode. The CNAP has larger amplitude than the SNAP and thus may be easier to record.

The amplitude and conduction velocity along nerves vary according to several factors:

- Upper limb nerves conduct faster than lower limb nerves (50 m/s upper limb, 40 m/s lower limb).
- Conduction is faster proximally along a nerve.
- Certain nerves conduct faster than others.
- There is a reduction in velocity at lower temperatures (reduced by 1 m/s per 1°C temperature fall of skin temperature).
- Conduction velocity is related to myelination, with slower velocities in very old and very young people.

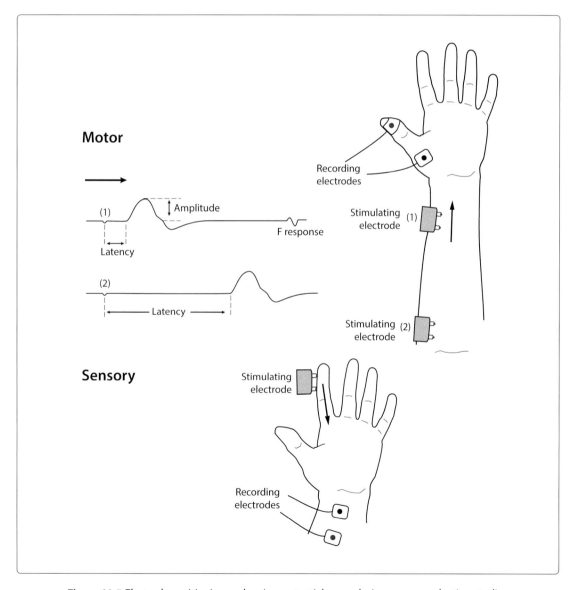

Figure 11.5 Electrode positioning and action potentials seen during nerve conduction studies.

In contrast to distal NCS, nerve conduction in the most proximal segments of the nerve is difficult to measure due to anatomical constraints; in this situation, late responses such as the **F response (wave)** and the **H reflex** are measured. These are low-amplitude responses with long latencies, including conduction in the proximal and distal sections of a nerve.

The **F response/wave** (F for foot where they were first described) shows late motor response and tests conduction of motor axons proximal to the stimulation site (the distal part of the impulse gives rise to the CMAP). Part of the impulse conducts proximally to the anterior horn cells depolarizing the axon hillock, causing it to backfire. This leads to an additional muscle depolarization that does not cross any synapses and can be thought of as an 'echo'. It is **useful in detecting early proximal nerve lesions**. A prolonged F response latency with normal peripheral motor nerve conduction would imply slowing over proximal motor fibres at the plexus or root level, **useful for assessing if nerve roots are intact in brachial plexus injuries**. The F response may be abnormal immediately after nerve root injury, even when the EMG is normal. However, multiple roots innervate muscle, and so an abnormal F response is present only with multiple severe motor root compromise, e.g. Guillaine–Barré syndrome, and extensive proximal neuropathies such as plexopathies.

The **H reflex** is the electrophysiological equivalent of a **deep tendon reflex**. It is elicited by a submaximal stimulation of Aα afferent fibres from muscle stretch receptors that enter the dorsal horn and synapse with alpha motor neurons, resulting in a motor response on completion of the monosynaptic reflex arc (apart from in the soleus muscle). The H reflex can be difficult to record, which limits its applicability. It is absent or delayed in polyneuropathies and radiculopathies, but it may also be absent in patients over 60 years of age.

Somatosensory evoked potentials (SSEP) can also be used to **investigate proximal lesions** and for **spinal cord monitoring**. Surface electrodes are used to stimulate a mixed nerve. The resultant evoked potential from the CNS can be recorded at a specific site such as Erb's point in the supraclavicular fossa or more proximally, from the skin overlying the cervical vertebrae and from the scalp overlying the sensory cortex. The pattern of abnormality may be used to diagnose the level of injury.

One of the most common examples of the application of NCS is for suspected carpal tunnel syndrome (CTS). Motor studies consist of a **stimulating electrode** placed over the median nerve proximal to the carpal tunnel; a **recording electrode** placed over a muscle in the hand supplied by the median nerve (abductor pollicis brevis, APB); an **indifference electrode** placed a few centimetres away; and a **ground electrode** placed over an inactive muscle. The stimulus is turned on until a threshold CNAP is recorded, and the current is then increased to supramaximal to ensure that all the motor units are activated.

In CTS, sensory latency studies are more sensitive than motor studies and are included for completeness. Routine testing for CTS also includes stimulation of the ulnar or radial nerve for comparison. In severe cases of CTS, the sensory potentials may be absent, and motor studies are then essential to demonstrate delayed conduction. In general, NCS are abnormal in 60% of patients with CTS. Indications for surgery based on NCS include prolonged distal motor latency, denervation of the APB and absence of a median digital SNAP. Normative data for NCS of the median and ulnar nerves are shown in *Table 11.4*.

Table 11.4 Normative data for common nerve-conduction studies in the upper limb

Nerve	F wave (ms)	Distal latency (ms)	Amplitude	Velocity (m/s)
Median (motor conduction)	‹32	‹4	›5 mV	›50
Median (sensory action potential)			›5 µV	›50
Ulnar (motor conduction)	‹32	‹3	›5 mV	›50
Ulnar (sensory action potential)			›5 µV	›50

EMG involves insertion of a needle electrode into a muscle and then recording the resting electrical activity and the activity after voluntary contraction. Under normal conditions when the muscle is at rest, electrical activity is minimal. When the muscle contracts, the needle records the MUAP, which represents the sum of all of the activity in the muscle fibres innervated by a particular motor unit. Abnormalities shown by EMG include abnormal recruitment patterns (neuropathic where there is axon loss and myopathic with diseased muscle) and spontaneous activity.

The timing of NCS and EMG affects the results obtained, reflecting the degree of injury and the extent of recovery. The patterns, with respect to nerve injury, are shown in *Table 11.5.*

Table 11.5 Nerve conduction and electromyographic (EMG) changes seen with varying degrees of nerve injury

Injury	SNAP / CNAP	Conduction velocity	EMG
Conduction block (neurapraxia)	↓ Amplitude proximal, normal	Conduction block at injury site / Preserved below level of the injury	No/sparse fibrillations / MUAP firing at rapid rates / Reduced interference pattern
Degenerative lesion, favourable prognosis (axonotmesis)	Absent ↓	Absent / Normal if present	Fibrillations / ↓ interference pattern / ↑ firing rate of MUAP
Degenerative lesion, unfavourable prognosis (neuronotmesis)	Absent	Absent	Fibrillations / No voluntary MUAP

MUAP: motor unit action potential.

Summary

An understanding of the anatomy and physiology of nerves is important in the diagnosis of nerve injury, prediction of resultant recovery and performing a repair if necessary.

Viva questions

1. Draw a cross-section of a nerve. Describe its structure and how this may vary along its course.

2. Classify nerve injuries. What does 'axonotmesis' mean? What is the mode of degeneration? What affects speed of recovery? What is the value of the Tinel sign?

3. What is the pathology of carpal tunnel syndrome?

4. Interpret a nerve conduction study.

5. What are the F wave and the H reflex? What is their clinical significance?

Further reading

Birch R. *Peripheral Nerve Injuries: A Clinical Guide*. Springer, 2013.

Maggi, SP, Lowe, JB, Mackinnon, SE. Pathophysiology of nerve injury. *Clin Plastic Surg* 2003;**30**(109):26.

Mallik A, Weir AI. Nerve conduction studies: essentials and pitfalls in practice *J Neurol Neurosurg Psychiatry* 2005;**76**:ii23–ii31.

12 Skeletal Muscle

Mike Fox, Steve Key and Simon Lambert

Structure

Skeletal muscle cells are of mesodermal origin. Mature cells are known as **myotubes** or **muscle fibres**. They are differentiated multinucleated cells formed by cytoplasmic fusion of immature mononucleated myoblasts. In muscle growth, these mononucleated precursor cells also fuse to the myotubes, adding to both the ends and the side of the cell. Muscle fibres vary in size and length between the sexes and between muscle groups. Individual fibres span the full length of the muscle they form. Fibres in muscles that have a precision requirement, such as the small muscles of the hand, tend to be smaller than in power muscles, such as the quadriceps, reflecting their contractile protein content. The fibre size is also related intimately to the innervation of the muscle, further illustrating the link between fibre size and function. Muscle fibres are bounded by a plasma membrane, the **sarcolemma**, and have a cytoplasm termed the **sarcoplasm**.

All cells have genes coding for contractile proteins. In non-muscle cells, these proteins have a role in cell motility and cytoskeletal adaptation. In skeletal muscle cells, contractile proteins are present in great numbers, forming around 80% of the cell volume; they are arranged in highly organized **thick** and **thin filaments** that are grouped into multiple longitudinally orientated **myofibrils** within each fibre, with the cell nuclei marginalized. By convention, muscle fibres are termed mature when nuclear marginalization is seen. Cell nuclei are congregated particularly densely at the neuromuscular junction.

Many muscle fibres grouped together are termed **fascicles** (**Figure 12.1a**). In turn, groupings of fascicles give structure to the muscle itself. The fascicle is the smallest unit of structure visible to the naked eye. It is the ability of the fascicle to contract that determines the character of the muscle.

In muscle, support cells and connective tissue run between fibres. **Endomysium** surrounds individual fibres, **perimysium** encloses the fascicles and **epimysium** surrounds the muscle in its entirety. These connective tissues are composed primarily of collagen types I, III, IV and V, and form a continuous membrane around and within the muscle belly.

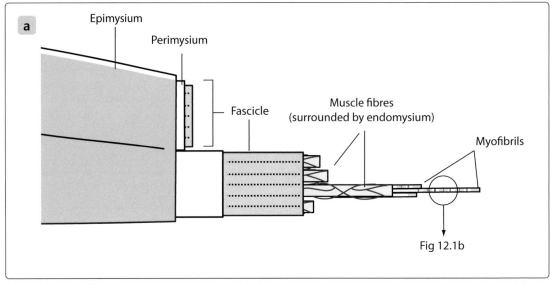

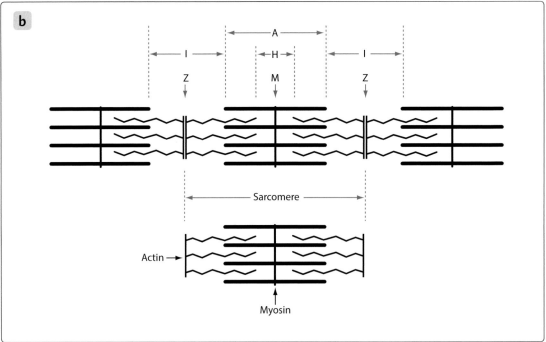

Figure 12.1 Structure and microscopic appearance of skeletal muscle.

Ultra-structure

The major contractile proteins in skeletal muscle are **actin** and **myosin**. The grouped functional unit of these filaments is termed the myofibril. Myofibrils are longitudinally segmented into functional contractile units called sarcomeres (**Figure 12.1b**), which are visible under electron microscopy. Sarcomeres are 2–2.5 μm in length and 1 μm in diameter when not contracted, and are connected longitudinally throughout the length of each myofibril. They are the fundamental contractile units whose length vary with muscle activity, but also show variation along the length of the myofibril. Sarcomeres in the myotendinous junction tend to be shorter. This may have a pretensioning or protective role.

The striations visible on either light or electron microscopy correspond to the contractile protein components:

- **Myosin related**
  - **A-bands** represent the myosin filaments (**anisotropic** on light microscopy).
  - **H-bands** correspond to the central myosin filament segment where there are no interdigitating actin filaments.
  - **M-lines** represent the connections between adjacent **myosin** filaments in their central region. These are termed the **M-band proteins**.
- **Actin related**
  - **I-bands** represent actin filaments in adjacent sarcomeres where there is no overlap with myosin filaments (**isotropic** on light microscopy).
  - **Z-discs** represent the attachment between adjacent sarcomeres within the fibril, and anchor the actin at the end of each sarcomere (from Zwischen = between [German]).

The arrangement of actin and myosin filaments is that of a hexagonal lattice in the centre of the sarcomere, i.e. each myosin filament is bounded by six actin filaments. This hexagonal arrangement becomes squarer towards the end of each sarcomere, i.e. at the Z-discs.

Other important proteins have a role in maintaining the structure of the sarcolemma, such as dystrophin (absent in Duchenne's muscular dystrophy). As a group, these proteins are termed **structural proteins**, as they maintain the overall architecture of the sarcomere during contraction.

Contractile proteins

Actin

Actin is a globular protein (molecular weight 42,000) that is a chief constituent of the **thin filaments** of the sarcomere (**Figure 12.2**). Other proteins that constitute the thin filament are **tropomyosin** and **troponin** subunits (troponin C, troponin T, troponin I).

Tropomyosin extends across seven actin subunits and blocks the binding sites of the myosin head until unblocked by calcium binding to the troponin C subunit. The activated troponin C subunit counteracts the inhibitory effect of the troponin I subunit. Troponin T assists troponin C binding to tropomyosin.

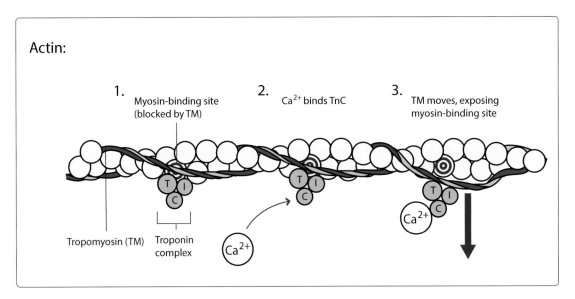

Actin:

1.
Myosin-binding site
(blocked by TM)

2.
Ca²⁺ binds TnC

3.
TM moves, exposing
myosin-binding site

Tropomyosin (TM)   Troponin
complex

Figure 12.2 Diagram of actin (thin) filament and the effect of calcium to expose binding site (see later). Ca²⁺: calcium; TM: tropomysin; TnC: troponin C.

Myosin

Myosin molecules have six distinct subunits: two heavy chains and four light chains. The light chains are of uncertain function in humans. The heavy chains have distinctive parts; one part articulates with actin filaments, the **S1 segment** or **globular head** forming the **cross-bridge**; the other part, the **S2 segment**, forms the **flexible neck**, which moves to allow articulation of the S1 head segment. The myosin molecules form the **thick filaments** (**Figure 12.3**).

Muscle cell membranes

Sarcoplasmic reticulum

Surrounding each myofibril is an intracytoplasmic membranous sac called the sarcoplasmic reticulum (**Figure 12.4**). This membrane serves as a repository for calcium, which is released to stimulate contraction. It forms terminal cisternae where it is adjacent to the transverse (T)-tubules. **Ryanodine receptors** on the terminal cisternae are the calcium channels that are opened by mechanical conformational change through their connection to T-tubule membrane proteins.

T-tubules

The sarcolemma of each muscle fibre gives off multiple invaginations at the junctions of the A- and I-bands. These T-tubules span the diameter of the muscle fibre, passing between the fibrils to carry the depolarization of the surface membrane deep inside the cell (**Figure 12.4**). Voltage-sensitive membrane proteins in the T-tubule, known as **modified dihydropyridine**

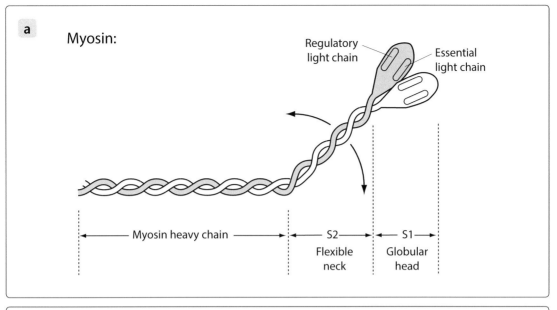

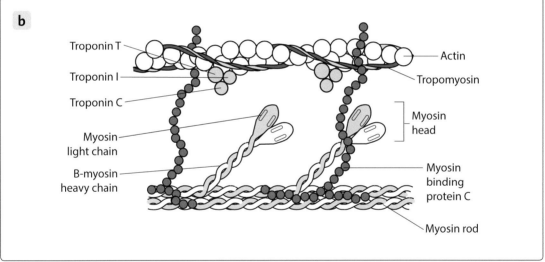

Figure 12.3 a Structure of the myosin (thick) filament; b: overview of the structures involved in cross bridging in skeletal muscle filaments

receptors, are mechanically coupled with **ryanodine receptors** of the sarcoplasmic reticulum. Depolarization of the T-tubule membrane causes a conformational change in these voltage-sensitive channels that, through its mechanical connection, opens the ryanodine receptor channel of the sarcoplasmic reticulum to cause calcium release and initiate contraction: the process of **excitation–contraction coupling**.

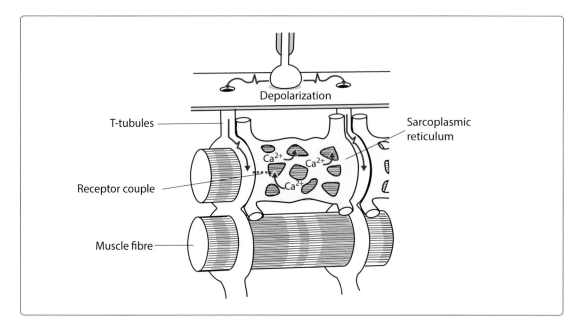

Figure 12.4 Surface depolarization flows down T-tubules, in turn affecting voltage sensitive channels that cause calcium to be released into the sarcomere.

Vascular supply of muscle

In mammalian muscles, vascular architecture follows a relatively constant pattern. A main, rapidly branching artery enters the muscle and creates a series of arcades. As in peripheral nerve, from these arcades, arterioles penetrate the sheath surrounding the fascicle. In muscle this is the perimysium. The arterioles enter obliquely or at right angles to the muscle fibres and then run parallel. The terminal capillaries are associated with muscle fibre nuclei.

Attachments of skeletal muscle

The contractile activity of the myofibrils must be transmitted to the bone for the muscle to act. The Z-discs of peripheral myofibrils are connected to the sarcolemma by a protein matrix, while at the ends of the cell the actin is directly inserted into a dense sarcolemma-bound protein matrix, rather than Z-discs. The sarcolemma itself sends protein microfibrils to adhere intimately with the collagen of the supporting connective tissues, the endomysium, perimysium and epimysium. The attachment to the bone can be direct or indirect, via tendons, aponeuroses or fascia, and is essentially the same in either case: collagen of the muscle's surrounding membranes or the indirect attachment is continuous with that of the periosteum, itself firmly adherent to the bone through dense **Sharpey's fibres**, which are thick collagenous extensions sent deep in to the bone's cortex.

The myotendinous junction

Tendons, aponeuroses and deep fascia are similar in their structure. Fascicles of mainly type I collagen are arranged longitudinally and are intimately connected with the collagen of the muscles' supporting membranes. The myotendinous junction is the area where insertion of every skeletal muscle fibre into its tendon occurs. This area has a specific morphology, which is adapted to its function. Specific features include shorter sarcomere lengths, greater number of organelles per cell (indicating greater synthetic ability), and a high degree of membrane folding into finger-like processes at the end of each fibre, which interdigitate with extracellular membrane collagens. The last of these increases resistance to stress by increasing surface area and reducing the angle of the force vector applied. The net result is that the junction is very strong.

Function

Innervation of skeletal muscle

Muscle develops with its motor nerve supply. Initially, each developing muscle fibre is multiply innervated by several axons. As the muscle develops, all but one of the axons lose their synaptic connection with the fibre. Each fibre is therefore innervated by a single motor neuron while, conversely, each motor neuron innervates multiple fibres via its axons. Because of the seemingly random establishment of the dominant axon to the fibre in development, muscle fibres lying next to each other are not usually innervated by the same parent motor neuron. A single motor neuron and all of the muscle fibres that it innervates are termed a motor unit.

Control of muscle contraction is by recruitment of motor units. A single contraction of an individual fibre is generally an 'all-or-none phenomenon'. Similarly, activity of a motor neuron will result in activation of the whole motor unit. For the whole muscle, therefore, contraction is dependent on the number of motor units activated and the size of those motor units. Smaller motor units are activated first, allowing fine control where small precise contractions are required. In muscles whose main purpose is a precision function, rather than power, the fibres are smaller and divided into numerous smaller motor units enabling finer gradation in recruitment and therefore control.

In addition to motor innervation, proper control of skeletal muscle function also requires a sensory supply. There are many free sensory nerve endings but also specialized sensory receptors known as **muscle spindles** containing **intrafusal** muscle fibres. Afferent signals from the muscle spindle are related to both absolute change in length (**nuclear chain fibres**) and rate of change in length (**nuclear bag fibres**). Along with Golgi tendon organs and Paciniform receptors found in joint capsules, these receptors provide important sensory feedback regarding the position and activity of the limb to guide motor control.

The neuromuscular junction

In the motor neuron, depolarization at the axon terminal produces an influx of Ca^{2+} through N-type voltage-sensitive channels. Increased concentrations of intracellular Ca^{2+} are believed to act through binding **synaptotagmin**, leading to fusion of preformed vesicles containing **acetylcholine (ACh)** with the pre-synaptic membrane. Acetylcholine released into the synaptic cleft binds to post-synaptic **nicotinic** ACh receptors (nAChR) on the sarcolemma (**Figure 12.5**). The nAChR is a non-specific monovalent cation channel, opened by binding ACh. The resulting Na^+ influx causes depolarization of the muscle fibre membrane known as the **end-plate potential**.

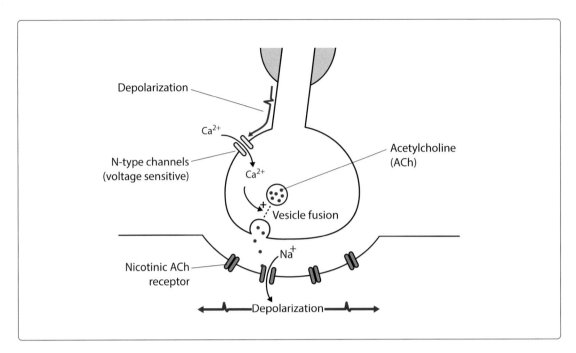

Figure 12.5 The neuromuscular junction. Calcium ions affect vesicle fusion via synaptotagmin binding.

Depolarization is dependent on the amount of ACh released into the synaptic cleft. Depolarization is also dependent on the rate of release of ACh into the cleft, as it is broken down rapidly by cholinesterases from the post-synaptic membrane. When the end-plate potential exceeds its threshold, an action potential will be initiated within the muscle fibre by activation of voltage-gated Na^+ channels. This muscle fibre action potential propagates through the sarcolemma in an identical manner to the nerve action potential.

Sliding filament contraction mechanism and force generation

Muscle contraction is produced by shortening of sarcomeres within the activated fibre. When viewed microscopically there is a reduction in length of the I- and H-bands within the contracted sarcomere. The length of the A-band, however, remains unchanged. Sarcomere contraction is produced by the thin filaments, and therefore the attached Z-discs at each end of the sarcomere, being pulled centrally toward the M-line by the thick filaments. The maximum possible shortening is produced when the I-band has been eliminated completely and the Z-discs are adjacent to the thick filaments of the A-band (**Figure 12.6**).

The cross-bridge theory was propounded by Huxley in 1957. In this theory, the filaments of myosin and actin move relative to each other because of an oscillating binding site on the myosin molecule, which binds to the actin molecule at differing rates. At the molecular level, the following sequence occurs (**see Figure 12.2**):

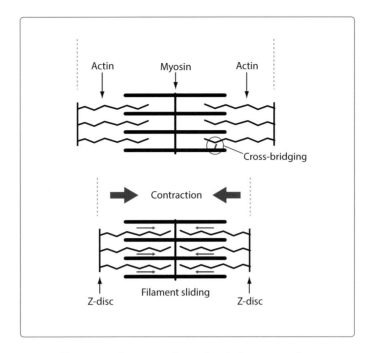

Figure 12.6 Sarcomere shortening during contraction.

- End plate depolarization at the neuromuscular junction causes action potential to propagate through sarcolemma and T-tubules (**Figure 12.4**).
- Voltage-sensitive modified dihydropyridine receptors on the T-tubule open ryanodine receptor channels in sarcoplasmic reticulum through mechanical linkage.
- Ca^{2+} released from sarcoplasmic reticulum into sarcoplasm.
- Ca^{2+} binds troponin C (**Figure 12.2**).
- Activated troponin C displaces inhibitory troponin I from site on tropomyosin/actin complex.
- Via coupling with troponin T, tropomyosin undergoes conformational change to expose myosin binding sites on actin.
- Myosin head forms cross-bridge with actin.
- Upon binding actin, S1 head segment rotation pulls thin filament toward M-line resulting in force generation.
- Myosin cross-bridge disengages from actin by adenosine triphosphate (ATP)-dependent mechanism, and returns to rest position.
- Myosin head produces new cross-bridge and continues cyclic force generation until stimulus ends (**Figure 12.7**).
- Ca^{2+} is returned to sarcoplasmic reticulum by ATP-dependent pumps.
- Muscle relaxation occurs by restoration of sarcoplasmic Ca^{2+} concentration and ATP-dependent disengagement of actin–myosin cross-bridges.

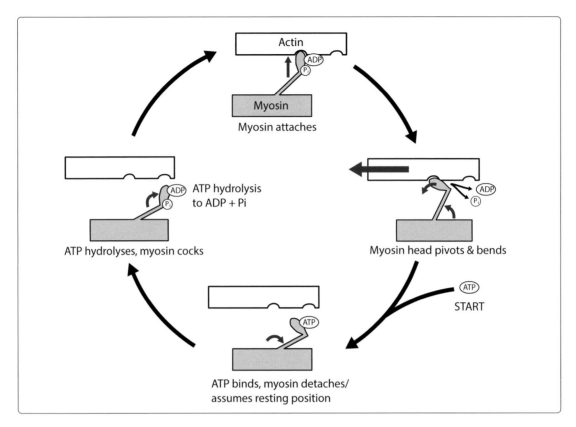

Figure 12.7 Cross-bridge cycling. ADP: adenosine diphosphate; ATP: adenosine triphosphate.

Force, speed and power of contraction

The **force** of a muscle at any given length is proportional to the cross-sectional area of the muscle. The more sarcomeres there are acting in parallel to each other, the higher the force generated. The force generated by a given muscle is also dependent on starting length. This is explained by the differing degree of overlap between the thick and thin filaments when the muscle is stretched, and therefore the number of actin–myosin cross-bridges that are able to be produced.

The **velocity** of muscular contraction is related to the length of the muscle. Upon stimulation of a muscle, all sarcomeres contract at the same time. For a long muscle, there will be a greater change in length per unit time, i.e. the greater the muscle velocity. The sarcomeres act in series. For a muscle of given length, contraction velocity is also dependent on the load being moved.

The **power** of a muscle is the product of its force and velocity. Short fat muscles produce high force but low maximum velocity. Long thin muscles produce low force but high maximum velocity. These represent opposite ends of the spectrum. Note that it is possible that both types of muscle could generate the same amount of power.

Although a single fibre twitch is essentially an all-or-none event, multiple rapidly repeated muscle stimulations can result in an increase in contraction strength, known as **frequency summation**. This is because calcium is released from the sarcoplasmic reticulum more rapidly than the pumping mechanisms return it; the sarcoplasmic calcium concentration remains elevated between stimulations and gradually increases, promoting increased cross-bridge formation. At a sufficiently high frequency, calcium will remain at supramaximal concentrations between stimulations and a continuous smooth contraction of maximal force will be produced, a state known as **tetanization**. In normal physiological activity, such frequencies are not achieved however, and smooth contraction is produced by asynchronous motor unit recruitment. The phenomenon of **treppe** occurs when the contraction strength of a muscle that has been inactive for a long period increases to its normal plateau over the course of about 10–50 twitches. This is also believed to be due to a gradual release of sequestered calcium back to normal functional levels, and is observed physiologically.

Types of muscle contraction

- **Isotonic** – muscle **tension is constant** throughout the range of motion, length changes.
- **Isometric** – muscle tension is generated while **length remains constant**.
- **Isokinetic** – muscle contracts maximally at a **constant velocity** throughout the range of movement.

Muscle contraction associated with change of length (i.e. isotonic or isokinetic contractions) may be either **concentric**, when the muscle shortens with contraction, or **eccentric**, where the external load exceeds the muscle force generated so the muscle lengthens during contraction.

Muscle fibre types

Muscle fibres in humans are of three main types. The types differ from each other in their size, speed and resistance to fatigue. These characteristics are a function of their relatively aerobic or anaerobic metabolism:

- **Type 1** – **slow oxidative fibres**:
  - slow contraction velocity – low myosin ATPase activity;
  - high concentration of myoglobin (red in colour);
  - high concentration of mitochondria;
  - high capillary density;
  - oxidative;
  - very fatigue resistant;
  - low force generation – small diameter fibres.
- **Type 2a** – **fast oxidative fibres**:
  - fast contraction velocity – high myosin ATPase activity;
  - intermediate myoglobin concentration;
  - high mitochondria concentration;
  - intermediate capillary density;
  - oxidative and glycolytic;
  - fatigue-resistant;
  - high force generation – large diameter fibres.

- **Type 2b – fast glycolytic fibres**:
  - very fast contraction velocity – high myosin ATPase activity;
  - low myoglobin concentration (relatively white in colour);
  - low mitochondria concentration;
  - low capillary density;
  - glycolytic;
  - fatiguable;
  - very high force generation – large diameter fibres.

A mixture of fibre types is found within a particular muscle, and reflects the function of the muscle. The pattern of activity imposed on the muscle is the single most important factor in fibre type expression. All fibres within a single motor unit are of the same type. Athletes who train extensively for endurance can reach proportions of up to 80% of type 1 fibres in their muscles.

Other muscle fibre types have also been described in smaller quantities. These probably represent interim fibre types that have not had sufficient stimulus to differentiate fully.

Injury

Mechanism of injury

Muscle cell damage by, for example, physical trauma leads to release of inflammatory mediators and damaged cellular components. The resulting inflammatory cascade ultimately produces proteolytic enzymes and reactive oxygen intermediates that cause further damage. In addition, damage to intracellular membranes and failure of ATP-dependent pumping mechanisms cause raised intracellular calcium concentrations. Calcium-activated enzymes, such as **protease** and **phospholipase**, in turn further damage the cell structure from within.

The inflammatory reaction, however, also liberates the mediators that initiate the repair process. Macrophages infiltrate and phagocytose the damaged portions of muscle fibre, eventually leading to scar tissue deposition. Limited regeneration is possible by proliferation of residual myoblasts.

Modes of muscle injury

Muscle injury can be considered in terms of location and cause:

- Direct physical trauma:
  - muscle belly tear;
  - muscle laceration;
  - musculotendinous junction injury;
  - crush injury and rhabdomyolysis;
  - delayed onset muscle soreness (DOMS): defined as soreness that develops 24–72 hours following intense exercise and associated with measurable muscle weakness. The pain occurs mainly at the myotendinous junction. It has been shown to be associated with intramuscular damage but is readily reversible. Connective tissue breakdown products such as hydroxyproline can be identified in the urine.

- Ischaemic damage and compartment syndrome.
- Denervation: after lower motor neuron injury, fibres of the affected motor units undergo atrophy, with a downregulation of myosin and actin synthesis, decrease in cell size and resorption of myofibrils. If reinnervation fails to occur within about 2–3 months, the fibres undergo fibrosis and fatty infiltration, with reduced capacity for functional recovery even if reinnervation subsequently occurs. Beyond 1–2 years there is no possibility for functional return. Disuse also results in atrophy due to lack of stimulation, but fibrosis and fatty infiltration do not occur because tonic stimulation is maintained. Recovery is therefore possible if use of the muscle is regained. Upper motor neuron injury similarly does not result in fibrosis, due to tonic stimulation by lower motor neurones.
- Metabolic injury: malignant hyperpyrexia – is a skeletal muscle reaction to inhalational anaesthetics or suxamethonium, with prolonged contraction of muscle, leading to catastrophic metabolic tissue disintegration. Most cases are due to autosomal dominant mutations in ryanodine receptors, resulting in massive intracellular calcium release. The extreme metabolic activation leads to excessive oxygen consumption, hyperthermia, metabolic acidosis and cell damage through failure of ATP-dependent pumping mechanisms and lytic enzyme activity. Potassium is released first, and therefore there is a risk of cardiac arrhythmias, followed by massive myoglobin load, leading to renal failure if the patient survives the initial insult.

Muscle damage may also result from acquired or congenital myopathies, muscular dystrophy, infection and neoplasia.

Repair

Muscle needs a blood supply and stimulation in the form of a nerve supply. Repair thus relies on rapid re-establishment of a vascular supply and innervation. In a complete muscle belly transection, the distal portion of muscle wastes rapidly. Muscle regeneration can occur without a nerve supply, but permanent muscle atrophy will develop if reinnervation fails. Note the following:

- The more proximal the belly tear, the worse the prognosis, as more bulk is denervated.
- Muscle laceration results in dense fibrous scar tissue formation. Myotubes regenerate across scar tissue in small numbers only. Partial lacerations predictably have better functional outcomes than complete belly lacerations. A complete laceration in the midsubstance can recover to only around 50% of the previous force that was generated by the muscle.
- Partial denervation recovers by axon sprouting from adjacent intact motor neurones (**Figure 12.8**). The result is larger motor units, but a reduction in the number of motor units, such that strength recovers at the expense of precise control. The reinnervated muscle fibres change type to match those of their new motor unit.

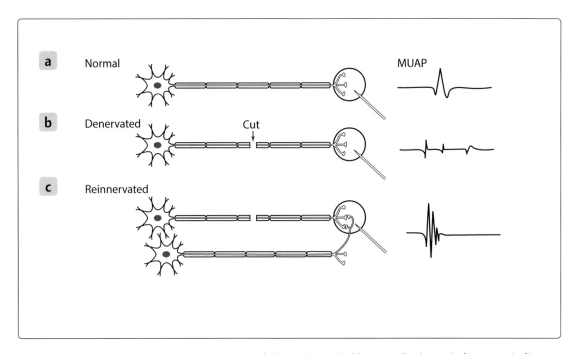

Figure 12.8 a: Normal motor unit action potential (MUAP) recorded by a needle electrode from muscle fibres within its recording area; b: after denervation, single muscle fibres discharge spontaneously, producing fibrillations and positive sharp waves; c: when reinnervation by axon sprouting has occurred, the newly formed sprouts conduct slowly, producing temporal dispersion (i.e. prolonged MUAP duration) and MUAP polyphasicity. The higher density of muscle fibres within the recording area of the needle belonging to the enlarging second motor unit results in an increased-amplitude MUAP.

Muscle tears

These have been poorly studied to date. Animal studies suggest that tears tend to occur near the myotendinous junction, with a segment of adjacent muscle avulsed when stretched to failure. They may be complete or incomplete. Immobilization accelerates granulation tissue formation. Immobilization in a lengthened position decreases contractures and helps to maintain strength.

Electrodiagnosis in muscle injury

Electromyography (EMG) is the recording of electrical activity in skeletal muscle. Needle electrodes are inserted into the muscle to be studied. The electrode records any spontaneous activity within the muscle at rest and the signal given by the firing of motor units when the muscle is activated. There is generally no spontaneous activity at rest in a healthy muscle after the needle has been inserted. The patterns of motor unit activity (seen as the **motor unit action potential, MUAP**) are related to the nerve supply to the muscle in question: the size of the MUAP is proportional to the number of muscle fibres innervated by the motor neuron(s) being stimulated, while injury to the motor nerve supply results in abnormal patterns of MUAP (**Figure 12.8**).

Summary of findings in motor nerve injury

Denervation:

- Spontaneous activity due to increased sensitivity to ACh:
  - acute denervation: sharp waves;
  - chronic denervation: fasciculations.

Reinnervation:

- Early:
  - reduced amplitude motor action potentials, longer duration;
  - poor recruitment.
- Late:
  - large amplitude, stable, consistent firing motor action potentials;
  - good recruitment of units gives polyphasic signal.

Viva questions

1. Describe the basic structure of skeletal muscle.

2. What is the mechanism of contraction of skeletal muscle?

3. What are the events that occur at the neuromuscular junction?

4. What different types of skeletal muscle fibre do you know of?

5. How does injured muscle heal?

Further reading

Beiner JM, Jokl P. Muscle contusion injuries: current treatment options. *Am Acad Orthop Surg* 2001;**9**:227–37.

Jarvinen TA, Jarvinen TL, Kaariainen M, Kalimo H, Jarvinen M. Muscle injuries: biology and treatment. *Am J Sports Med* 2005;**33**:745–64.

Kirkendall DT, Garrett WE, Jr. Clinical perspectives regarding eccentric muscle injury. *Clin Orthop Relat Res* 2002;**403**:S81–9.

Lieber RL, Friden J. Clinical significance of skeletal muscle architecture. *Clin Orthop Relat Res* 2001;**383**:140–51.

Peterson GW, Will AD. Newer electrodiagnostic techniques in peripheral nerve injuries. *Orthop Clin North Am* 1988;**19**:13–25.

a

13 | Basics of Bone

Peter Bates, Bjarne Moller-Madsen, Ali Noorani and Manoj Ramachandran

Function

Bone is a specialized connective tissue that performs **three main functions**:

- **Reservoir of calcium and phosphate:** Bone is the primary reservoir of calcium and phosphate in the body.
- **Haemopoiesis**: The haematopoietic marrow located in cancellous bone supplies the body's cells, tissues and organs with erythrocytes, leukocytes and platelets.
- **Protective and mechanical:** Bone has a protective and mechanical role in supporting the body's tissues, protecting the soft internal viscera and providing sites of attachment for the muscles that effect body movement and locomotion.

Structure

Woven (immature) bone

In rapidly formed woven bone, **collagen fibres** are aligned randomly and have **no lamellae** (see below), making the bone weaker but more flexible than lamellar bone. This irregular arrangement affords it **isotropic** characteristics, i.e. it has uniform properties in all directions, independent of the direction of load application. Woven bone exhibits a rapid rate of deposition and turnover, with more cells per unit volume than lamellar bone. It is found in the **embryonic** and **neonatal skeleton**, the **metaphyseal region of growing bones** up to age 4 years and in the **fracture callus** of children. It is absent in the normal adult but appears in the early hard callus following fracture. It is also found in **pathological bone**, e.g. in tumours, Pagetic bone and osteogenesis imperfecta.

Lamellar (mature) bone

Lamellar bone forms the structural component of **cortical** and **cancellous** bone with **stress-orientated collagen fibres** contributing to its **anisotropic** characteristics. **Osteoblasts** lay down collagen matrix in microscopic thin-layered sheets called **lamellae**. Within each lamella, collagen fibres run parallel to each other. Fibres in adjacent lamellae run at oblique angles to each other (**herring-bone structure**), with cement lines separating the lamellae. Lamellar bone is composed predominantly of matrix with a small cell population of osteocytes (trapped osteoblasts) encased within bony **lacunae** and resting **bone-lining cells** (with osteoblastic potential) covering the bony surfaces.

Cortical (compact) bone

Cortical bone is a subtype of lamellar bone and comprises 80% of the adult skeleton forming the envelope of cuboid bones and the diaphyses of long bones. Lamellae are laid down as concentric rings forming tubular lamellar systems called osteons or **Haversian systems,** which are approximately 50 μm in diameter (**Figure 13.1**). Individual osteons are aligned along lines of force (usually parallel with the long axis of the bone). Each osteon has a central neurovascular channel (**Haversian canal**) surrounded by five to seven concentric layers (lamellae) of bone matrix. Rings of trapped osteocytes intercommunicate via gap junctions within channels called **canaliculi,** which spread out radially from the central canal like spokes of a wheel. **Cement lines** separate osteons, with neither canaliculi nor collagen fibres crossing them, forming areas of relative weakness along which cracks may propagate.

A second system of canals called **Volkmann's canals** penetrates and runs perpendicular to the long bone axis, connecting the inner and outer surfaces of the bone. These canals carry blood vessels to and from the Haversian systems. At the periosteal and endosteal surfaces, lamellae run parallel to the surface, forming **circumferential** and **endosteal lamellae.**

Cortical bone is denser and has a higher Young's modulus of elasticity (around 20 GPa) than cancellous bone (around 1 Gpa). Cortical bone is also **more resistant to bending and torsion.**

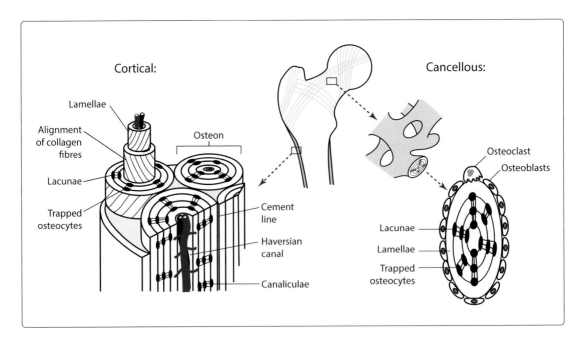

Figure 13.1 Cortical and cancellous bone lamellar structure. In cortical bone, the lamellae are arranged in concentric rings around Haversian canals. In cancellous bone, they are arranged as layers within the trabeculae, which are themselves aligned along lines of force.

Cancellous (trabecular) bone

This is another form of lamellar bone and is found mainly in the metaphyses and epiphyses of long bones and centrally in cuboid bones (**Figure 13.1**). It has a three-dimensional lattice of interconnecting trabeculae, which are aligned along axes of mechanical stress, enclosing elements of the bone marrow. Each of the trabeculae is made up of parallel sheets of lamellae. Osteocytes, lacunae and canaliculi in cancellous bone resemble those in cortical bone. However, Haversian systems are not present in cancellous bone. Cancellous bone has eight times the metabolic turnover rate of cortical bone due to its large surface area. It is less dense, less elastic and less strong than cortical bone.

Periosteum

This circumferential connective tissue covering bone is responsible for growth in bone diameter (appositional growth) and therefore is more prominent in children. It has two layers: an **inner cambial layer**, which is loose, vascular and osteogenic, and an **outer fibrous layer**, which is more structural, less cellular and continuous with joint capsules. With age, periosteum thins and has less osteogenic capability.

Cells and matrix

Bone is a composite material consisting of cells (10%) within a matrix (90%) that has both inorganic and organic components.

Cells

Osteoblasts

These are bone-forming cells derived from **undifferentiated mesenchymal stem cells** in marrow, which produce osteoid (or bone matrix) containing type I collagen, depositing it on pre-existing mineralized surfaces (known as the **mineralization front**). Osteoblasts line the surfaces of bone, have great **synthetic capacity** (abundant rough endoplasmic reticulum, Golgi apparatus and mitochondria) and show high **alkaline phosphatase** activity. Cell differentiation is mediated by a large number of bone morphogenetic proteins (BMPs), growth factors and cytokines. Osteoblasts have **three fates**: they may become **inactive bone-lining cells**, surround themselves with matrix and become **osteocytes** or disappear from the site of bone formation as a result of **apoptosis**.

Osteocytes

Osteoblasts that become entrapped by calcified bone matrix are known as osteocytes. They comprise 90% of the bone cell population and interconnect with other bone cells via long cytoplasmic processes in the canaliculi. They are important in **controlling calcium** and **phosphorus metabolism**, responding to chemical stimuli such as parathyroid hormone (PTH) and calcitonin, and also to **mechanical** and **electrical potential stimuli** (which may be the basis of Wolff's law and of the electromechanical effects on fracture healing).

Bone-lining cells

These flat cells lying on the surface of bone possess cytoplasmic extensions that penetrate bone matrix and **communicate with osteocytes**. They are considered **inactive osteoblasts** that may be reactivated to become osteoblasts during periods of new bone formation. They are also thought to have a **gatekeeper function**: when stimulated by PTH, they undergo cyclic adenosine monophosphate (cAMP) mediated morphological changes that expose the bone surface and allow osteoclasts to start resorption.

Osteoclasts

Mononuclear osteoclast precursor cells (preosteoclasts) arise from the haematopoietic macrophage and monocyte stem cell line. They may be found in the marrow and circulating blood. When stimulated, these cells proliferate and fuse to form **large multinucleated osteoclasts**, typically having 3–20 nuclei and large numbers of mitochondria and lysosomes and producing acid phosphatase. Osteoclasts resorb bone within pits or depressions known as **Howship's lacunae** on endosteal and periosteal surfaces of bone. In dense cortical bone, they lead to osteonal **cutting cones** that tunnel through the bone, creating resorption cavities. On completing their resorptive activities, they may divide into mononuclear cells that can be reactivated to form new osteoclasts.

When lying on the bone surface, their contact area has a **ruffled (brush) border** (Figure 13.2) that increases surface area from membrane in-foldings, which binds to the bone surface via integrins, sealing the area. A low pH is produced beneath this layer (via the carbonic anhydrase system, adenosine triphosphate (ATP)-dependent proton pumps and the Na$^+$/H$^+$; exchange system), which dissolves the inorganic apatite crystals. Acidic proteolytic lysosomal enzymes,

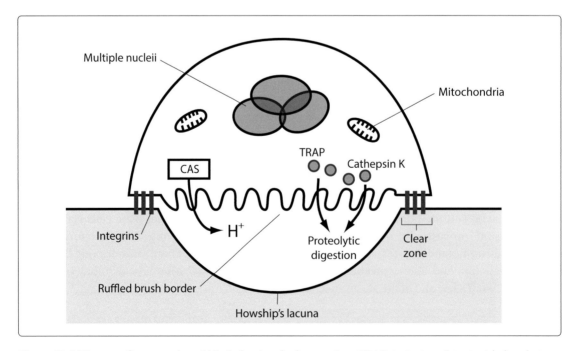

Figure 13.2 Diagram of an osteoclast. CAS: Carbonic anhydrase system; TRAP: tartrate-resistant acid phosphatase.

such as the tartrate-resistant isoenzyme of acid phosphatase (TRAP), and cysteine proteinases, such as the cathepsins, then hydrolyse the organic matrix components. Control of osteoclast function is related closely to that of osteoblasts.

Lack of osteoclast activity is implicated in osteopetrosis, while overactivity is found in Paget's disease.

Bone remodelling unit

A **bone remodelling unit** (BRU) is an area of bone remodelled by a set of osteoblasts, osteoclasts and stromal supporting tissue. In normal bone, formation matches resorption with continual turnover of bone. Osteoclast precursors are activated to form osteoclasts, which resorb bone. This is followed by reversal, whereby osteoblast precursors are activated to form osteoblasts, which lay down osteoid (collagen and non-collagenous proteins). The osteoid subsequently undergoes mineralization to form bone.

Bone matrix

The **inorganic matrix (60%) resists compressive forces**, while **the organic matrix (40%) resists tensile forces**.

Inorganic matrix

This is composed mainly of calcium phosphate crystals, analogous to calcium hydroxyapatite $[Ca_{10}(PO_4)_6(OH)_2]$, and is responsible for the **compressive strength of bone**. The formation of solid calcium phosphate crystals (known as **mineralization**) occurs as a result of phase transformation of soluble calcium and phosphate within specific hole and pore zone regions of the collagen fibrils in the organic matrix of bone, with progressive mineral deposits eventually occupying all of the available space within the fibrils. **Osteocalcium phosphate (brushite)** is also found in bone.

In addition, the inorganic matrix serves as a reservoir for approximately **99% of the body's calcium, 85% of the body's phosphorus** and **40–60% of the total body sodium and potassium**. Bone also contains numerous impurities, such as strontium, lead and fluoride.

Organic matrix

Collagen (type I), constituting 90% of the organic matrix, consists of a triple helix of two alpha 1 chains and one alpha 2 chain (with a repetitive GlyXY sequence, where glycine is in the first position and X and Y are often proline and hydroxyproline) arranged in a quarter-staggered structural array producing single fibrils (see Chapter 8). After synthesis in osteoblasts and fibroblasts, the alpha chains are modified by hydroxylation of lysine and proline residues; **hydroxyproline** is therefore a good indicator of **bone turnover**. The modified alpha chains are exported from the cell; pro-collagen extensions are removed from the chains (**procollagen** is a good indicator of **bone formation**, along with collagen telopeptides, e.g. carboxy-terminal (CTX). Finally, cross-linkages form between adjacent triple helices; **cross-linked collagen-derived peptides**, e.g. pyridinoline and deoxypyridinoline, are therefore a good indicator of bone breakdown. Collagen is primarily responsible for the **tensile strength** of bone. Small amounts of collagen types V and XI are also found in bone.

Note that in addition to the **bone resorption markers** mentioned above, bone formation can be assessed with pro-collagen type I pro-peptides, e.g. carboxy-terminal extension peptide (**P1CP**) and amino-terminal extension peptide (**P1NP**) along with bone-specific **alkaline phosphatase** and **osteocalcin** (see below).

Mineralization in immature bone (e.g. during preliminary ossification of cartilage and fetal bone) occurs as a result of alkaline phosphatase activity in mineralizing vesicles, derived from osteoblasts or chondroblasts, which breaks down pyrophosphate (an inhibitor of mineralization) and initiates mineralization. In **mature bone**, the more important mechanism is the deposition and propagation of apatite crystals in the **hole zones** that exist between the ends of fibrils and the **pore zones** that lie between the sides of fibrils of collagen.

Other organic constituents of bone include:

- **Bone-specific proteoglycans**: involved in mineralization, organization of collagen fibres and binding of growth factors.
- **Non-collagenous matrix proteins**:
  - **osteocalcin**: produced by osteoblasts and involved in the control of osteoclasts (gene on chromosome 1);
  - **osteonectin**: secreted by osteoblasts and platelets for regulation of mineralization (gene on chromosome 5);
  - **osteopontin** (bone sialoprotein I): a non-bone-specific cell-binding protein anchoring osteoclasts to the mineralized matrix (gene on chromosome 4);
  - **bone sialoprotein II**: bone specific (gene on chromosome 4);
  - **others**: e.g. thrombospondin (important in cell attachment) and serum proteins (in same concentration as serum but with increased albumin).
- **Growth factors and cytokines**:
  - **BMP 1–17**: members of the transforming growth factor beta (TGF-beta) family of multifunctional molecules;
  - **insulin-like growth factor** (IGF) I and II;
  - **interleukins** 1 (IL-1) and 6 (IL-6).

Blood supply

The skeletal system receives 5–10% of cardiac output. Individual long bones have **three interactive circulatory systems** (**Figure 13.3**), all of which communicate in the adult. In the child, the metaphyseal–epiphyseal system separates when the ossific nucleus is formed.

Nutrient artery system (high-pressure system)

A major artery of the systemic circulation enters the **mid-diaphysis** through a nutrient foramen. Once in the medullary canal, it divides into **ascending** and **descending** arteries or arterioles, which anastomose with metaphyseal vessels and directly penetrate the **endosteal surface**, supplying the inner two-thirds of the cortex. In the child, these vessels end on the metaphyseal side of the physis, contributing to the process of endochondral ossification. At the microscopic level, arterioles run in Volkmann's canals with branches to the Haversian systems, draining into venules and then into the central venous sinus and out via the nutrient vein.

Metaphyseal–epiphyseal system

The periarticular vascular complex penetrates the thin cortex and supplies the **metaphysis, physis** and **epiphysis**. The metaphyseal vessels anastomose with the medullary and epiphyseal arteries after growth plate fusion. In epiphyses with large articular surfaces, such as the radial and femoral heads, vessels enter the bone between the articular cartilage and the physis, making the supply relatively tenuous.

Periosteal system (low-pressure system)

Capillaries enter at the sites of **major muscle attachments**, normally supplying the outer third of the cortex. This is the dominant system in the child and is responsible for circumferential growth.

These three systems are interconnected, and each is able to become the dominant supply if another is damaged. The normal direction of flow is **centrifugal** (inside to out), but if the endosteal system is damaged, e.g. after intramedullary reaming, the periosteal system becomes dominant and the flow becomes **centripetal** (outside to in). Note that the venous system is normally centripetal in nature.

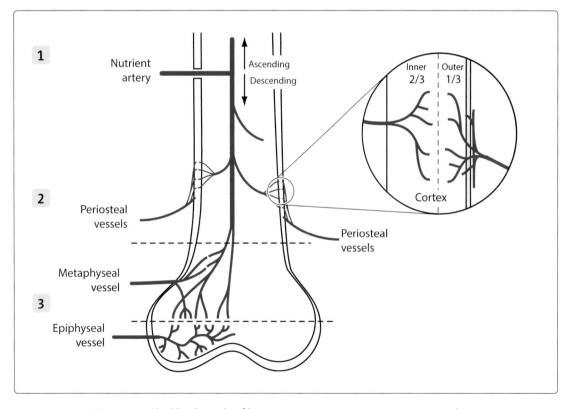

Figure 13.3. The blood supply of bone. 1: nutrient artery system; 2: periosteal system; 3: metaphyseal–epiphyseal system.

Bone metabolism

Serum calcium levels and bone mineral homeostasis are related intimately and controlled by the synchronized actions of vitamin D3 metabolites, PTH, calcitonin and other hormones. Feedback mechanisms play an important role in regulating plasma calcium and phosphate levels.

Calcium

Ninety-nine per cent of total body calcium is sequestered in bone, leaving 1% circulating in the extracellular fluid. Intracellular calcium levels are negligible in comparison. Calcium is also important for **nerve, muscle** and **hormone** function and in **clotting**.

Plasma calcium (less than 1% of total body calcium) is 50% free and 50% bound, mainly to albumin, and is maintained at a level between 2.2 and 2.6 mmol/L. Calcium is absorbed from the duodenum via **active transport**, mediated by calcium-binding protein and ATP, and regulated by 1,25-dihydroxycholecalciferol [1,25(OH)$_2$-vitamin D3] and via passive diffusion from the jejunum.

Ninety-eight per cent of the calcium filtered in the kidneys is reabsorbed, 60% of this process occurring in the proximal convoluted tubules. A small amount of calcium is also excreted in stools. The three calcitropic hormones and other paracrine factors govern the extracellular calcium levels and the flow in and out of cells.

Dietary calcium deficiency produces a progressive loss of bone mass. In elderly people, the renal hydroxylation of 25(OH)-vitamin D3 is reduced, leading to lower levels of active vitamin D3 and an increased dietary requirement for calcium (*Table 13.1*).

Table 13.1 Recommended daily intake of calcium

	mg/d
Children <10 y	600
10–25 y	1400
25–65 y	750
Lactation	2000
Postmenopausal women and fracture healing	1500

Phosphate

Phosphate is a key component of bone mineral, with 85% of total body stores being found in bone. Phosphate also functions as a metabolite and as a buffer in enzyme systems. It circulates unbound in the plasma. The daily requirement of phosphate is 1–1.5 mg/day. Dietary intake is usually sufficient.

Regulators of calcium and phosphate metabolism

Vitamin D (active metabolites)

These **naturally occurring steroids** are either **ingested** in the diet from fish oils, such as cod liver oil, and plants or activated in the skin by **ultraviolet** (UV) light (see below). They **enhance calcium and phosphorus absorption** across the small intestine via promotion of synthesis of a calcium-transporting protein and **enhance osteoclastic resorption** from bone. The overall effect is to **increase serum levels of calcium and phosphate**. Vitamin D metabolites also inhibit PTH release.

The activation process occurs as follows (**Figure 13.4**): UV light on the skin transforms 7-dehydrocholesterol to cholecalciferol (vitamin D3). One hour of direct sunlight produces the daily requirement in people with paler skin types, but the process takes longer on darker skin. Vitamin D3 is subsequently hydroxylated in the liver to 25-hydroxycholecalciferol [25(OH)-vitamin D3] (an inactive form). Serum 25(OH)-vitamin D3 is the most accurate indicator of body vitamin D stores.

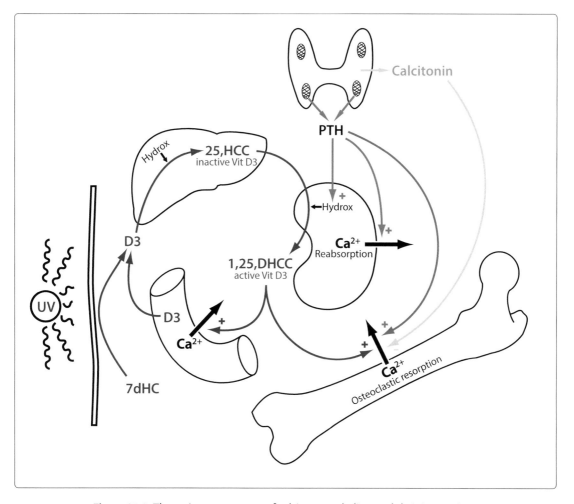

Figure 13.4. The major components of calcium metabolism and their interactions.

Further hydroxylation of 25(OH)-vitamin D3 occurs in the mitochondria of the proximal convoluted tubular cells of the kidney to 1,25-dihydroxycholecalciferol [1,25(OH)$_2$-vitamin D3] (the active form of vitamin D). Activation is in response to raised levels of PTH or decreased levels of serum calcium or phosphate. Decreased PTH levels or raised calcium or phosphate results in conversion of the active form to the inactive 24,25(OH)$_2$-vitamin D3.

Parathyroid hormone

This is an 84-amino acid peptide secreted by the **chief cells** of the four parathyroid glands in response to changes in extracellular calcium via a recently identified calcium-sensing receptor. PTH is secreted in response to decreased serum calcium and phosphate. Its production is inhibited by elevated serum calcium or 1,25(OH)$_2$-vitamin D3. PTH has numerous effects, including the following:

- **In the kidney**:
  - stimulation of hydroxylation (activation) of 25(OH)-vitamin D3 in the proximal tubules, leading to indirect intestinal effects;
  - increasing reabsorption of filtered calcium in the kidney;
  - promotion of urinary excretion of phosphate from the kidney.
- **In bone**: stimulation of osteoclasts and their precursors, producing bone resorption.
- **Overall effect**: serum calcium levels are increased and phosphate levels are decreased.

Calcitonin

Calcitonin is a 32-amino acid peptide secreted by the parafollicular C-cells of the thyroid gland. Calcitonin is secreted in response to elevated serum calcium and inhibited by decreased serum calcium. Calcitonin directly inhibits osteoclasts (which have calcitonin receptors). Its effects include reduction of cellular motility, retraction of cytoplasmic extensions and reduction in ruffled border size. This produces a transient decrease in serum calcium.

Other hormones and growth factors

- **Oestrogen**: inhibits bone resorption and therefore prevents bone loss. Also inhibits bone formation and so does not increase bone density.
- **Corticosteroids**: reduce gastrointestinal absorption and increase renal excretion of calcium, thus inhibiting bone matrix formation, causing hyperparathyroidism and leading to rapid bone loss. Patients on corticosteroids should be given calcium and vitamin D, with or without bisphosphonates.
- **Thyroid hormones**: increase bone turnover, favouring bone resorption (seen in hyperthyroidism).
- **Growth hormone**: produces a positive calcium balance by increasing gut absorption.
- **Insulin**: type I diabetes, if poorly controlled, may lead to bone loss.
- **Growth factors**:
  - IL-1, IL-6 and tumour necrosis factor alpha (TNF-alpha;) stimulate proliferation of osteoclast precursors;
  - IGF activates osteoblasts and is produced by osteoblasts;
  - TGF activates osteoblasts; also stimulates osteoclastic precursors *in vitro*.

Physiological changes with age

Normally, bone mass increases up to a peak between 16 and 25 years, after which there is a normal physiological loss of bone mass over time for both men and women of 0.3–0.5% per year. Thus, calcium balance is positive in the first three decades of life, after which it becomes negative.

Women have an increase in bone loss (up to 2–3%) at the menopause, but after the first post-menopausal decade the rate of bone loss is equivalent for both men and women.

Viva questions

1. What is the structure of bone?
2. What cells are found in bone? What are their functions?
3. What does the matrix of bone contain?
4. How does remodelling of bone occur?
5. How is calcium regulated in the body? What is the contribution of bone?

Further reading

Boskey AL, Posner AS. Bone structure, composition, and mineralization. *Orthop Clin North Am* 1984;**15**:597–612.

Buckwalter JA, Cooper RR. Bone structure and function. *Instr Course Lect* 1987;**36**:27–48.

Buckwalter JA, Glimcher MJ, Cooper RR, Recker R. Bone biology: I. Structure, blood supply, cells, matrix, and mineralization. *Instr Course Lect* 1996;**45**:371–86.

Forriol F, Shapiro F. Bone development: interaction of molecular components and biophysical forces. *Clin Orthop Relat Res* 2005;**432**:14–33.

Posner AS. The mineral of bone. *Clin Orthop Relat Res* 1985;**200**:87–99.

14 Bone Injury, Healing and Grafting

Peter Bates, Andrea Yeo and Manoj Ramachandran

Introduction

In this chapter, we review the key facts concerning fracture biomechanics and healing, and bone grafting and banking.

Fracture biomechanics

Bone can be subjected to compressive, tensile, bending and/or torsional forces. Fractures can be classified according to the nature of their causative force.

Repetitive force

Stress fractures may result from cyclical loading with forces below the ultimate strength of the bone. Micro-damage may occur with each cycle of loading, with microscopic cracks forming along cement lines. The bone fails if the crack propagation moves faster than the reparative processes of internal (primary) remodelling and periosteal callus formation.

Single force

A single application of force produces a fracture pattern characterized by the nature of the application of force (**Figure 14.1**). Forces may be either direct or indirect. **Indirect forces** may act either along the length of the bone, as in spiral fractures, or via the soft tissues, as in avulsion fractures of the patella and olecranon.

Cortical bone is stiffer than cancellous bone and tolerates less strain before fracture. Cortical bone fractures at an *in vitro* strain of 2%, while cancellous bone fractures at an *in vitro* strain of 75%. **Cortical bone is anisotropic** and is **strong in compression but relatively weak in tension and shear**. Therefore, the areas where tensile and shear stresses are greatest fail first.

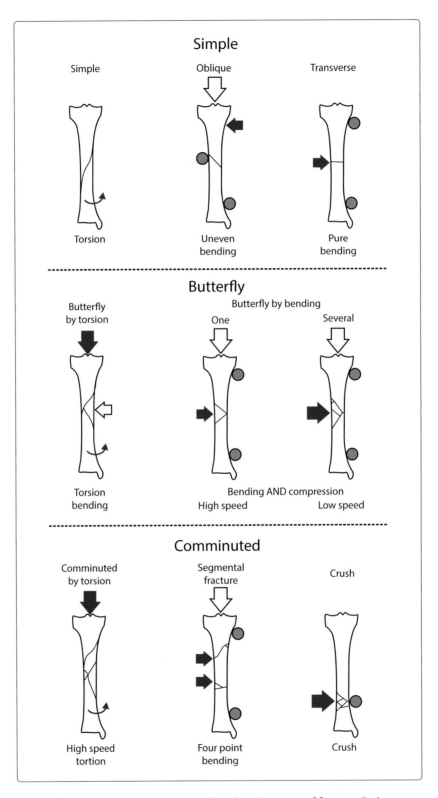

Figure 14.1. Fracture pattern is related to the nature of force applied.

The rate of application of force determines the energy (E) transferred:

$$E = 1/2\,m\,v^2$$

where m is the mass and v is the velocity.

Thus, the energy imparted increases as the square of the velocity of the injury. Bone is **viscoelastic**, i.e. its biomechanical properties vary with the rate of application of load. Bone is stiffer, stronger and more brittle when loads are applied at a higher rate. With rapid loading, bone absorbs more energy than when loaded more slowly, and this energy is released as it fractures. Therefore, as the energy or velocity increases, the more comminuted the fracture is likely to be and the more extensive is the soft tissue injury associated with it. High-energy and high-velocity injuries and injuries associated with extensive soft-tissue damage have significantly longer times to healing and higher complication rates.

The type of fracture produced by forces acting on bone is dependent on five key factors:

- Load.
- Rate.
- Direction.
- Bone properties, e.g. shape, anatomical area, quality of bone.
- Soft-tissue forces.

Pure compression forces are rare in the skeleton but lead to shear forces, and often on to fractures at 45° to the compressive load. Shear lines are formed by buckling of lamellae and oblique cracking of osteons, which occurs first at areas of stress concentration in the bone, e.g. vessels or resorption spaces, leading to **oblique fractures**. **Uneven bending forces** also create oblique fractures.

Tensile (pulling) forces tend to arise at soft-tissue insertions to cancellous bone, producing **transverse fractures** due to debonding of cement lines and pulling out of osteons, e.g. olecranon, patella and medial malleolus. Note that percentage lengthening to fracture with tensile strain is 2% for cortical bone and more than 75% for cancellous bone, although the stress required to fracture is higher for the former.

Pure bending forces result in **transverse fractures** from tension on the convexity and compression on the concavity , with the neutral axis moving towards the fracture. A **bending wedge (butterfly) fragment** may occur on the compression (concave) side, especially with high-energy injuries. With **combined bending and compression**, the bending force causes a transverse crack in tension and the compression force causes an oblique fracture, resulting again in a **bending wedge** or **butterfly fracture**.

Torsional forces cause **spiral fractures** with two components: one spiral fracture line around the circumference of the bone at approximately 45° to the horizontal caused by a failure in tension perpendicular to the crack, and a vertical line linking the proximal and distal ends of the spiral due to shear failure (the latter probably initiating the fracture). If **torsion and compression** are combined, then a **spiral wedge fracture** results.

Four-point bending, such as a car bumper striking a tibia, creates segmental fractures.

Fracture healing

Fracture healing shares many similarities with soft-tissue healing, but it is unique in its ability to heal completely without scar formation. Complete fracture healing is dependent on its biology (i.e. adequate vascularity) and mechanical stability.

Perren's strain theory of fracture healing

To comprehend the stages of fracture healing, Perren's strain theory must first be understood. Fracture healing is dependent on its strain environment. After any form of fixation or immobilization, a fracture that is loaded will undergo some degree of movement or strain.

Fracture gap strain is defined as the relative change in the fracture gap (ΔL) divided by the original fracture gap (L). Strain at a fracture site is therefore decreased with increased fracture gap or greater surface area, such as in metaphyseal fractures (larger bone diameter) and in multifragmentary or segmental fractures (where the overall strain is shared among the individual fragments).

The degree of interfragmentary strain appears to govern the cellular response and therefore the type of tissue that forms between the fracture fragments. Each of these tissues is able to tolerate a different amount of strain:

- **Granulation tissue**: up to 100%.
- **Fibrous connective tissue**: up to 17%.
- **Fibrocartilage**: 2–10%.
- **Lamellar bone**: 2%.

Therefore, immediately following a fracture, the strain is high, stimulating granulation tissue formation; but as the strain decreases with time, cartilage and then bone form (soft and subsequently hard callus).

In the presence of **absolute stability** (compression plating or rigid external fixation), if the fragments are in intimate contact, then the fracture site strain is so low as to inhibit callus formation and allow direct (primary) Haversian remodelling. If fragments are fixed rigidly but a gap is present, then primary bone healing (cutting cones) may not be able to bridge the gap. The lack of strain may inhibit callus formation and secondary healing, predisposing to non-union.

In the presence of **relative stability** (splint immobilization, intramedullary fixation or bridge plating), the more strain-tolerant cartilaginous callus is required to stiffen the fracture site before hard woven bony callus forming and replacing it (secondary healing). A larger strain produces a bigger callus.

In the presence of **complete instability**, callus is unable to form because the strain is too much for it to tolerate. The more strain-tolerant fibrous tissue forms, creating a hypertrophic non-union.

Primary (direct cortical, osteonal or Haversian) bone healing

This type of healing only occurs when there has been **anatomical reduction** and **interfragmentary compression**, leading to **absolute stability** (no motion between fracture surfaces under functional load). The process is very intolerant of strain (movement) at the fracture site (interfragmentary strain should be <2%).

However, even under conditions of interfragmentary compression, the biomechanical micro-environment differs within the fracture site and influences the process by which bone is produced. Full congruency between the fragment ends is never achieved. Instead, contact and compression are achieved in circumscribed zones (**contact points**), separated by areas where fragment ends are separated by small **gaps**. For example, a compression plate applied across a transverse fracture will generate compression and hence improved contact in the cortex under the plate; conversely, the far cortex becomes the tension side with a small gap produced.

Direct bone healing therefore takes two forms: contact healing and gap healing. In contact healing, bone union and remodelling occur simultaneously whilst in gap healing, they are sequential steps.

In the **first few days**, there is minimal activity in areas of direct contact (**contact healing**); whilst new blood vessels grow into any small gaps that exist (**gap healing**), and mesenchymal cells differentiate into osteoblasts, laying down lamellar bone in small gaps and woven bone in large gaps. Both gap and contact healing differ from secondary bone healing by the absence of resorption of the fracture ends or the formation of callus.

Subsequently, osteoclasts form cutting cones (**Figure 14.2**) that tunnel across the fracture site wherever there is contact between the bone ends or a minute gap. This leaves a path for blood vessels and osteoblasts to follow in their wake, laying down lamellar bone in the form of new osteons. This process of newly formed osteons bridging the gap may take many months and may be difficult to see on an X-ray. This is the same process as the **remodelling phase (stage IV)** of secondary bone healing.

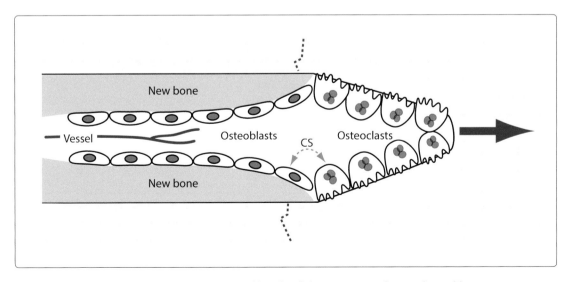

Figure 14.2 Cutting cone. CS, cytokine signals between osteoclasts and osteoblasts, which includes factors such as RANK-Ligand (RANKL).

Secondary (callus) bone healing

This process occurs in the presence of **relative stability** (some controlled motion between fracture surfaces under functional load) and is characterized by the formation of an intermediate callus prior to bone formation (**Figure 14.3**). Strain or movement at the fracture site stimulates secondary healing by two discrete processes:

- **Periosteal bony callus (intramembranous ossification)**: multipotent cells in the periosteum differentiate into osteoprogenitor cells, which produce bone directly without first forming cartilage. This hard callus forms early on at the periphery of the fracture site, providing there has not been extensive periosteal stripping.
- **Fibrocartilaginous bridging callus (endochondral ossification)**: this process occurs simultaneously between the adjacent bone ends and involves the formation of fibrocartilage that becomes calcified and is then replaced by osteoid or woven bone. This process also occurs within the surrounding soft tissues.

Secondary healing is arbitrarily divided into three overlapping stages: **inflammation, repair** and **remodelling** (*Table 14.1*). The passage through different stages of increasing tissue stiffness and strength eventually leads to a biomechanical environment permitting bone formation and union (see Perren's strain theory). The amount of callus produced depends on the stability of the fracture and increases with decreasing stability.

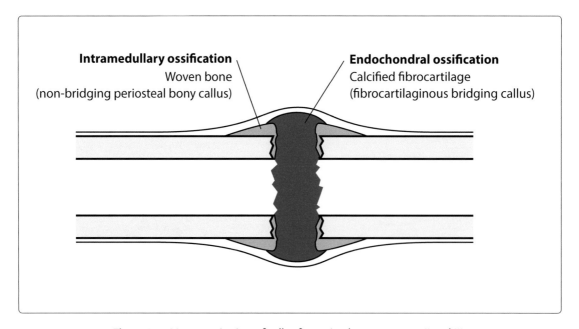

Figure 14.3 Macroscopic view of callus formation between stages II and III.

Table 14.1. Stages of callus formation

Stage	Timescale	Order of events
Stage I Haematoma and inflammation	Up to 1 week	**Haematoma** from ruptured blood vessels forms a fibrin clot. Damaged tissue and degranulated platelets release signalling molecules, growth factors and cytokines
		Migration of inflammatory cells into the haematoma occurs, responding to local growth factors and cytokines (IL-1, IL-6, TGF-β superfamily including BMPs, PDGF, FGF, IGF)
		Proliferation, differentiation and matrix synthesis as haematoma is replaced by granulation tissue. There is capillary in-growth (angiogenesis), recruitment of fibroblasts, mesenchymal cells and osteoprogenitor cells. The periosteum plays an important role in this process
		Cell types involved include polymorphonuclear neutrophils, macrophages and then fibroblasts
		At the necrotic bone ends, bone resorption is mediated by osteoclasts and removal of tissue debris by macrophages
Stage II Soft callus	1–4 weeks	Increased cellularity with proliferation, differentiation and neovascularization
		Callus is a combination of fibrous tissue, cartilage and woven bone
		Intramembranous (bony/periosteal) callus is a primary callus response: Type I collagen (osteoid) is laid down from periosteal osteoblasts in the cambium layer as periosteal bony callus or woven bone. This is hard callus, but it does not bridge the fracture
		Endochondral (fibrocartilaginous/bridging) callus is a bridging external callus: Multipotential cells differentiate to form chondroblasts and fibroblasts within the granulating callus that produce the type II cartilaginous and fibrous elements of the matrix (chondroid). Chondroblasts then calcify the chondroid matrix they have produced, creating calcified fibro-cartilage or soft callus
		Medullary callus: This is a later process and can slowly unite the fracture if external callus fails
Stage III Hard callus	1–4 months	Calcified soft callus is then resorbed by chondroclasts and invaded by new blood vessels. These bring with them osteoblast precursors that produce the bony (type I) elements of the matrix (osteoid) and then mineralize it to form woven bone
		Soft calcified chondroid callus becomes hard mineralized osteoid callus. Bony bridging continues peripherally as subperiosteal new bone formation. At this point the fracture is united; it is solid and painless on movement
Stage IV Remodelling	Up to several years	Once the fracture has united, the hard callus is remodelled from woven bone to hard, dense lamellar bone by a process of osteoclastic resorption, followed by osteoblastic bone formation. The medullary canal reforms at the end of this process
		This is the same mechanism as for direct cortical, osteonal or primary bone healing, seen following fracture fixation with absolute stability
		Bone assumes a configuration and shape based on stresses acting on it (Wolff's law)
		Electrical fields may play a role in Wolff's law, with osteoclastic activity being predominant on the electropositive tension side of bone and osteoblastic activity on the electronegative compression side

BMP: bone morphogenetic protein; FGF: fibroblast growth factor; IL: interleukin; IGF: insulin-like growth factor; PDGF: platelet-derived growth factor; TGF: transforming growth factor.

Fracture healing concepts

There are several concepts in fracture healing that govern whether a fracture unites or not. The traditional biomechanical concept of anatomical reduction and rigid fixation may still hold true for certain fracture types (e.g. intra-articular fractures); however, newer concepts that focus more on the biology of a fracture have surfaced in recent years.

The concept of '**biological osteosynthesis**' emphasizes the role of soft tissue integrity in bone healing and a 'less than rigid' fixation of fractures. The goals of biological fracture fixation are to restore the overall length and alignment of the bone whilst minimizing manipulation of fracture fragments. This principle governs the surgical techniques of minimally invasive plate osteosynthesis (MIPO) and circular frame fixators; whilst newer devices like the dynamic locking screw or far cortical locking screw allow for micro-motion and a less rigid construct. Construct stiffness can be further decreased by increasing the implant's working length or decreasing the number of screws.

The outcome of bone repair may be thought of as a balance between **anabolic** (bone forming) and **catabolic** (bone resorbing) responses, both of which are governed by mechanical, biological (e.g. growth factors and cytokines) and pharmacological (e.g. bone morphogenetic proteins [BMPs], parathyroid hormone [PTH], non-steroidal anti-inflammatory drugs [NSAIDs]) stimuli. The anabolic response produces the sequence of steps that results in the bridging of the fracture by new bone, whilst the catabolic action is an essential component of remodelling of bone during the later stages of repair. Excessive or dysregulated catabolism may, however, impede union.

Similarly, the '**diamond concept**' for biological enhancement of fracture healing pays heed to mechanical stability, osteoprogenitor cells, growth factors and an adequate scaffold to create a 'biological chamber' active enough to support efficiently all the necessary physiological processes for successful union. This theory provides a conceptual framework of what parameters and co-factors a clinician should contemplate when optimizing the bone repair process.

Factors influencing fracture healing

Several factors influence fracture healing (*Table 14.2*).

Non-union

This is defined as **lack of healing** of a fracture within the expected time, which varies with the bone involved, e.g. distal radial fractures are expected to heal by 6 weeks, scaphoid fractures by 8 weeks, tibial fractures by 16 weeks and femoral fractures by 16 weeks.

Clinical union is defined by the absence of tenderness or motion at the fracture site with no pain on loading, while **radiological union** is defined as the presence of visible bridging trabeculae on three out of four cortices on X-rays.

In normal fractures, a certain amount of time is required before bone healing can be expected to occur. This normal time may vary according to age, bone involved, level of the fracture and associated soft tissue injury. **Delayed union**, by definition, is present when an adequate period

Table 14.2. Factors affecting fracture healing

Local	Systemic
Degree of soft tissue trauma	Smoking (affects osteoblast function)
Associated neurovascular injury	Diabetes mellitus
Degree of bone loss	Nutrition
Degree of immobilization	Age
Open fracture or presence of infection	Drugs (steroids, NSAIDs)
Local pathological lesion (e.g. tumour)	Hormones
Type of bone fractured (e.g. tibia, 3–4 months; metacarpal, 4–6 weeks)	Associated head injury (enhances fracture healing)
Site of fracture (metaphysis versus diaphysis)	
Interposition of soft tissue or inadequate reduction	

NSAIDs: non-steroidal anti-inflammatory drugs.

of time has elapsed since the initial injury without achieving bone union, taking into account the above variables.

Hypertrophic non-union

A good blood supply but excessive strain at the fracture site prevents progression of the callus to form bone. These usually require biomechanical stabilization to allow callus progression to bone to occur.

Atrophic non-union

A poor blood supply may be due to soft-tissue damage, periosteal stripping and/or fracture comminution, which may occur at the time of injury or during the exposure for internal fixation. A fracture fixed with rigid fixation (zero strain) and with the fragments distracted will also lack stimulation of callus formation. Atrophic non-unions are more likely to heal following stabilization and biological enhancement.

Bone grafting

Definition

Bone grafting is the use of any implanted material that alone or in combination with other materials promotes a bone-healing response by providing **osteogenic, osteoconductive** or **osteoinductive** activity to a local site. Bone grafts have **mechanical** (providing support) and **biological** (stimulus for bone formation) functions. An ideal bone graft material is one which has osteogenic, osteoinductive and osteoconductive abilities, which is readily available in a range of quantities at low cost and has minimal toxicity and morbidity associated with its use. No bone graft material currently available meets all of these requirements.

Indications

- **Provision of structural stability**: i.e. massive proximal femoral grafting in revision total hip arthroplasty for the reconstruction and/or replacement of skeletal defects.
- **Stimulation of bone formation**: bone grafting in spinal fusions where the graft improves the fusion rate but does not provide any mechanical support, even in the short term.
- **Enhancement of fracture healing**:
  - **acute**: for mechanical or biological reasons, e.g. in comminuted fractures with bone loss;
  - **non-union**: usually for biological reasons.

Properties of bone grafts

Osteogenicity

The graft contains **living precursor cells** that are capable of **differentiation** into bone. Osteogenesis occurs independent of the host bed, i.e. the graft may survive and incorporate successfully, even in a fibrotic, previously irradiated bed.

Osteoconduction

The graft provides a **three-dimensional scaffold** that supports in-growth of capillaries, perivascular tissues and osteogenic cell precursors. The surface of the scaffold allows attachment, division and differentiation of cells and ultimately remodelling. The graft does not have to be biological in order to possess osteoconductive properties. The effectiveness of an osteoconductive material is dependent on factors such as porosity and surface roughness.

Osteoinduction

The graft provides a **biological stimulus** that stimulates mitosis and differentiation of undifferentiated mesenchymal cells into osteoprogenitor cells with the capacity to form new bone. The graft has the ability to promote bone formation at non-skeletal sites and may be added to osteoconductive compounds, but the condition of the host bed is critical. Note that demineralized bone graft has potent osteoinductive properties as it contains several bone BMPs, insulin-like growth factors 1 (IGF-I) and 2 (IGF-II), acidic and basic fibroblast growth factors (FGFs), interleukins, granulocyte colony-stimulating factor (G-CSF) and granulocyte/macrophage colony-stimulating factor (GM-CSF).

Genetics of bone grafts

Autografts

Tissue is harvested from and implanted into the **same individual**. Examples include cancellous, cortical and vascularized grafts and bone marrow.

Allografts

Tissue is harvested from one individual and implanted into **another individual of the same species**. The host is likely to mount an immune response to the cells of a fresh allograft and, therefore, the graft is processed in order to remove immunogenic cells, decreasing the risk of both immune response and transmission of infection. Allografts can be classified according to following:

- **Anatomy**: cortical, cancellous, corticocancellous.
- **Processing**: fresh, frozen, freeze-dried, demineralized bone matrix.
- **Sterilization method**: sterile processing, irradiated, ethylene oxide.
- **Handling properties**: powder, gel, paste/putty, chips, strips/blocks, massive.

Xenografts

Tissue is harvested from one species and implanted into a **different species**. Unfortunately, a vigorous immune response precludes the use of most preparations. Examples include Kiel bone (defatted and deproteinated xenograft, which has a decreased immune response), processed xenograft with autologous bone marrow and processed bovine collagen (biocompatible flexible substrate material, which is a component of several bone graft preparations).

Dangers of bone grafts

- **Autografts**: donor site morbidity (scar, haematoma, infection, pain).
- **Allografts**:
  - disease transmission: both microbiological (e.g. risk of human immunodeficiency virus [HIV] transmission is 1 in 1.5 million, hepatitis C is 1 in 60,000 and hepatitis B is 1 in 100,000) and pathological (e.g. 8% of femoral head allografts have histological evidence of disease such as malignant and benign tumours, such as osteomas);
  - immune sensitization (see below).

Specific graft types

The properties of common bone grafts and bone graft substitutes are shown in *Table 14.3*.

Table 14.3 Properties of common bone grafts and bone graft substitutes

	Immunogenicity	Osteogenic	Osteoconductive	Osteoinductive	Structural	Vascularized
Autograft						
Bone marrow	–	++	–	+	–	–
Cancellous	–	++	++	+	+	–
Cortical (early)	–	+	+	+	++ (early)	–
Vascularized	–	++	+++	+	++	+++
Allografts						
Cancellous	+	–	++	+	+	+
Cortical	+	–	++	+	++	++
Demineralized	+	–	++	++ (BMPs)	–	–
Bone graft substitutes						
Calcium phosphates	–		++		+	+

BMPs: bone morphogenetic proteins; –: none; +: weak; ++: moderate; +++: strong.

Bone grafts

Cortical or cancellous bone grafts may be used. Autologous cancellous bone is considered the 'gold standard'. These may be:

- **Autografts**:
  - harvested and implanted within the same individual, usually fresh and containing a living cell population and associated cytokines and growth factors;
  - problems with donor site morbidity (scar, haematoma, infection, pain) and limited supply;
  - vascularized autografts (e.g. fibula) have significant donor site morbidity but heal like fractures with no initial resorption (cells retain their viability). They are technically difficult to perform but allow rapid union. These grafts are best for **irradiated tissues** and for **large tissue defects**.
- **Allografts**:
  - donor is from the same species;
  - no donor site morbidity;
  - large amounts available;
  - high infection rate (10–12%);
  - cell population is destroyed.
- **Xenografts**:
  - donor from a different species (porcine, bovine);
  - seldom used.

Graft incorporation

This is the process by which invasion of the graft by host bone occurs, such that the graft is replaced partially or completely by host bone. Initial stages of the inflammatory response (with or without a specific immune response), revascularization and osteoinduction are similar for cortical and cancellous bone, but the latter stages of osteoconduction and remodelling are different. The process of incorporation is also different for autografts and allografts. Allograft incorporation is slower and is accompanied by a variable amount of inflammation as a result of the host immune response to the graft. As there is always some genetic disparity, the host accepts most allografts, albeit reluctantly, and incorporates them, although a few may be rejected if there are strong genetic differences. Note that frozen allografts incorporate better than fresh allografts (due to the presence of fewer immunogenic cells) and that allografts can sensitize patients, limiting the options for subsequent organ transplants (less likely with frozen compared with fresh allograft; more likely if more than one bone donor used).

Cancellous graft incorporation

Autogenous non-vascularized cancellous grafts incorporate initially in a manner similar to that for cortical grafts, undergoing an **inflammatory response**. Subsequently, the process is similar to callus formation, with formation of an initial bony scaffold and subsequent remodelling, with all cancellous graft eventually being replaced by **creeping substitution**:

- **Phase 1**: vascular in-growth, chemotaxis and invasion/differentiation of multipotent stem cells. As **revascularization is rapid**, surface osteocytes survive.

- **Phase 2**: osteoblasts (whose formation is induced by factors within the graft) lay down new bone on the scaffold of dead trabeculae, with simultaneous osteoclastic resorption (**creeping substitution**). This leads to early increase in density on X-rays and an associated transient increase in strength.
- **Phase 3**: osteoclast/osteoblast remodelling of the trabeculae along lines of force, with associated **decreased radiodensity**.

Allogenic grafts undergo a similar process, but with a more marked inflammatory phase and less predictable and possibly incomplete incorporation.

Since there is prompt formation of new bone on to the dead scaffold, cancellous grafts achieve early structural strength.

Cortical graft incorporation

Autogenous non-vascularized cortical grafts, after an initial but much slower process of inflammation and revascularization, incorporate in a different manner to cancellous grafts. All donor bone has to be removed before appositional bone formation occurs.

Osteoclastic resorption via cutting cones into the graft has to precede osteoblastic bone formation. Therefore, 40–60% of mechanical strength is lost in the first 3–6 months and returns fully only over 1–2 years. Initial incorporation occurs at the **host–graft junction** via endochondral bone formation. Subsequently, there is new **appositional bone formation** by in-growth of new osteons, following the new blood vessels. In contrast to cancellous grafting, the entire graft is not incorporated and there is no remodelling phase.

Allogenic grafts undergo a similar process, but more slowly and with less overall in-growth. Rarely, allografts may undergo immunogenic destruction following a massive inflammatory response.

Vascularized grafts are autogenous and incorporate in a manner analogous to fracture repair, as similar biological and mechanical conditions prevail. The cells retain their viability.

Factors affecting incorporation

- **Modification of inflammatory response**: use of indomethacin delays response.
- **Mechanical environment of graft**: inadequate mechanical stability of graft leads to formation of granulation tissue and fibrosis.
- **Quality of host bed**: abundance and competence of progenitor cells affects incorporation. Host bed may be deficient in cells if:
  - previous infection;
  - poor vascularity;
  - previous irradiation;
  - immunocompromised host.

Osteochondral allograft

The cartilage component also induces an **immune response** and, therefore, tissue typing is required. Survival of cartilage may be improved by immersion in glycerol or dimethyl sulphoxide. These grafts are used increasingly in tumour surgery.

Bone graft substitutes

- **Cell-based**, bone marrow aspirate contains osteogenic precursors, but this is an inefficient method as most of what is obtained is red blood cells. Modern culture techniques allow mesenchymal stem cells to be isolated from a bone marrow aspirate and cultured *in vitro*, expanding the number of cells. These may be incorporated into osteoconductive grafts.
- **Factor-based**, e.g. BMP-7 and BMP-2 are now produced and sold commercially. Platelets are a rich source of signalling molecules (e.g. platelet-derived growth factor [PDGF], vascular endothelial growth factor [VEGF] and epidermal growth factor [EGF]). Platelet-rich plasma as an autologous additive to bone grafts has been used predominantly in maxillofacial surgery, theoretically supplementing the levels of growth factors.
- **Calcium phosphates:**
  - **bulk**, e.g. tricalcium phosphate (which undergoes partial conversion to hydroxyapatite *in vivo*), hydroxyapatite and combinations of the two. These materials degrade at a very slow rate;
  - **injectable**, e.g. Norian SRS: injectable paste of inorganic calcium and phosphate used to fill bone voids after acute fractures, which hardens in minutes and is osteoconductive. Eventually resorbed and replaced by host bone.
- **Calcium carbonates**, e.g. Biocora™: chemically unaltered marine coral that is resorbed and replaced by bone.
- **Coralline hydroxyapatite**, e.g. Pro-Osteon™: calcium carbonate skeleton undergoes a thermo-exchange process to convert this into calcium phosphate.
- **Calcium sulphate**, e.g. Osteoset™: osteoconductive calcium sulphate pellets.
- **Silicon-based**, e.g. bioactive glasses, glass-ionomer cement: used as delivery systems for osteoinductive compounds.
- **Synthetic polymers**, e.g. polylactic acid and polyglycolic acid: problems include the production of acidic degradation products.
- **Ceramic composites**, the primary inorganic component of bone is hydroxyapatite, and calcium phosphate-based ceramics attempt to mimic this material, e.g. Collagraft™: calcium–collagen graft material – an osteoconductive composite of hydroxyapatite, tricalcium phosphate and collagen used as a bone graft substitute or expander, mixed with autologous bone marrow to provide cells and growth factors.

Osteoinductive agents

Growth factors act as osteoinductive signalling molecules but may have other effects, as detailed below. Some, such as BMPs, are gaining popularity in the clinical arena.

Transforming growth factor-beta

- Super-family of growth factors found in platelets and many cell types.
- Broad range of activity within bone and fracture callus.
- Induces synthesis of type II collagen and proteoglycans.
- Stimulates proliferation/differentiation of osteoblasts and other cell types.
- Stored in bone matrix and released during resorption.

Bone morphogenetic proteins

- Family of at least 20 glycoproteins able to stimulate ectopic bone formation.
- BMPs 2–7 and BMP 9 have been found to possess independent osteoinductive activity.
- Induce differentiation of mesenchymal cells to osteogenic lineages.
- BMP 2 and BMP 7 (OP-1) have been approved for clinical use, such as in tibial non-union.

Fibroblast growth factor

- Mitogenic for many cell types.
- Released from endothelial cells.
- Stimulates angiogenesis and callus formation.

Platelet-derived growth factor

- Potent chemotactic activity following fracture.
- Released from platelets and monocytes after trauma.
- Stimulates deoxyribonucleic acid (DNA) synthesis.

Bone banking

As human bone grafts are available in only limited quantities, bone banks have been set up to provide bone to institutions that require it. The following principles apply to the process of bone banking:

Donor consent

- **Living donors**: consent is needed in order to cover retrieval, testing and access to medical records.
- **Cadavers**: the prerequisite is lack of objection from the next of kin.

Donor screening

- **Medical and behavioural history**: this helps to pick up certain donors that may need to be excluded, e.g. intravenous drug abuse. The history is usually obtained from the next of kin for living donors and from general practitioner notes for cadavers.
- **Blood tests**: performed for hepatitis B and C, HIV, syphilis and Rhesus status.

A dedicated practitioner is required to counsel patients who are to be donors.

Exclusion criteria

- HIV.
- Hepatitis B and C.
- Malignancy.
- Systemic disorders that may compromise biological or biomechanical integrity of graft, e.g. rheumatoid arthritis, autoimmune disease, long-term steroid treatment.
- Diseases of unknown origin, e.g. Alzheimer's disease, Creutzfeldt–Jakob disease, multiple sclerosis.

Allograft processing

Allografts are processed to remove superfluous proteins, cells and tissues in order to decrease immune sensitization and disease transmission. Processing also allows better graft preservation. Techniques may include:

- **Physical debridement** of unwanted tissue.
- **Ultrasonic processing** with or without pulsatile washes to remove remaining cells and blood.
- **Ethanol treatment** to denature cell proteins and reduce bacterial and viral load.
- **Antibiotic soak** to kill bacteria.
- **Irradiation** to sterilize tissue, particularly if contaminated or if not processed in a sterile manner (but this affects collagen and alters mechanical strength).
- **Demineralization**, produced by acid extraction of allograft cortical bone. Demineralized bone matrix (DBM) contains type 1 collagen, which provides the osteoconductive scaffold for osseous in-growth; and osteoinductive growth factors like BMPs, FGF, IGF, PDGF and transforming growth factor-β (TGF-β).

Allograft preservation

Preservation techniques include the following:

- **Fresh**:
  - most immunogenic.
- **Fresh-frozen** at -70°C:
  - has least impact on mechanical strength;
  - decreases immunogenicity;
  - preserves BMPs.
- **Lyophilized** (freeze-dried):
  - least immunogenic;
  - lowest likelihood of disease transmission;
  - BMP depleted;
  - may structurally weaken during rehydration.

Examples of products available from bone banks

- **Fresh-frozen femoral head**: a whole femoral head, retrieved from a living donor, which is unprocessed and greater than 50 g in weight. Available only frozen, and supplied only to hospitals that collect fresh-frozen femoral heads for tissue services when limited stock available.
- **Cancellous cubes**: approximately 1 cm³ in volume. Available freeze-dried and irradiated in packs of five.
- **Cortical struts**: struts of cortical bone from femoral shafts that are cut to various lengths from 2 to 22 cm. Available as freeze-dried or frozen and sterilized by gamma-irradiation.
- **Massive bone allografts**: grafts prepared with articular cartilage and soft tissue removed. Available frozen and irradiated. A small stock of proximal and distal femora and proximal tibiae is normally maintained.

Augmenting fracture healing

In addition to the use of bone grafts, bone-graft substitutes and osteoinductive agents, other techniques used to enhance fracture healing include the following:

Systemic enhancement

Several systemic approaches to enhance fracture healing have been hypothesized, but none of them are in routine clinical use. Examples include IGF-I and IGF-II, growth hormone, PTH, vitamin D3 and prostaglandins.

Distant skeletal injury

Injury to bone marrow enhances bone healing at distant sites. Corticotomy in a long bone has a stimulatory affect on fracture healing elsewhere in the same bone.

Electromagnetic fields

Piezoelectric currents are produced within bone as the collagen fibres are deformed. **Streaming potentials** (electrokinetic currents) are produced as charged constituents of extracellular matrix flow past the mineral phase of bone as it is deformed. The underlying effects of electromagnetic fields (EMs) on cellular responses are not well understood, but *in vitro* exposures of osteoblasts to EMs stimulates the secretion of numerous growth factors including BMPs, TGF-β, and IGF-II, influencing normal bone modelling and remodelling. Clinical devices use electromagnetic induction waveforms to try to reproduce these potentials and so speed up or augment fracture healing.

Low-intensity pulsed ultrasound

There is good evidence that low-intensity pulsed ultrasound (LIPUS) can affect gene expression, stimulate chondroblast and osteoblast activity, enhance blood flow and accelerate or augment fracture healing. Pressure waves from ultrasound may also stimulate differentiating bone lining cells along the edges of a fracture. There is NICE guidance on the use of LIPUS in the management of delayed union and non-union.

Mechanical methods

Controlled axial micromotion has been shown to enhance the healing of tibial fractures, using either intramedullary devices or external fixators.

Summary

Table 14.4 summarizes the advantages and disadvantages of different types of bone grafts and bone-graft substitutes.

Table 14.4. Advantages and disadvantages of bone graft and bone graft substitutes

	Advantages	**Disadvantages**
Autograft	Non-immunogenic No disease transmission Rapid incorporation	Donor site morbidity Limited amounts available
Allograft	More available No donor site morbidity	Allograft immunogenic (fresh ‹ frozen ‹ freeze-dried) Disease transmission Slow incorporation
Fresh	No preservation required	Availability and need may not coincide
Frozen	Simple technique Reduced immunogenicity	Expensive Needs to be transported frozen
Freeze-dried	Easily transported Stored at room temperature	Expensive Structurally weak Less completely incorporated
Xenograft	Unlimited amounts	Immunogenic No osteogenesis unless autograft added
Kiel bone	Reduced immunogenicity	
Bone graft substitutes	Unlimited amounts No disease transmission Biocompatible Osteoconductive Biodegrades No donor site morbidity	Brittle No osteoinduction

---

Viva questions

1. How do fractures heal?
2. What factors affect fracture healing?
3. What are the indications for the use of bone allografts? Are there any precautions to consider?
4. What types of bone graft do you know of? What are their pros and cons?
5. How are allografts processed?

Further reading

Einhorn TA. Enhancement of fracture healing. *J Bone Joint Surg Am* 1995;**77**:940–56.

Giannoudis PV, Einhorn TA, Marsh D. Fracture healing: the diamond concept. Injury 2007;**38**(Suppl. 4):S3–6.

Khan SN, Cammisa FP, Jr, Sandhu HS, et al. The biology of bone grafting. *J Am Acad Orthop Surg* 2005;**131**:77–86.

Little DG, Ramachandran M, Schindeler A. The anabolic and catabolic responses in bone repair. *J Bone Joint Surg Br* 2007;**89**:425–33.

NICE. Low intensity pulsed ultrasound to promote fracture healing. Interventional Procedure Guidance 374 (issued Dec 2010). http://www.nice.org.uk/nicemedia/live/12408/52076/52076.pdf.

Stevenson S, Emery SE, Goldberg VM. Factors affecting bone graft incorporation. *Clin Orthop Relat Res* 1996;**324**:66–74.

Termaat MF, Den Boer FC, Bakker FC, Patka P, Haarman HJ. Bone morphogenetic proteins: development and clinical efficacy in the treatment of fractures and bone defects. *J Bone Joint Surg Am* 2005;**87**:1367–78.

15 | Intervertebral Disc

Will Aston, Alexander Montgomery and Rajiv Bajekal

Introduction

This chapter outlines the structure and function of the intervertebral disc, its biomechanical function and relevance in clinical practice. This level of knowledge is appropriate to the general orthopaedic surgeon.

Embryology

Development of the vertebral column and discs begins in the pre-cartilaginous mesenchymal stage at **week 4** of gestation. The **vertebral body** is formed from sclerotome cells migrating to surround the notochord (**Figure 15.1**). The **intervertebral disc** is formed by contributions from the mesenchymal cells and the **notochord** (which forms the **nucleus pulposus**). The **annulus fibrosus** later surrounds the nucleus pulposus with its circular fibres. A secondary cartilaginous

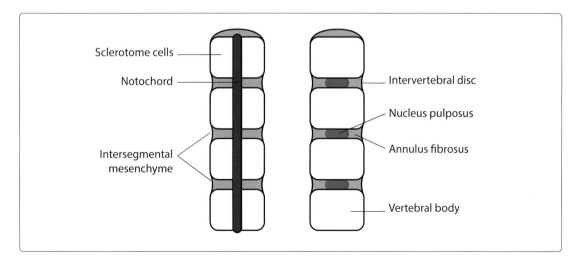

Figure 15.1 Embryological development of the spine from sclerotome cells.

joint between the two vertebral bodies is formed (also known as an **intervertebral symphysis**). Notochord remnants can persist to give rise to **chordomas** in the lumbosacral region and the base of the skull (incidence 1 in 1,000,000). The **vertebral arch** is formed from mesenchymal cells surrounding the neural tube (**Figure 15.2**). The **costal processes**, which later form the ribs, are formed from mesenchymal cells in the vertebral wall. The pre-cartilaginous stage preceeds the **cartilaginous** (week 6) and **bony stage** in the formation of the vertebral column and ossification centres (week 8).

Anatomy

The developed intervertebral disc consists of a tough outer layer (annulus fibrosus) and a soft inner core (nucleus pulposus). The anatomy of the discs vary according to the spinal level. The physiological function of the disc is to **redistribute compressive load, resist tensile, rotational** and **shear forces** and contribute to **vertebral height**.

Annulus fibrosus

The annulus fibrosus (outer layer) consists of **lamellae**, which are densely packed concentric layers of predominantly **type I collagen** orientated at about 30° to the horizontal, in alternating directions. This gives it **high tensile strength** and **resists distractive and shear forces** (**Figure 15.3**). The annulus contains **water** (60% outer, 70% inner annulus), **proteoglycans** and **elastin fibres**, with a high collagen to proteoglycan ratio. It contains **fibroblast-like cells**, which are responsible for producing type I collagen and proteoglycans. **Sharpey's fibres** link the outer annulus to the vertebral end plate forming the **ring apophysis**. The fibrocartilaginous part of the end plate is formed from the inner annulus, which covers the inferior and superior aspects of the disc. Type II collagen and water increase in proportion from the outer annulus towards the inner annulus and transition zone.

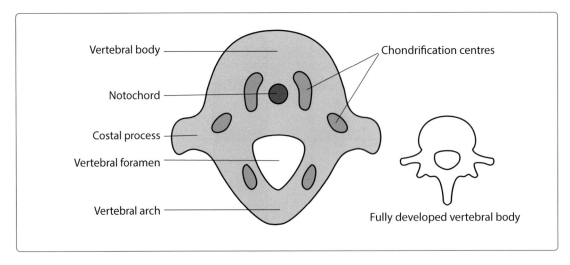

Figure 15.2 The developing spine in axial section.

The **function** of the annulus fibrosus is to contain the radial bulge of the central nucleus pulposus, enabling uniform distribution and transfer of compressive loads between the vertebral bodies. It distends and rotates, facilitating joint mobility.

Nucleus pulposus

The nucleus pulposus represents the inner layer encased by the annulus fibrosus. It consists of **notochordal cells** present at birth, which gradually disappear and are replaced by **chondrocyte-like cells** (present only in adults). These chondrocyte-like cells produce type II collagen and proteoglycans and survive in hypoxic conditions. **Water** (88%) and **type II collagen** are present in a mucoprotein gel rich in polysaccharides. A **proteoglycan matrix** with central hyaluronan filaments and multiple aggrecan molecules (stabilized by link proteins) give it **viscoelasticity, stiffness** and **resistance to compression** through its **hydrophilic** interaction with water. Unlike the annulus, it has a low collagen to proteoglycan ratio.

The **function** of the nucleus pulposus is to maintain vertebral height (**Figure 15.4**) and resist compression through the hydrophilic proteoglycan matrix, ensuring an **even force distribution** to the annulus and vertebral end plates. The vertebral end plate and annulus both contain and restrain the force of the nucleus.

Vertebral end plate

The vertebral end plate consists of **hyaline cartilage in children** and is **highly vascularized**. This decreases dramatically over the first year and by the third decade there are essentially no blood vessels present, increasing the predisposition to degeneration.

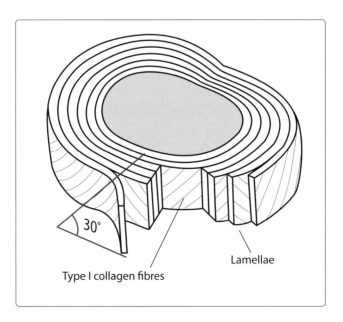

30°

Type I collagen fibres

Lamellae

Figure 15.3 Annulus fibrosus with its concentric lamellae. Collagen fibres are orientated at 30 degrees to horizontal in alternating directions.

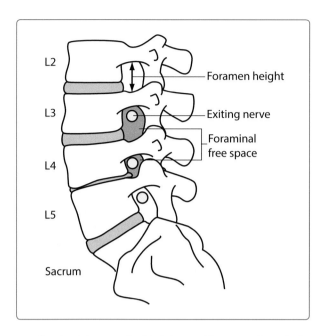

Figure 15.4 Importance of maintaining vertebral height, avoiding neuroforaminal narrowing and nerve root compression. L: lumbar.

The **most superior and inferior regions of the intervertebral discs in a mature adult** are the **cartilaginous vertebral end plates (Figure 15.5)**. They form a 1 mm thick junction between the annulus and the vertebral body. The end plate adjacent to the annulus is primarily composed of **collagen fibres** that are continuous with the disc. The end plate adjacent to the osseous vertebral body however, is primarily made up of **hyaline cartilage**. This latter portion is less adherent, and more prone to separation during trauma. Its **susceptibility to horizontal shear forces** is due to the lack of fibrillar connection with the collagen of the vertebral subchondral bone. The longitudinal ligaments attach to the vertebral bodies and to the intervertebral discs both anteriorly and posteriorly. In the **elderly**, the end plate consists of calcified cartilage.

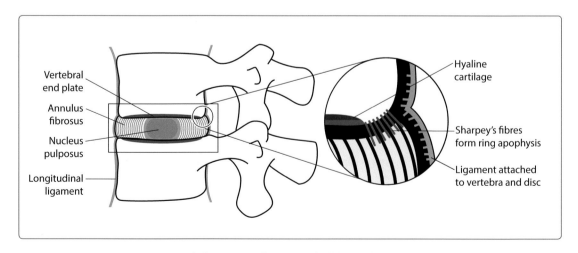

Figure 15.5 Detailed structure of intervertebral disc and vertebral end plate.

Comparative disc anatomy

The height of the discs in the coronal plane increases from the peripheral edges to the centre, appearing as a **biconvex shape** that becomes about 11% larger per segment from cephalad to caudal (from the cervical spine to the lumbosacral articulation).

In the **lumbar and cervical spine** the discs are thicker in the anterior portion contributing to lordosis. L5/S1 is the thickest disc with L4/5 being the largest and most avascular disc. In the **thoracic spine** the discs are uniform in height, and are thicker caudally (possibly allowing greater movement). The thoracic spinal curvature is due to the shape of vertebral bodies.

Nerve supply

In the normal disc, only the **outer annulus** has nerve fibres. In the degenerate disc, extensions of nerve endings enter the nucleus pulposus. The **sinovertebral nerve** (dorsally) and the **sympathetic chain** (ventrally) supply the disc. **Paravertebral muscle** innervation is highly connected to the intervertebral disc (**Figure 15.6**). **Neuropeptides** thought to be involved in **sensory transmission** in the disc are substance P, calcitonin gene-related peptide, vasoactive intestinal polypeptide, and C-flanking peptide of neuropeptide Y (CPON).

Blood supply

The intervertebral disc is **almost completely avascular**, with the capillaries terminating at the vertebral end plates. **Nutrition** reaches the nucleus pulposus by **diffusion** through the **porous central concavity of the end plate** and the porous-permeable solid matrix. The annulus is not porous enough to allow diffusion, but may have some remnant supply from that initially present during development. The disc is supplied by distal branches of the **interosseous arteries** that supply the vertebral body (**Figure 15.7**). **Glycolysis** is the primary means of cellular energy metabolism due to the relatively anaerobic environment. In the **degenerate disc**, normal anastomotic arteries on the anterolateral surface are obliterated and replaced by small, **tortuous arteries**. These changes occur prior to the degenerative process, implying it may be due to ingrowth of vessels from osteophytes.

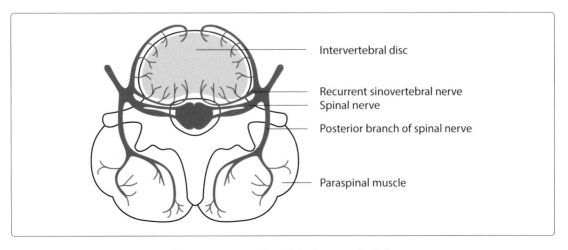

Intervertebral disc

Recurrent sinovertebral nerve
Spinal nerve

Posterior branch of spinal nerve

Paraspinal muscle

Figure 15.6 Innervation of the intervertebral disc.

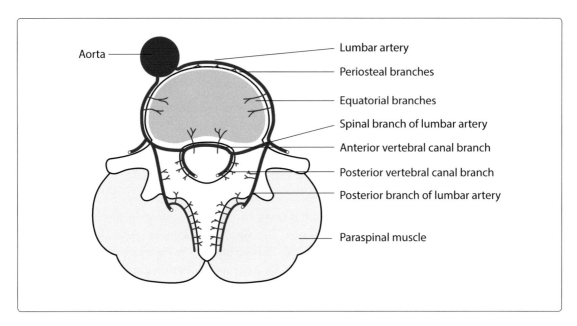

Aorta

Lumbar artery

Periosteal branches

Equatorial branches

Spinal branch of lumbar artery

Anterior vertebral canal branch

Posterior vertebral canal branch

Posterior branch of lumbar artery

Paraspinal muscle

Figure 15.7 Arterial supply of the vertebral body and intervertebral disc.

Biomechanical properties

The **viscoelastic properties** of the disc arise from **hydrostatic pressure in the interstitial fluid**, the **Donnan osmotic pressure** (repulsive forces between fixed negative charges on proteoglycans and also forces arising from freely mobile interstitial counter-ions such as sodium and calcium) and the loose framework of the **porous-permeable collagen–proteoglycan matrix**. These properties are also present in the inner annulus and permit large deformations in response to load, creating intradiscal fluid flows that dissipate energy and viscoelastic creep.

Viscoelasticity ensures that the disc demonstrates **creep** (deformity over time) and **hysteresis** (energy absorption with repetitive axial compression). This property decreases with time. The **biphasic theory** for soft-hydrated biological materials is demonstrated in disc. This is equally applicable to meniscus, articular cartilage, tendon and ligament. The **biphasic phenomenon** for discs relates to the **hoop stresses** generated during compression in the outer layers of the annulus, in comparison with the inner layers, which deform and act as shock absorbers. The **annulus fibrosus** has the **highest tensile stress** whereas the **nucleus pulposus** has the **highest compressive stress**.

Diurnal physiological changes

Intradiscal pressure is lowest when lying supine (sleep), intermediate when standing and highest when sitting and flexed forward with weights in the hands. When you carry a weight, the closer the object is to the body, the lower the pressure.

During sleep, the disc height is restored by the in-flow of water into the discs. Prolonged periods of axial loading (standing, walking) cause interstitial water to be squeezed out of the discs, causing a decrease in height and therefore bulging of the annulus. The latter phenomenon explains why most disc herniations occur in the morning when the disc is loaded on upright posturing.

Herniated nucleus pulposus

Herniation of the nucleus pulposus (**Figure 15.8**) through a **defect in the annulus fibrosus** most often occurs at the insertion of the outer annulus into the vertebral body, where the stresses and motion are greatest. This leads to either bulging of the annulus or herniation of nuclear material, causing spinal cord, thecal or nerve root compression. Symptoms from a herniation mostly resolve with time (90% of patients with painful disc herniations are pain free at 3 months). They are most common in the lumbar and cervical spine.

Nuclear material extrusion is associated with a significant **inflammatory response**. Disc injury results in an increase in the pro-inflammatory molecules, **interleukin-1 (IL-1), IL-8, and tumour necrosis factor (TNF)-alpha**. Macrophages respond to nuclear material in the canal, with substance P (which is associated with pain) also detected. Radicular pain is initially caused by inflammation of the nerve. This explains the lack of correlation between the size of the disc herniation and symptoms. It also explains why most symptoms resolve following activity restriction and anti-inflammatory medication.

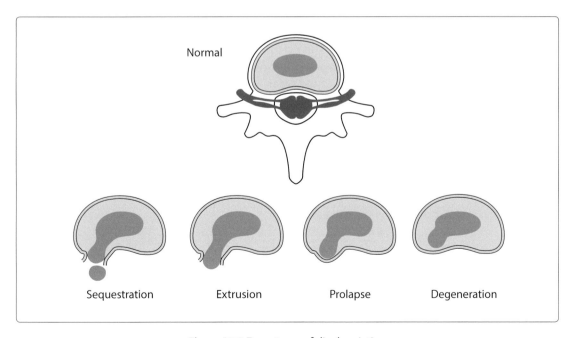

Figure 15.8 Four stages of disc herniation.

Several factors seem to influence the occurrence of herniated nucleus pulposus. **Increases in disc pressure** result from prolonged standing, high mechanical axial loading, chronic coughing and other stresses on the disc. Sitting without lumbar support causes an increase in disc pressures, and **driving** poses a significant risk due to the combination of sitting, vibrations from the road and lifting heavy loads after driving (truck drivers). **Smoking** is a risk factor in the epidemiology of lumbar disc herniations and has been documented to decrease the oxygen tension in the avascular disc.

Intervertebral **disc degeneration** may result in radial tears and leakage of the nuclear material, which leads to neural toxicity. The subsequent inflammatory response often results in neural irritation causing radiating pain without numbness, weakness or loss of reflex, even when neural compression is absent.

Disc degeneration

Disc degeneration occurs due to **pathological** and **non-pathological** (age-related) processes in the disc.

Pathological processes

Smoking and atherosclerosis play a role through a decrease in nutrient supply in the capillaries. **Body weight** and axial disc area are associated with an accelerated degenerative process. **Occupational risks** such as exposure to vibrations and heavy manual labour lead to end plate damage. Patients that are symptomatic have been found to have a **decreased diffusion rates** across the endplate compared to those that are asymptomatic.

The role of **genetic predisposition** is being increasingly recognized as a risk factor. Patients who are diagnosed with herniated discs before the age of 21 years are four to five times more likely to have a significant family history of disc herniation and similar magnetic resonance imaging (MRI) disc degeneration appearances have been noted in monozygotic twins. Genetic variations exist in the degree of synthesis and breakdown of structural components of the disc. Collagen IX encoding genes (*COL9A2, COL9A3*), genes encoding type I collagen (COL1A1-Sp1 binding site), Sox 9 (regulates the genes for **aggrecan**), vitamin D receptor gene and matrix metalloproteinase (MMP)-3 gene are some of those being studied for possible association with disc degeneration.

Degeneration seems to be initiated by an **increase in matrix degradation factors** (like TNF-α, and IL-1) and MMPs, with a **reduction in tissue inhibitors**. The increase in growth factors triggers a reparative process, albeit a poor one.

Non-pathological (age-related) processes

Two key normal processes that occur with natural disc degeneration are **reduced proteoglycan content** within the disc (hence increasing dehydration) and **decreased end plate permeability** (hence decreased metabolic exchange). Type II collagen molecules are replaced by the **denser type I collagen** molecules in the nucleus. These type I molecules tend to cross-link and form even denser tissue that further **inhibits exchange of nutrients and metabolic waste**. By the sixth to seventh decades, the entire disc (apart from the fibrotic outer annulus) often becomes stiff fibrocartilage.

The **annulus**, composed of fibrous connective tissue in infancy, becomes **increasingly hyalinized** with collagen fibres in the first year. By the **third decade** of life the annulus starts showing **fissures**, and by the **fourth decade** an increasing ratio of cell death to cellular proliferation occurs. This leads to an **invasion of vasculature through the clefts and tears**.

The **nucleus** shows **gradual replacement of the notochordal cells with chondrocytes** in the second decade. Subsequent decades show the occurrence of **clefts**, which leads to the formation of **fibrous tissue** later in life. Increased cross-links give the older discs a yellow colour. Matrix synthesis also decreases with aging.

The **end plate** has vasculature up to the third decade. It gets thinned with formation of clefts and fissures in the fourth decade and finally is replaced by fibrocartilage in the sixth decade. The end plates tend to show the earliest changes. The decrease in end plate vasculature in the teens may be the critical factor leading to loss of nutrients and oxygen for the nucleus, leading to further degeneration.

The **blood supply** of the periphery of the disc gradually declines with the onset of adulthood. This is compounded by calcification of the cartilaginous end plates, accumulation of degraded matrix macromolecules and decrease in matrix water concentration, all of which serve to interfere with **nutrient convection and diffusion**.

Stages of degeneration

The degenerative process can be divided into three main stages: **dysfunction, instability** and **restabilization**.

Dysfunction involves outer annular tears and separation of the end plate, cartilage destruction and facet synovial reaction. The **instability** stage follows, in which disc resorption and loss of disc space height occur. An initial weakness of the annulus spreads to lead to global disc degeneration, loss of restraint of the nucleus and inability of the disc to oppose extrinsic forces. This results in bulging, herniation and decreased disc height. Facet capsular laxity may follow, leading to subluxation. In the stage of **restabilization**, the progressive degenerative changes lead to facet hypertrophy and ligamentum buckling, osteophyte formation and stenosis.

Disc repair

Injury to the disc causes an **inflammatory cascade** that leads to build up of lactic acid, increased secretion of proteolytic enzymes, decreased proteoglycan production, decreased hydration and cell apoptosis. Intervertebral discs have a very **limited capacity to heal** following injury. The outer portion of the annulus is vascularized and heals through an inflammatory process. There is an insufficient quantity or quality of collagen to replace any structural damage. Inflammatory tissue that lacks the tensile strength of collagen may form from large tears.

Pain from a degenerate disc

The complex processes that occur during degeneration of the disc may account for the variability in symptomatic response. Following the influx of **inflammatory mediators** into the annulus, there is **proliferation of nerves and blood vessels** deeper into the disc, allowing for nociception in areas with no prior innervation. Influx of inflammatory mediators, such as **TNF, substance P** and **interleukins** can lead to the symptoms of pain from the degenerating disc.

MRI of the disc

A normal disc has a high signal on T2-weighted imaging in the nucleus. The signal characteristics of the disc in T2-weighted MRIs reflect changes caused by aging or degeneration. The brightness of the nucleus has been shown to correlate directly with the proteoglycan concentration, but not with the water or collagen. Other MRI findings associated with degeneration include disc space narrowing, herniation, stenosis, facet hypertrophy and ligamentum buckling, rotational changes on axial views (indicating possible scoliosis) and scoliosis on coronal views. Changes in the signal intensity of the adjacent vertebral body marrow are described as Modic changes.

Recent advances in the understanding of intervertebral disc biology have led to increasing interests in the development of biological treatments aimed at disc regeneration. Growth factors, gene therapy, stem cell transplantation and biomaterials-based tissue engineering may, in the future, allow for intervertebral disc regeneration by overcoming the limitations of the self-renewal mechanisms.

Viva questions

1. What type of joint is present between two vertebrae?
2. What is the function of an intervertebral disc?
3. How does the microscopic anatomy of the disc relate to its function?
4. What is an annular tear, and how does it differ from herniation?
5. Disc degeneration inevitably occurs with age. What changes occur during this process?

Further reading

Boos N, Weissbach S, Rohrbach H, et al. Classification of age-related changes in lumbar intervertebral discs: 2002 Volvo Award in basic science. *Spine* 2002;**27**:2631–44.

Buckwalter JA. Aging and degeneration of the human intervertebral disc. *Spine* 1995;**20**:1307–14.

Gruber HE, Hanley EN, Jr. Recent advances in disc cell biology. *Spine* 2003;**28**:186–93.

Kadow T, Sowa G, Vo N, Kang JD. Molecular basis of intervertebral disc degeneration and herniations: What are the important translational questions? *Clin Orthop Relat Res* 2015;**473**(6):1903–12.

Kaplan KM, Spivak JM, Bendo JA. Embryology of the spine and associated congenital abnormalities. *Spine* 2005;**5**:564–76.

Roberts S. Disc morphology in health and disease. *Biomed Soc Trans* 2002;**30**:864–9.

16 Basic Concepts in Biomechanics

Manoj Ramachandran and Paul Lee

Introduction

The workings of the musculoskeletal system, although complex, can be understood using basic laws of mechanics. A working knowledge of biomechanics is essential for the orthopaedic surgeon. Material and fluid mechanics are dealt with in Chapters 17 and 25, respectively.

Biomechanics is the branch of science dealing with the action and effects of internal and external forces on living biological systems using the principles and techniques of engineering and mechanics. Biomechanics involves the study of:

- **Statics**: study of forces acting on rigid bodies in equilibrium, either at rest or moving at a constant velocity.
- **Dynamics**: study of forces acting on rigid bodies in motion, of which there are three subtypes:
  - **kinetics**: study of forces acting on a rigid body and the resulting motion;
  - **kinematics**: study of motion of a rigid body with no concern of the forces that cause the motion;
  - **kinesiology**: study of human movement.

Background

Since early civilizations, humans used their body parts and environmental elements to define measurements, and the British (or Imperial) system evolved similarly. For example, the yard (Saxon word gird) was originally the circumference of a person's waist, but later the distance from King Henry I's nose to the end of his thumb. Subsequently, standard references were used by royal decrees, and the yard was defined as the length of a permanent measuring iron stick during King Edward I's reign; in 1824, a brass bar with a gold button at each end was legalized by the British Parliament as the standard yard.

In 1790, during the French Revolution, the French Academy of Sciences established the metric system. The metre was defined as one ten-millionth of the distance from the North Pole to the equator on a line passing through Paris, with other linear measurements being decimal fractions of the metre. Although Napoleon renounced the metric system in 1812, the system was later adopted as the international standard and formalized as le Systéme International d'Unitès (SI units) in 1960 (*Table 16.1*). Definitions of base units nowadays have become more sophisticated, e.g. the metre was defined as the wavelength of radiation emitted from the krypton-86 atom and then redefined in 1983 as the distance travelled by light in a vacuum in 1/299,792,458 of a second.

SI units

SI units consist of three groups:

- **Base units**, e.g.:
  - metre (m) for length;
  - kilogram (kg) for mass;
  - second (s) for time.
- **Derived units**, e.g.:
  - area (m^2);
  - volume (m^3);
  - speed (m/s);
  - acceleration (m/s^2);
- **Derived units with special names**, e.g.:
  - force ($kg\,m/s^2$) = newton (N);
  - moment (Nm).

Table 16.1 Conversion of Imperial to SI units

Unit	SI Imperial Conversion		
Length	Metre (m)	Foot (ft)	1 ft = 0.3048 m
Mass	Kilogram (kg)	Pound-mass (lbm)	1 lbm = 0.454 kg
Temperature	Celsius (°C)	Fahrenheit (°F)	°F = (9/5) × °C + 32
Time	Second (s)	Second (s)	1 s = 1 s
Force	Newton (N = kg × m/s²)	Pound-force (lbf) = (1 lbm × g [where g = acceleration due to gravity])	1 lbf = 4.448 N
Pressure	Pascal (Pa = N/m²)	Pounds per square inch	1 psi = 6895 Pa
Energy	Joule (J = N × m)	Foot pounds (Ft-lb)	1 ft-lb = 1.356 J
Power	Watt (W = J/s)	Horsepower (hp)	1 hp = 7457 W

Note that there are two broad types of unit: scalar and vector. **Scalar units** have magnitude but no direction, e.g. length, mass, time, area, volume, speed. **Vector units** have both magnitude and direction, e.g. acceleration, force, moment. Velocity is a vector as it has both magnitude (speed) and direction. Vectors, in addition to **magnitude** (length of the vector) and **direction** (head of the vector in degrees), are also characterized by their **point of application** (tail of the vector) and **line of action** (orientation of the vector).

Newton's laws

The unit of force was named after the English scientist Sir Isaac Newton (1642–1727), whose work on gravitation was allegedly inspired by an apple falling from a tree on to his head (interestingly, 1 N is approximately equivalent to the weight of a medium-sized apple, i.e. approximately 0.1 kg, and is defined as a force magnitude capable of producing an acceleration of 1 m/s² to a rigid body with 1 kg of mass). Newton's fundamental equations of physical laws are key to understanding biomechanics as related to human movement.

Newton's first law (inertia)

A body at rest will remain at rest, and a body in motion will remain in motion at a constant velocity in a straight line. This requires the sum of the external forces acting on the body to be zero (i.e. the body is in equilibrium), and so static analysis can be performed with the help of the equations $\Sigma \mathbf{F} = \mathbf{0}$ (sum of forces is zero) and $\Sigma \mathbf{M} = \mathbf{0}$ (sum of moments is zero).

Newton's second law (action)

A body with a non-zero net force will accelerate in the direction of the force, the magnitude of the acceleration being proportional to the magnitude of the force ($\mathbf{F} = m\mathbf{a}$). This is useful for dynamic analysis.

Newton's third law (reaction)

For every action, there is an equal and opposite reaction. The forces of action and reaction are equal in magnitude but in the opposite direction. This law is important for free-body analysis and understanding ground-reaction forces.

Trigonometry

A basic knowledge of trigonometry is helpful in biomechanical analysis. The mnemonic **sohcahtoa** is helpful in remembering that for the angle θ in **Figure 16.1**:

- $\sin\theta$ = opposite/hypotenuse;
- $\cos\theta$ = adjacent/hypotenuse;
- $\tan\theta$ = opposite/adjacent.

It also helps to remember the following approximations:

- sin 30° = cos 60°; approx 0.5;
- sin 45° = cos 45°; approx 0.7;
- sin 60° = cos 30°; approx 0.9.

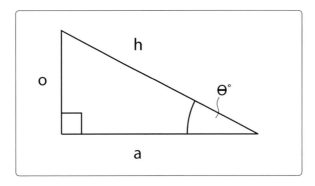

Figure 16.1. Basic trigonometry. a: adjacent; o: opposite; h: hypotenuse.

Moment of force

Force

A **force** is a **mechanical disturbance** or **load** that acts on a body. In its most basic form, a force can either be a push or a pull. Forces can be **external** to the human body (e.g. gravity, ground reaction, air resistance) or **internal** to the human body (e.g. joint contact and shear forces, muscle contraction forces, tendon forces, capsuloligamentous constraint forces). As forces are vectors, they are usually represented by a **boldface** letter or a letter with an arrow, or bar over it. Vectors can be resolved into their component vectors in the x, y and z planes, which are mutually perpendicular Cartesian coordinate axes:

$$\mathbf{F} = (f_x, f_y, f_z)$$

Use of the Pythagorean theorem allows the magnitude of the force F, denoted by |F|, to be calculated:

$$|\mathbf{F}|^2 = F_x^2 + F_y^2 + F_z^2$$

Two forces can be added using the parallelogram method (or graphic) of vector addition, where the two vectors are represented pictorially as two sides of a parallelogram and a third arrow is drawn along the diagonal (**Figure 16.2**).

We can also add vectors by connecting the tail of one vector to the tip of the other (tail-to-tip method).

When three forces act upon a body, and the body is in equilibrium, the three forces can be drawn to scale in their correct directions to form a closed triangle. This is useful, because when the magnitude and direction of two of the forces are known and the triangle is drawn to scale, the third force can be calculated with ease.

Moment

The **moment** of force is the effect of a force at a perpendicular distance from an axis, which results in rotational movement and angular acceleration.

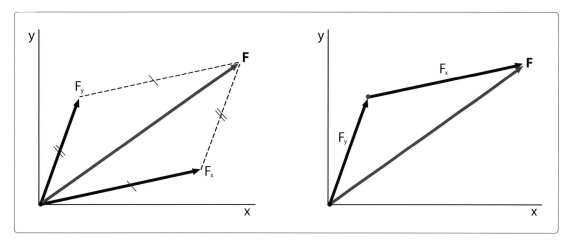

Figure 16.2. Parallelogram of vector addition.

$$M_O = Fd$$

where M_O is the moment of force about axis O, **F** is the magnitude of the force and **d** is the moment arm or perpendicular distance from the axis of rotation to the line of force.

The **magnitude** of a moment is known as **torque**. Torques generated by the body translate skeletal flexor and extensor muscle contraction into rotational movements of limbs about joints.

Levers

In essence, the musculoskeletal system is a collection of lever systems linked together. There are three types of lever systems in the body. The difference lies in where the **fulcrum** (i.e. the **joint**) and applied **forces** (F) are in relation to the **load** (L) (**Figure 16.3**):

- **First-class lever**: the fulcrum lies in **between** the applied force and the load. Mechanical advantage is gained by increasing the force arm length in relation to the load arm length. An example is the atlanto-occipital joint as the fulcrum, with the weight of the head as the load and the counter-force being applied by the erector spinae muscles. An everyday example is the use of a pair of scissors.
- **Second-class lever**: the fulcrum is at **one end** of the lever, with the applied load force at the other end and the load in between. The force arm length is always greater than the load arm length. An example is the act of standing on one's toes, with the toes as the fulcrum, the weight of the ankle offering resistance being the load, and the counter-force being applied by the calf muscles. An everyday example is the use of a nutcracker.
- **Third-class lever**: the fulcrum is at **one end of the lever, but the load is at the other end**, with the applied force in between. The load arm length is always greater than the force arm length, and so a greater force is needed to move the load. This is the most common type of lever found in the human body. An example is the elbow joint as the fulcrum, with the load being any object held in the hand and the elbow flexors providing the counterforce. An everyday example is using a shovel.

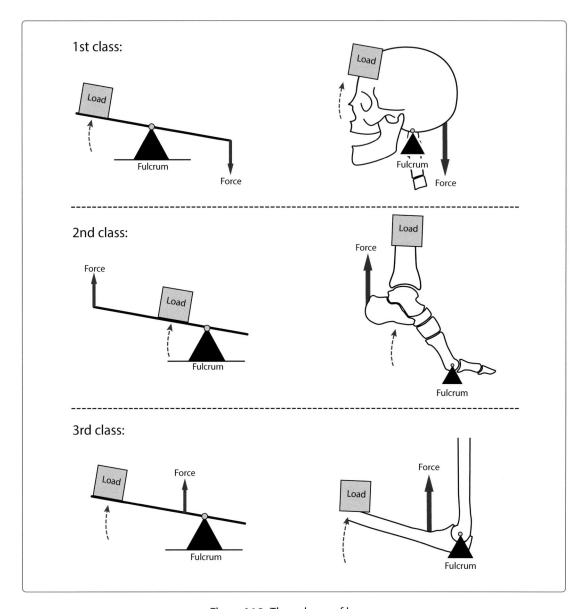

Figure 16.3. Three classes of lever.

Force couple

The final basic concept is that of a **couple**, which is a moment created by **equal, non-collinear, parallel** and an **oppositely directed pair of forces**, e.g. the effect of two hands on a steering wheel or two fingers twisting off a bottle cap. Note that collinear forces act along the same line. A couple is a free pure moment vector with no resultant force. Couples are useful for understanding the effects of muscle action about joints, for example upper trapezius and serratus anterior on scapular rotation.

Statics

Static equilibrium

From Newton's first law (inertia), an object is in **static equilibrium** if the sum of all the forces acting on it is balanced (i.e. no linear acceleration occurs, as $\Sigma F = 0$) and all the moments acting on it are balanced separately from the forces (i.e. no angular acceleration occurs, as $\Sigma M = 0$). Balance of forces is termed **translational equilibrium**, since forces will translate the object, while balance of moments is termed **rotational equilibrium**, since moments will rotate the body. The best way to state the required balance of forces and moments is to break down the force balance equations into their x, y and z components. The resulting equations for forces ($\Sigma F_x = 0$, $\Sigma F_y = 0$, $\Sigma F_z = 0$) and moments ($\Sigma M_x = 0$, $\Sigma M_y = 0$, $\Sigma M_z = 0$) can be used to solve for unknown forces and moments in a given plane. Biological systems are rarely in equilibrium, but static analysis is a useful tool in estimating unknown musculoskeletal forces that balance the known forces in a system at rest.

In **statically determinate** systems, the number of unknown forces and moments is equal to the number of equations available (six equations in three dimensions – force equilibrium in the x, y and z directions and moment equilibrium in the x, y and z axes), thus allowing the unknown forces to be calculated. In **statically indeterminate systems**, there are more unknowns than available equations, and therefore there are no unique solutions. Unfortunately, in orthopaedic biomechanics, the latter situation is prevalent when determining muscle and joint forces, as a large number of muscles span each joint. Approaches to this problem include reduction and optimization methods, the former being used more commonly in order to reduce the number of unknowns to equal the number of equations, e.g. the concept of a **single equivalent muscle** allows forces around a joint to be calculated. A common line of action first represents a group of muscles, e.g. elbow flexors, the moment arm and angle of pull are estimated, and finally, assuming that a single equivalent muscle generates the net joint moment, the muscle force can be calculated as:

Muscle force (F) = net moment (M_0)/moment arm (d)

Static analysis

Static analysis by **free-body diagram** is a method of determining the forces and moments acting on a body by isolating that body part and ensuring that it is in static equilibrium. As forces and moments are vectors, they must sum up to zero in each of three perpendicular directions. Therefore, in the x, y and z dimensions, there are six equations of equilibrium (see above), allowing a maximum of six unknowns to be solved.

A number of assumptions are involved in free-body analysis in order to estimate important joint or muscle forces:

- The musculoskeletal system model assumes that the **bones are rigid rods** (they do not stretch, compress or deform, regardless of the forces and moments acting on them) and the **joints are rigid frictionless hinges**.
- There is **no antagonistic muscle action**.
- The **weight** of the body is concentrated at the exact **centre of the body mass**.

- Only **external forces** and moments acting on the free body are usually considered. **Internal forces are assumed to cancel each other out**.
- Muscles are assumed not to exert compressive forces and, therefore, **act only in tension**.
- The line of action of the muscle is along the centre of **cross-sectional area of muscle mass**.
- Joint reaction forces are assumed to be only **compressive**, as tensile forces would lead to loss of contact of the joint surfaces.
- The joint acts as only a **hinge**, ignoring other possible axes of rotation and translation.

Examples of free-body diagram analysis can be found in the relevant chapters on the biomechanics of individual joints. For rigid bodies subjected to concurrent forces (where all forces intersect at one point), when these forces are joined from tip-to-tail in any sequence, all the force vectors must form a closed polygon. This **static analysis by graphical method** can be used to solve for unknown forces within a concurrent force system.

Dynamics: kinetics

Basic concepts

Work (W) is the product of force acting along the direction of displacement (only components parallel to the displacement) and the displacement of a rigid body in motion. The unit of work is the newton-metre (Nm) or joule (J), i.e. work = force × distance. **Energy** is the ability to perform work and is measured in joules or newton-metres. Using the law of conservation of energy, energy is neither created nor destroyed but instead is transferred from one type to another (i.e. the sum of all energies is constant). It is important to understand the following:

- **Potential energy (E_p)**: the potential of a body to do work due to its position (e.g. height) or configuration (strain energy), i.e. stored energy.
- **Kinetic energy (E_k)**: the amount of work required in order to stop a body moving at velocity v or to move a body from rest to velocity v. For a rigid body with mass m, $E_k = 1/2mv^2$. It is assumed that no energy is dissipated through friction (f), which is the opposing force created by two bodies as they slide over each other.

Power (P) is the work done per unit time and is measured in joules per second, or watts. **Momentum** (L) is equal to the product of a body's mass and velocity, i.e. $L = mv$. **Mass moment of inertia** (I) is the tendency of a rigid body to resist rotation (as opposed to pure mass, which tends to resist translation). The mass moment of inertia depends on the magnitude of the mass and its geometric distribution. The further the mass is distributed from its centre of rotation, the larger the mass moment of inertia.

Kinetic analysis

In general, **direct dynamic problems** (DDP) predict motion of rigid bodies from known forces, while **inverse dynamic problems** (IDP) involve the calculation of forces from known motions.

In a dynamic (non-equilibrium) situation, the forces acting on a rigid body will accelerate the body (i.e. increase its velocity). **Linear forces** cause linear acceleration ($\sigma F = ma$), while **moments about an axis of rotation** cause angular acceleration ($\sigma M = I\alpha$ where α is the angular acceleration). These equations can be used to solve for unknown forces and moments acting on rigid bodies in motion, similar to equations of equilibrium in static analysis.

In reality, calculating forces and moments for the human body is far more difficult, as the accelerations of different parts of the body must be taken into account. The body is usually divided into segments linked together (**link-segment model**), and the forces, moments and accelerations of each segment are calculated separately from distal to proximal, either using mathematical equations (**indirect method**) or using devices such as accelerometers, magnetic tracking systems and optoelectronic motion analysis systems (**direct method**).

Dynamics: kinematics

Joint kinematics

Degrees of freedom (DOF) are defined as the number of independent modes of motion in a joint. In two dimensions, a free joint has three DOF: translation in x direction, translation in y direction and rotation in z direction. A free joint in three dimensions would have six DOF: three in translation and three in rotation along the x, y and z axes. Closely packed hinge joints (e.g. the ulno-humeral joint) have one DOF, universal joints have two DOF, and ball-and-socket joints (e.g. the hip) have three DOF, all in rotation.

There is a direct relationship between DOF and joint constraint forces. In two dimensions, the total number of DOF and constraint forces is three (i.e. one DOF has two associated joint constraint forces); for example, in the sagittal plane, the proximal interphalangeal joint has one DOF (flexion-extension) and two constraint forces (axial compression and palmar-dorsal shear). In three dimensions, the total number of DOF and constraint forces is six; for example, the wrist joint has two DOF (flexion-extension and radial-ulnar deviation) and four constraint forces (axial compression, medial-lateral shear, volar-dorsal shear and axial rotational torque).

Pure linear, or **translational**, motion of a rigid object occurs when all points on that object move the same distance. However most musculoskeletal joints do not articulate in a pure translational motion but in a **rotational motion** where one point on a bone remains stationary (the **centre of rotation or COR**), and all other points rotate around this point (**Figure 16.4**). For three-dimensional motion, the COR would be replaced by an axis of rotation, and there could also be translation along this axis.

Joint kinematics are even more complex, as joints undergo two kinds of motion:

- **Gross joint motion**: used to study joint function and to calculate forces and moments passing through the joint centre under dynamic conditions.

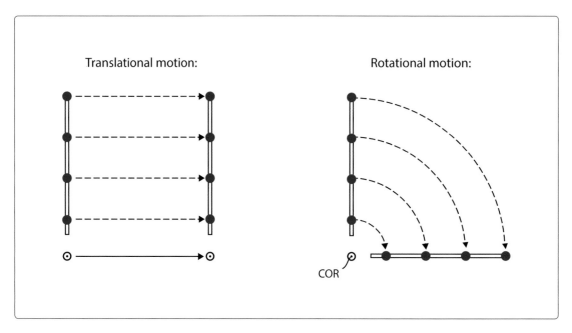

Figure. 16.4 Translational vs. rotational motion. COR: centre of rotation.

- **Articulating surface motion**: of three types, although a combination of all three is found in most anatomic joints (**Figure 16.5**):
  - **rotation**: the circular body rotates on a flatter surface;
  - **rolling**: contact points on circular and flat surfaces constantly change but remain at a constant zero velocity, i.e. no slip occurs. The circular surface undergoes a relative motion of translation and rotation on the flat surface. As the contact point changes constantly, this type of motion leads to the least amount of wear;
  - **gliding**: pure translation, in which one surface is flat and the contact point on the circular surface does not change (like it does on the flat surface).

Rigid-body kinematics

The position of a moving object (again assumed to be a rigid body) can be defined relative to a reference frame, usually in the x–y plane. Two reference points are sufficient to define an object's position in the x–y plane at a given time (three points are need for a three-dimensional position). If these two points are moving in the same direction, translation occurs. If the two points are moving in two different directions, both translation and rotation occur. **Linear velocity** is denoted v (units of m/s), while **angular velocity** (i.e. rotational velocity) is denoted by ω (units of radians/s). The motion of any rigid body can be defined by a combination of translation and rotation. Further knowledge of rigid-body kinematics is beyond the level expected for any exit examination.

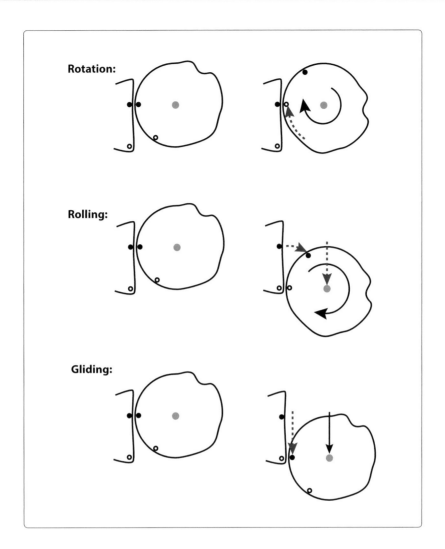

Figure 16.5. Three types of articulating surface motion.

Viva questions

1. What are the three Newton's physical laws relevant to orthopaedics?
2. What is a force?
3. What is a moment?
4. Draw a free-body diagram of the x joint (where x can be any large joint in the human body).
5. What are the assumptions made when performing free-body analysis?

Further reading

Burstein AH, Wright TM (eds). Fundamentals of Orthopaedic Biomechanics. Baltimore, MD: Williams & Wilkins, 1994.

Cochrane GVB. A Primer of Orthopaedic Biomechanics. New York, NY: Churchill Livingston, 1982.

Fung YC (ed). Biomechanics: Mechanical Properties of Living Tissues, 2nd edn. New York, NY: Springer-Verlag, 1993.

Mow VC, Hayes WC (eds). Basic Orthopaedic Biomechanics, 2nd edn. New York, NY: Lippincott-Raven, 1997.

Nordin M, Frankel VH (eds). Basic Biomechanics of the Musculoskeletal System, 2nd edn. Philadelphia, PA: Lea and Febiger, 1989.

Oatis C (ed). Kinesiology: Mechanics and Pathomechanics of Human Movement, 2nd edn. New York, NY: Lippincott Williams & Wilkins, 2008.

17 Biomaterial Behaviour

Subhamoy Chatterjee, Toby Baring and Gordon Blunn

Introduction

In order to describe biomaterials accurately, we must understand the basic concepts of material behaviour. In this chapter, we describe the basic concepts of stress, strain, strength, deformation and failure as applied to biomaterials. For the purposes of any orthopaedic examination, you should be able to reproduce a stress–strain curve and explain its salient features. You should also be able to explain the mechanics of bending and torsional forces on simple constructs such as plates and nails. The concepts of tribology (friction, lubrication, corrosion and wear) are covered in Chapter 25.

Basic principles

All materials can be described by their stress–strain behaviour. The force applied can be compressive, tensile, bending or shear, and in many cases the mechanical properties can vary according to the direction in which forces are applied. For example, cortical bone, due to the columnar structure of its osteons, is extremely strong in axial loading (compression) but is not as strong against transverse forces (bending).

Stress = force applied to a material per unit area

Materials that behave identically, irrespective of the direction of the applied force, such as most orthopaedic metals, alloys, polymers and woven bone, are termed **isotropic**. However, almost all living tissues, including cortical bone and some composite biomaterials, display directionally-dependent behaviour and are termed **anisotropic**.

Tensile stresses occur when two forces pull away from each other along the same line, while **compressive stresses** occur when two forces push towards each other along the same line.

When a material is subjected to a force, strain is the change in length of a material with respect to its original length. Technically, strain has no units, as it is normalized with respect to the original length. Commonly, however, stress is referred to either in millimetres per millimetre or as a percentage. Strain is a relative measure of the deformation of a body as a result of loading.

Strain = change in length/original length

However, strain does not take into account the cross-sectional area of the material being tested. So, in order to characterize a material more completely, we combine the properties of stress and strain in terms of a stress–strain curve that eliminates the variables of initial material length and material cross-sectional area. Stress–strain curves, however, are still different for anisotropic materials, as the curve varies according to the direction of the force applied. **Young's modulus** (Thomas Young was a physician before turning his mind toward physics), or the **elastic modulus**, is found by **dividing the stress by the strain over the linear portion of the stress–strain curve**. As a result, the Young's modulus for an isotropic material is constant. Note that the units of Young's modulus are Newtons per square metre and in Système International (SI) units 1 N/m^2 is equal to 1 pascal (Pa).

Summary

- **Stress = force per unit area applied (N/m^2).**
- **Strain = change in length with respect to original length.**
- **Young's (elastic) modulus E = stress/strain (N/m^2).**
- **Isotropy: material behaves similarly in all directions of application of force.**

The Young's modulus for common materials is shown in *Table 17.1*. A useful approximation is shown next to the true figures. The modulus is the constant, which quantifies the **linear relationship between stress and strain over the linear portion of the graph**. This relationship is known as **Hooke's law**.

Table 17.1 Young's modulus of common orthopaedic materials

Material	Young's modulus (GPa)	Approximate values
Cartilage	0.02	0.02
Tendon	0.4	0.5
Cancellous bone	0.005–1.5	1
UHMWPE	1.2	1
PMMA bone cement	2.2	2
Cortical bone	12–24	20
Titanium alloy	110	100
Stainless steel	190	200
Cobalt chrome	210	200

PMMA, polymethylmethacrylate; UHMWPE, ultra-high-molecular-weight polyethylene.

Stress–strain curve

A typical stress-strain curve for a ductile material is shown in **Figure 17.1**. Key features are described below.

Elastic portion

Here, the stress-strain relationship is linear and Hooke's law is obeyed. The Young's modulus can be determined from the gradient of the line in this region of the graph. All the deformation present in this portion of the graph is **elastic**, i.e. recoverable. The stiffness of the material increases as the gradient of the line becomes steeper. Note that a linear elastic material is insensitive to the rate of loading.

Plastic portion

At this point in the graph, further deformity is no longer recoverable, i.e. it is **plastic**. This commences at the **yield point** (where there is a dramatic increase in strain with little increase in stress) and then a region where **strain hardening** occurs. The **yield stress** is defined as the **stress necessary to produce a specific amount of permanent deformation**, i.e. 0.002 (**0.2%**). Note that in orthopaedics, the proportionality limit, the elastic limit (which is a little further along the curve, where Hooke's law is not obeyed, beyond the elastic limit but where elastic recovery can occur) and yield stress are all very close together and so are taken to be the same, i.e. the yield point.

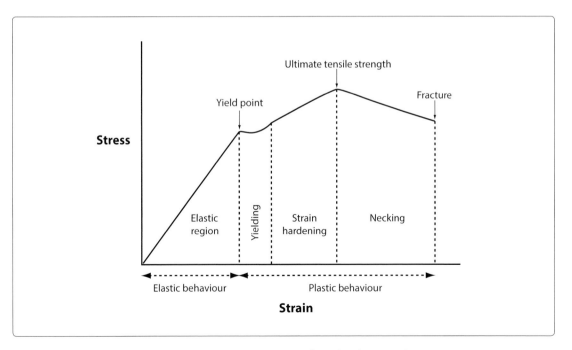

Figure 17.1 Stress–strain curve for a ductile material.

Where the graph ends abruptly, the material's integrity is breached and it is therefore fractured. The stress level at which this happens is termed the **fracture stress**. Sometimes this almost coincides with the maximum amount of stress the material can withstand before which fracture is imminent, and is termed the **ultimate tensile stress**.

Other terms

- **Ductility**: ductile materials undergo a large amount of plastic deformation before failure, e.g. metals.
- **Brittleness**: brittle materials **do not deform plastically but display elastic behaviour right up to failure**, e.g. ceramics. In brittle materials, the yield stress is almost equivalent to the fracture stress.
- **Stiffness: deflection under a given load**. The steeper the stress–strain curve, the stiffer the material. The less steep the curve, the more flexible the material.
- **Strain energy: area under the stress–strain curve**. Combines recoverable strain energy (elastic region of the curve) and absorbed strain energy (plastic region of the curve).
- **Toughness: amount of energy per unit volume that a material can absorb before failure**. This value is also related to the area under the stress–strain curve. When comparing brittle and ductile materials with the same ultimate tensile strengths, the brittle material is less tough, as it has less area under its stress–strain curve.
- **Strength**: a somewhat imprecise term that can be said to represent the degree of resistance to deformation of a material. **A material is strong if it has a high ultimate tensile strength**.
- **Hardness: surface property of a material; ability of a material to resist scratching and indentation on the surface**. Its value is not determined from the stress–strain curve, but it does influence the durability and machinability of the material.

Stress–strain curve lexicon

- **Gradient of elastic region**: stiff if steep, flexible if shallow.
- **Extent of plastic deformation**: ductile if long, brittle if short.
- **Ultimate tensile strength**: strong if high, weak if low.
- **Area under the curve**: tough if large, not tough if small.

Fatigue failure and notch sensitivity

Fatigue failure refers to **failure of a material with repetitive loading at stress levels below the ultimate tensile strength**. It is worth knowing the *S–n* curve (**Figure 17.2**), where stress (*S*) on the y-axis is plotted against number (*n*) of cycles (millions) on the x-axis.

The **endurance limit** is defined as the **stress at which the material can withstand 10 million cycles without experiencing fatigue failure**. Clinically, total hip replacements operate above the endurance limit, while total knee replacements operate at the endurance limit, especially the polyethylene component, predisposing the latter to fatigue failure.

Notch sensitivity is the extent to which the **sensitivity of a material to fracture is increased by the presence of a surface inhomogeneity, e.g. cracks and scratches**. Ductile materials such as stainless steel have low notch sensitivity, while brittle materials such as ceramic and titanium have high notch sensitivity.

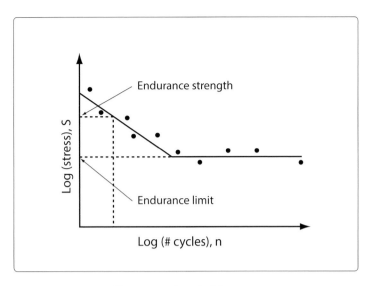

Figure 17.2 A typical S–n curve.

The above discussion is aimed at material properties. When discussing a structure, one must also consider the shape of the structure, along with forces applied and material properties. For example, **stiffness** refers to a material's ability to resist deformation, while **rigidity** refers to a structure's ability to resist deformation.

Time-dependent behaviour

The elastic behaviour discussed above does not always occur. Sometimes, there is time-dependent behaviour, termed **viscoelasticity**. Materials and structures such as cartilage, ligaments and intervertebral discs display such behaviour. **Viscous properties** are **time-dependent** and involve **non-recoverable deformation**; elastic properties are **time-independent** and involve **recoverable deformation**. Several phenomena characterize viscoelasticity, namely **creep, stress relaxation, time-dependent strain behaviour** and **hysteresis**.

When a material is loaded with a constant force there is an initial elongation (the elastic component), but in viscoelastic materials there is further continuous deformation over time (viscous component). This is termed **creep (time-dependent deformation in response to a constant load)** (**Figure 17.3a**).

If the material, after being loaded, is held at a specific strain (i.e. at a certain length), then the stress level required to maintain this strain decreases over time until equilibrium is reached. This is termed **stress relaxation (time-dependent decrease in load required to maintain a material at a constant strain)** (**Figure 17.3b**).

Time-dependent strain behaviour can be illustrated by the behaviour of plasticine. If we gradually pull apart a blob of plasticine, we create a long thin thread of plasticine before it eventually breaks into two. However, if we pull the blob apart quickly, then the plasticine breaks quickly. Note that the strength required to break the plasticine is higher when pulling

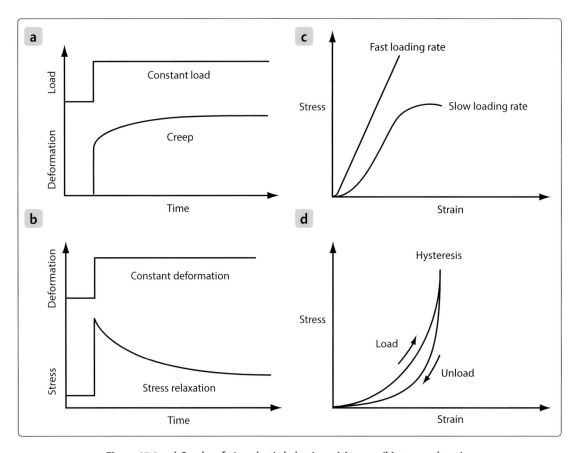

Figure 17.3a–d Graphs of viscoelastic behaviour. (a) creep (b) stress relaxation
(c) rate-dependent strain behaviour (d) hysteresis.

it apart quickly and less when trying to break the long thread after slowly pulling the plasticine apart. Translating this into mechanical terms, the rate of change of length of the plasticine (the strain rate) affects the behaviour. **The faster the strain rate, the higher the stress at a given level of strain (i.e. the material becomes stiffer).** Conversely, a low strain rate requires more time but less stress to fracture the material. This is shown graphically in **Figure 17.3c**.

Hysteresis refers to the stress–strain curve differing during loading and unloading (Figure 17.3d). Strain energy is lost between loading and unloading as heat, due to the internal friction within the material.

The underlying mechanisms responsible for viscoelastic behaviour are, first, **friction** internally, as micro-elements in the structure move against each other as a material is stretched, as described previously in the unfurling of collagen fibres. Second, the movement of interstitial fluid through a material that is a semi-porous matrix creates a **drag**, which produces viscoelastic behaviour. The femur exhibits features of viscoelastic behaviour in terms of stress relaxation. When implanting an uncemented femoral prosthesis in hip replacements tap down the prosthesis, wait a few seconds, tap it down again, wait a few seconds, and so on. As you taps down the prosthesis, circumferential hoop stresses are generated in the femur. If you now wait a few seconds, the femur exhibits stress relaxation and the hoop stresses diminish, so that you can continue tapping the prosthesis down. This technique reduces the risk of femoral fracture, as it limits the level of stresses generated during implantation.

Shear forces

Shear stresses occur when two forces are directed parallel to each other but not along the same line and are either pushing towards each other or pulling away. When applied to an object, these stresses will create a shearing force. As with linear forces, there is a relationship between shear stress and shear strain, and we can calculate a shear modulus, which gives an idea of a material's resistance to shearing forces:

Shear modulus = shear stress/shear strain

A useful rule of thumb is that the shear modulus is between 30% and 50% of the elastic modulus for most materials. It is worth noting that bone is weakest against shear forces, while it is strong in compression. When analysing forces acting on bone, note that in reality almost all the forces to which a bone may be subjected are a combination of tension, compression, bending, torsion and shear. As a result, bone tends to fail (fracture) in the shear component first. Analysing the forces on bone in a given situation is complex, and computer analysis is essential for calculating accurately the various force components.

Bending forces

Having introduced the concepts above, it is clear that in the body most forces are not pure tension or compression but a combination of the two. Bending forces are common in the skeleton, e.g. loading of the femur causes it to bend. In the case of the femur, it is bowed anteriorly. The shape is the result of the femur being subjected to loading forces, which cause the anterior surface to be put in tension and the posterior surface into compression. A simplified model of this is shown in **Figure 17.4**.

If we examine a cross-section of the beam, there is a graduation of stresses from extreme edges of the beam, where the compressive and tensile forces are the largest respectively, towards the centre of the beam (the mid-point of the cross-section), where there is no resulting force. The line of no force throughout the beam is termed the **neutral axis**.

In order to calculate the bending stress at any given point, we apply the following equation:

Bending stress = (applied force × distance from neutral axis)/second moment area of material

The **second moment area** (SMA) is a variable that describes the spatial distribution of a material within a structure. The type of material does not affect the SMA. The SMA is affected by the organization and shape of the material. Some basic shape types and formulae for SMAs are shown in **Figure 17.5**.

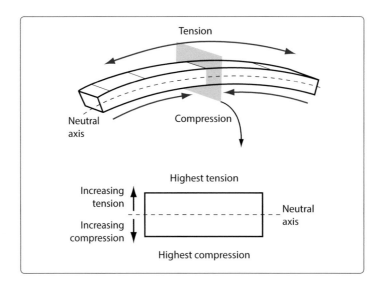

Figure 17.4 Bending forces as applied to a beam (longitudinal and cross-sectional views).

Note the following:

- **For materials with rectangular cross-sections, the perpendicular distance away from the neutral axis (h) has a third power effect on the SMA.**
- **For materials with a solid circular cross-section, the radius (which is the distance from the neutral axis) has a fourth power effect on the SMA.**
- **For materials with a hollow circular cross-section, the total SMA equals the SMA of the solid outer portion minus the SMA of the missing inner hollow portion.**

Using the formula to compare a pipe and a solid rod, it can be seen that for identical cross-sectional areas, the SMA is actually larger for the hollow pipe. As a result, the hollow pipe deforms less (is stronger) than the solid pipe of the same cross-sectional area. An example of this is that as bone ages, outward appositional growth enlarges the medullary canal and increases the overall girth of the whole bone. This increases the SMA and consequently the bone strength and resistance to fracture. This probably helps to offset the loss of bone strength from osteoporosis.

It is worth noting that the calculation of forces in bending does not take into account the nature of the material being tested but considers only its shape and size. However, once bending moments have been calculated, we can think about relevant materials that can withstand the forces applied.

Rigidity in bending is a particularly important concept when choosing metal plates for fracture fixation:

Bending rigidity = SMA × Young's modulus

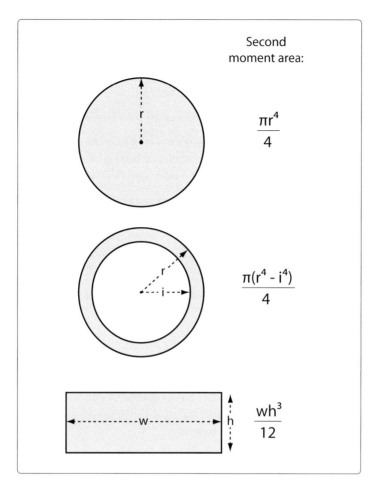

Figure 17.5 Common geometrical shapes and their second moment areas. h: height; i: inner radius; r: outer radius; w, width.

When defined in this way, rigidity incorporates both the nature of a material and its shape, size and structure. From this equation, some important conclusions can be derived. Choosing a material that is twice as stiff (i.e. double the Young's modulus), such as cobalt chrome over titanium, makes a plate of a given shape, size and structure twice as rigid. More importantly, working through the equations for a rectangular shaped plate, then doubling the thickness of the plate results in an increased SMA and consequently increased rigidity by the third power of the multiplying factor; i.e. doubling the plate thickness increases rigidity by 2^3 ($=8$).

Torsional forces

Equal and opposite shear forces, as applied to a cylinder constrained in space, cause the cylinder to twist. This is known as a **torsional** or **torque force**. If we substitute the cylinder for a tibia, then the following discussion can be applied to understanding how a skier sustains a spiral fracture in the tibia when the skis twist around. The twisting of the skis applies a torsional force.

Similar to bending forces, graduations of the torque force apply through the cylinder, from the surfaces edges, where the torque is maximal, to the centre of the cylinder, where the resultant force of the two opposite shearing forces is zero. A line connecting areas of zero net force throughout a structure is termed the **axis of twist**. The formula for calculating the shear stress force generated by the torque forces at any given point is:

Shear stress = (applied torque × distance from axis of twist)/polar moment of inertia

The polar moment of inertia, or **polar moment area** (PMA), similar to the SMA, is a variable parameter related to the size and shape of a structure but not the material from which it is constructed. **Figure 17.6** shows the formula for calculating the PMA for cylindrical shapes.

Returning to the skiing example, the ski tip is a long distance from the tibia of the skier. As a result of the long moment arm, the force applied to the tibia is high. Using the formula below for a hollow cylinder, we can calculate the order of magnitude of forces required to fracture the tibia. Again, the formula demonstrates that in terms of the dimensions of the cylinder, the radius (i.e. the distance from the axis of twist) affects the PMA to the fourth power.

The rigidity of materials to torsion is calculated in a similar way to that of bending rigidity:

Torsional rigidity = PMA × shear modulus

Torsional rigidity is a measure of the resistance of a material in a particular size and shape to torsional forces. From **Figure 17.6** we see that for a cylinder, the polar moment varies to the fourth power of the radius. Therefore, an intramedullary rod that is twice as thick has 2^4 (= 16) times the rigidity. If an intramedullary nail is either slotted or cannulated, the polar moment area will be decreased and therefore the torsional rigidity will be reduced significantly, whereas the bending rigidity will be affected only minimally.

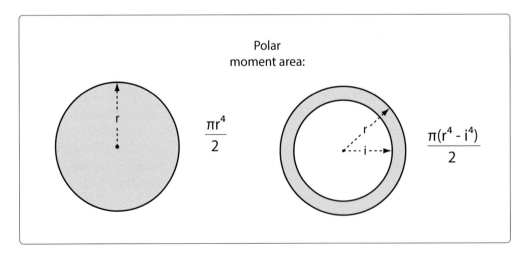

Figure 17.6 Cylindrical shapes and their polar moment areas. i: inner radius; r: outer radius.

Viva questions

1. Draw a stress–strain curve and describe how to calculate the Young's modulus.

2. What do you understand by the term 'fatigue failure'? Draw an S–n curve.

3. Explain how increasing the thickness of metal plates affects their rigidity.

4. Explain how your choice of solid or slotted nails affects the rigidity of the construct.

5. How does the phenomenon of creep govern your surgical technique of implanting uncemented femoral prostheses?

Further reading

Brinckmann P, Frobin W, Leivseth G. *Musculoskeletal Biomechanics.* Stuttgart, New York: Thieme, 2002.

Lucas GL, Cooke FW, Fris E. *A Primer of Orthopaedic Biomechanics*. New York, NY: Springer Science and Business Media, 1999.

Mow VC, Huiskes R (eds). *Basic Orthopaedic Biomechanics and Mechano-Biology*, 3rd edn. New York, NY: Lippincott-Raven, 2004.

Nordin M, Frankel VH (eds). *Basic Biomechanics of the Musculoskeletal System*, 3rd revised edn. Philadelphia, PA: Lea and Febiger, 2001.

Ozkaya N, Nordin M, Goldsheyder D, Leger D. *Fundamentals of Biomechanics: Equilibrium, Motion, and Deformation*. New York, Springer, MD: Williams & Wilkins, 2012.

Radin EL. *Practical Biomechanics for the Orthopedic Surgeon*, 2nd edn. New York, NY: Churchill Livingstone, 1992.

18 Biomaterials

Subhamoy Chatterjee, John Stammers and Gordon Blunn

Introduction

Biomaterials have an integral role in orthopaedic surgery. **Biomaterials** are defined as 'a **non-viable material used in a medical device intended to interact with biological systems**'. **Biocompatibility** is '**the ability of a material to perform with an appropriate host response in a specific application**'.

Clinical decision making in orthopaedics is influenced by an understanding of the types, compatibility, mechanical properties and processing of biomaterials available. Historically materials were selected for their **bioinert** properties. Bioinert materials produce **no host response to the material**. Bioactive, biodegradable and materials stimulating a molecular response have an increasing role in orthopaedic biomaterials.

There are four major classes of biomaterials: metals, polymers, ceramics and natural materials. Composites are the combination of two or more classes.

Metals
General properties of metal alloys

Metallic alloys are the combination of metallic and non-metallic elements. Specific properties such as corrosion resistance and mechanical properties are determined by the micro-structure. The strong metallic bonds result in stiff, ductile and hard properties. **Pure metals have a crystalline lattice micro-structure of metallic bonds with free circulating electrons.** There are three typical crystalline arrangements shown in **Figure 18.1a–c**.

The metallic bonds are stronger the closer the atoms are together in the higher density face-centred cubic and hexagonal close-packed crystalline arrangements. The crystalline arrangement, density, grain size and presence of defects affect strength. High grain sizes are associated with earlier fatigue and failure. Within the grain boundaries, imperfections known as **vacancies and dislocations** can occur, macroscopically seen as **scratches and voids**. The

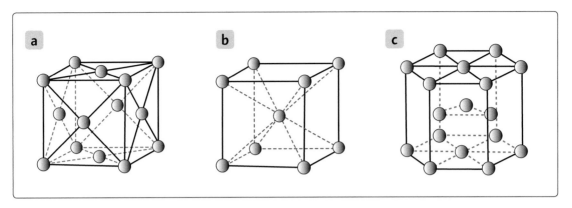

Figure 18.1 Common metal crystalline arrangements. a: Body-centred cubic; b: face-centred cubic; c: hexagonal close packed.

presence of non-metallic elements (solutes) within the crystal arrangement of metal atoms creates slight deformation in the crystal and resistance to the flow of crystal units against each other. This increases yield strength by increasing dislocations, which increases resistance to plastic deformation.

The electrochemically harsh saline environment within the body exposes implants to corrosion or the dissolution of metal within a solution (see Chapter 25). **Passivation** is a process to protect metals from corrosion by the forming of a surface oxide layer. Crevice corrosion is often due to mechanically-assisted corrosion, where the unreactive surface layer is damaged exposing the deeper reactive layer. Unwanted hard on soft metal-on-metal articulation, such as cobalt chrome on titanium in patients with failed polyethylene liners and micro-motion at the head neck taper in total hip replacements, are well-documented causes of catastrophic crevice corrosion. When selecting a combination of dissimilar metals, it is important that they have a low tendency to interact galvanically.

Many metals undergo **forging**, a manufacturing process to optimize material properties using pressure and it is classified as cold, warm or hot working, relative to its recrystallization temperature. **Cold working** increases the number and density of defects or dislocations by plastic deformation. Termed **strain hardening**, this increase in dislocations makes it difficult to further deform the material. Yield strength increases but ductility is reduced. **Hot working** is plastic deformation above the recrystallization temperature, reducing grain size, increasing homogeneity and ductility. Hot working enables larger deformations to be made without over-hardening or fracturing the material.

Common orthopaedic metal alloys

Stainless steel, cobalt chrome and titanium are alloys widely used in orthopaedic surgery; their composition, material properties, advantages and disadvantages are summarized in *Table 18.1*.

Table 18.1 Properties of common metal alloys

Alloy	Composition	Processing	Elastic modulus (GPa)	Yield strength (MPa)	Ultimate tensile strength (MPa)	Advantages	Disadvantages	Typical uses
Stainless steel **316L**	Iron 62%, chromium 18%, molybdenum **3**%, nickel **16**%, carbon **0.03**%, **L**=low carbon	Cold worked	190	792	930	Strength with cold working Ductile Biocompatible and cheap Chromium and carbon provides corrosion resistance Cheap	Prone to crevice, stress and galvanic corrosion Avoid in nickel allergy	Trauma-plates, screws Hip arthroplasty
		Annealed	190	331	586			
Titanium **6Al 4V**	Titanium 89%, aluminium **6**%, vanadium **4**%, others 1%	Cold worked	110	485	760	Excellent biocompatibility and bone integration through TiO_2 oxide layer Excellent resistance to corrosion (better than stainless steel) Ductile Reduced stress shielding due to lower Young's modulus Fatigue resistance Low artefact on MRI	Susceptible to wear Poor articulating surface without surface treatment Notch sensitivity Release of cytotoxic elements locally and systemically, such as vanadium	Plates, screws, intramedullary nails Stems of implants MRI-safe external fixators Articulating surfaces if hardened/ ceramised
		Annealed	116	896	965			
Cobalt chrome	Cobalt (34–61%), chrome (20–30%), molybdenum (6–10%), nickel (2.5–35%), carbon (0.02–0.35%), tungsten	F 75 Cast-annealed	210	448–517	655–889	Corrosion resistant (due to high chromium) Biocompatible Strength in articulating surfaces	Expensive Large head metal-on-metal total hip arthroplasty ion release	Bearing surfaces
		F799 Hot forged	210	448–1200	1399–1586			
		F562 Cold forged	232	1500	1795			

MRI: magnetic resonance imaging.

Stainless steel

Chromium provides stainless steel corrosion resistance by forming an oxide layer (Cr_2O_3). Stainless steels are classified based on their crystalline structure. 316L is austenitic steel with austenite, a face-centered cubic crystal, as the primary phase. They do not harden by heat treatment and are typically processed by cold working. Newer stainless steels replace nickel with nitrogen and manganese. Adding nitrogen reduces allergy from nickel and confers corrosion resistance and increased yield strength.

Cobalt chrome

Due to the poor wear resistance of stainless steel in metal-on-metal articulation, cobalt chrome was introduced with the McKee–Farrar prosthesis (1966) and is now routinely coupled with polyethylene. Both stainless steel (190 GPa) and cobalt chrome (220GPa) have a high elastic modulus relative to cortical bone (20–30 GPa) and therefore stress shielding of the adjacent bone can cause bone resorption and eventual loosening. The effects of stress shielding are reduced by implanting the stem with bone cement (polymethyl-methacrylate, [PMMA] 1.1–4.1 GPa).

Titanium

Titanium has an elastic modulus of 110 GPa and femoral stems do not suffer from stress shielding as much as stainless steel and cobalt chrome. As a result, titanium alloys are suited to intramedullary devices and uncemented femoral stems. Due to its relative softness, titanium is susceptible to particle-induced wear. As a result, titanium without further processing is not used as an articulating surface and certain cemented titanium stems have had high failure rates (e.g. 3M Capital hip).

Osseointegration and surface properties

Osseointegration is the 'holy grail' of uncemented arthroplasty systems, improving long-term behaviour. Stress shielding, loosening by wear particles, fatigue failure, corrosion and peri-prosthetic infection are reduced if bone grows onto the implant. Surface parameters such as roughness, wettability and electrostatic charges can be manipulated to optimize bone on-growth.

Early attempts to osseointegrate metal implants involved surface roughening by grit blasting, sintering titanium beads and porous coatings. Mechanically, these surfaces aided early primary stability and histologically bone formed near the surface, but they were not bioactive in that there were no covalent bonds between metal and bone. Hydroxyapatite (see Ceramics) and other bioglass ceramic coatings are bioactive and in the right mechanical environment, bonds form between implant and bone. Porous metallic foams of titanium or tantalum mimic cancellous bone in terms of porosity and elastic modulus (3 GPa). They have a high coefficient of friction providing good primary fixation, and their open weave mesh allows bone ingrowth around the mesh to provide long-term stability. These metallic foam augments have been particularly effective in revision surgery where large volume bone loss is encountered. Chemical coatings can infer bioactive properties. Future development of these metallic foams involves osseoinductive surfaces using proteins and peptides to mimic cell matrix receptors. Addition of growth factors and drug delivery coatings are also under development.

Polymers

Polymers, both synthetic and natural, are long-chain molecules of small repeating subunits. Ultra-high-molecular weight polyethylene (UHMWPE) and PMMA are the most commonly used, but examples of polymers in orthopaedics include small joint silicon arthroplasty, polymers in sutures and tissue engineering scaffolds.

Polymers are synthesized by either **condensation polymerization** or **addition polymerization**. PMMA and UHMWPE are formed by addition polymerization where an initiator, such as a free radical or catalyst, breaks the monomer double bond activating it to react with an adjacent monomer. This process continues through the propagation phase until termination.

Polymer development

The molecular structure, conformation and orientation of the polymers can have a major effect on the material properties of the material. Clinically this explains the mechanical performance between 1st to 3rd generation cementing techniques and the polyethylene used by Sir John Charnley in the 1970s, compared to the current vitamin E enriched highly cross-linked UHMWPE. Most polymers are semicrystalline containing a combination of tangled chains and no order (termed **amorphous** and **crystalline**) regions of three-dimensional highly organized repeating patterns at the molecular level (**Figure 18.2**).

Historically, the manufacture of high-density polyethylene used in arthroplasty is attributed to Karl Ziegler who invented the Ziegler Process. The process has been refined and now there are many variations to achieve clinical grade UHMWPE.

Ram extrusion is the process where pre-compressed powder resin is heated and pressurized into a rod.

Sheet compression moulding similarly uses heated powder as ram extrusion but the pressure is applied and held over a longer period of time, up to 24 hours, to increase homogeneity. The sheets undergo milling into the required shape.

The advantage of **direct compression moulding** over sheet compression moulding is that the resin is pressurized and heated in a single mould of the desired shape, avoiding the need for milling. The end result therefore has an extremely smooth surface.

Hot isostatic compression moulding is a multistage batch process, first cold compressing resin into a bar and then heating it under pressure in an inert atmosphere.

Post-production processing

Gamma irradiation not only sterilizes the material but improves cross-linking, which increases the hardness and reduces the wear rate. Oxidation is an unwanted process by gamma irradiation where free radicals are produced that bond with oxygen. Oxidized UHMWPE results in degradation and loss of mechanical properties resulting in greater wear. Manufacturers now sterilize UMWPE by irradiation in an inert atmosphere and package the final product in a vacuum or inert gas. Adding vitamin E, a natural antioxidant, to polyethylene is the latest technique to reduce oxidation in highly cross-linked polyethylene.

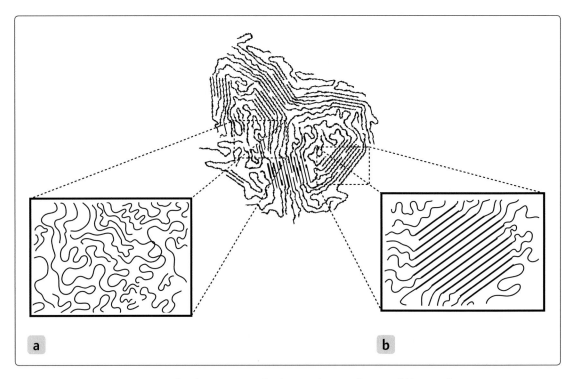

Figure 18.2 Molecular structure of polymers a) amorphous and b) crystalline.

Ethylene oxide and gas plasma are alternative methods of sterilization that do not produce the free radicals implicated in oxidation, but also do not produce highly cross-linked UHMWPE with its more desirable wear properties.

Annealing or the heating of the material and slow cooling in comparison to remelting provides improved fracture resistance in highly cross-linked UHMWPE.

The mechanical requirements of UHMWPE vary between hip and knee arthroplasty. Adhesive wear debris, osteolysis and aseptic loosening are seen in the hip, whereas abrasive wear, fatigue, fracture and delamination are greater problems in the knee. The trade-off of low wear to reduced strength of highly cross-linked polyethylene is favourable to the hip but not the knee.

PMMA

PMMA has been used in cemented joint arthroplasty for over 50 years. Historically its inert properties were realized during World War II where splinters of PMMA (as Flexiglass/Perspex) were used to make Spitfire aeroplane canopies that did not react in the eye. Primary fixation is provided by anchorage between the gaps of the implant and the trabecular bone. The components of PMMA bone cement are shown in *Table 18.2*.

Drawbacks to bone cement include:

- Large exothermic reaction where, particularly in thick layers of cement, thermal necrosis can occur, disrupting the cement bone interface.
- Unpolymerized monomer entering the blood supply producing fat embolism.
- Differences in stiffness of the implant, the cement and bone make it susceptible to fracture, generating cement particles that can induce an inflammatory response.
- Radio-opacifier and antibiotics reduce the mechanical properties.
- Antibiotics must be heat stable.

Gravius *et al.* (2007) reported that the greatest resistance to bending occurred in vacuum mixed cement, cured under pressure. Conversely, blood contaminated specimens had the lowest strength with air bubbles; antibiotic inclusions were also associated with fatigue cracks. *Table 18.3* summarizes the evolution of cementing techniques. In weight-bearing cement, the addition of more than 10% antibiotic powder to cement significantly reduces its mechanical properties. Antibiotics in liquid form should be avoided due to the associated decrease in mechanical strength.

Bioresorbable polymers

Bioresorbable implants reduce stress shielding, avoid the need for removal and enable post-operative imaging without metal artefact. The disadvantages are variable resorption rate, and therefore unpredictable mechanical properties, and iatrogenic non-specific foreign body reaction to the implant or degradation products. Newer bioresorbable polymers are under development to eliminate these disadvantages but there are no long-term clinical studies.

Table 18.2 Components of polymethyl-methacrylate (PMMA) bone cement

Powder	Role
Polymer	Polymethyl-methacrylate
Copolymers methacrylate-methylmethacrylate	Alter mechanical properties of cement
Barium sulphate or zirconium dioxide	Opacifier to visualize cement on radiography
Chlorophyll dye	Distinguish cement from bone
Antibiotics	Antimicrobial prophylaxis
Liquid	
Monomer	Methylmethacrylate monomer
N,N-dimethyl-p-toluidine (DMPT)	Initiator
Benzyl peroxide	Catalyst reacting with DMPT
Hydroquinone	Stabilizer preventing polymerization premixing
Dye	Distinguish cement from bone

Table 18.3 Evolution of cementing techniques

1st Generation	2nd Generation	3rd Generation
Hand mix	Hand mix, pack cement gun	Vacuum/centrifuge mixing
Leave cancellous bone	Remove cancellous bone	Remove cancellous bone
Femoral canal vented	Cement restrictor	Cement restrictor
Minimal canal preparation	Brush and pulse lavage	Brush and pulse lavage
Irrigate and suction canal	Irrigate, pack and dry canal	Irrigate, pack with adrenaline soaked gauze, dry
Finger insertion of cement	Cement gun injection	Cement gun and pressurizing
Manual stem positioning	Manual stem positioning	Proximal and distal stem centralizers

Degradation time depends on polymer crystallinity, porosity, molecular weight, monomer concentration and temperature. Biodegradability occurs in two stages. Water preferentially bonds to the amorphous phase chemical bonds, shortening the polymer chains. The crystalline regions continue to provide structural support. The second phase is enzymatic degradation accelerated by the acidic degradation products.

Sutures are the most commonly used bioresorbable polymer in orthopaedics and the strength retention and final resorption is important in deciding an appropriate suture (*Table 18.4*).

Ceramics

Ceramics are **inorganic compounds of metallic** and **non-metallic elements**. Unlike metals where electrons are freely circulating, in ceramics, electrons are either transferred (ionic bonds) or shared (covalent). These strong bonds, typically between positively charged metal ions and negatively charged non-metal ions, result in tightly packed atoms, sharing a similar polygranular structure to metals. Ceramics are **stiff** and **brittle**. The hardness and wear resistance for orthopaedic use requires high purity and homogeneity using fine powder compressed into casts before thermal processing. The **chemical inertness** and insolubility confer excellent biocompatibility compared to metal bearing surfaces. Strength is inversely proportional to porosity and grain size; however, heating reduces porosity but increases grain size. Despite modern processing, ceramics are brittle and this limits their role.

Broadly, there are two types of ceramics used in orthopaedics: bearing surfaces and bone-graft substitutes or osteoconductive surface coatings.

Common orthopaedic ceramics

Alumina (AL_2O_3) and **zirconia** (ZrO_2) are used in bearing surfaces. Alumina and zirconia share abrasion resistance, low friction and high wettability, resulting in a superior bearing surface. Alumina is particularly brittle and historically had a significant rate of fracture (up to 5%), but processing has reduced the grain size and increased density, reducing fracture risk. Zirconia requires a stabilizer, otherwise it is sensitive to phase changes that can cause micro-cracking and reduce its mechanical properties. Heat and resterilization need to be

Table 18.4 Common suture materials used in orthopaedics

Bioabsorbable suture	Construction	Strength retention	Absorbed by
Polyglactin 910 (Vicryl™)	Braided	14 days – 75% 21 days – 50% 28 days – 25%	56–70 days
Polyglactin 910 (Vicryl Rapide™)	Braided	5 days – 50% 10–14 days – 0%	42 days
Poliglecaprone (Monocryl 25™)	Monofilament	7 days – 50–70% 14 days – 20–40%	91–119 days
Polydioxanone (PDS ›3-0)	Monofilament	14 days – 80% 28 days – 70% 42 days – 60%	183–238 days

avoided as they can cause surface roughening. Zirconia had accelerated wear in ceramic-on-ceramic bearings and is only designed for ceramic-on-polyethylene use. The original zirconia was withdrawn but oxidized zirconium has improved fracture resistance and is used in femoral heads and total knee replacements. Due to the high Young's modulus of ceramics compared to cancellous bone, stress shielding can result in failure, particularly when used for the acetabular component.

Ceramic coatings, such as titanium niobium nitride (TiNbN) and titanium nitride (TiN), aim to combine the mechanical resistance of metals with the wear resistance of ceramics. There are limited long-term clinical studies with ceramic surface coatings.

Osteoblasts covalently bond to bone when in contact with some ceramics, glass–ceramics, and calcium phosphates, and therefore they are osteoconductive. A **hydroxyapatite layer (Ca10[PO4]6[OH]2)** has enabled bone on-growth to uncemented prostheses and has been in clinical use for almost three decades. The thickness of coating and processing to attach the hydroxyapatite is debated. If the layer is too thick, it risks fracturing off due to its brittleness. If too thin, it can dissolve before bone on-growth. Hydroxyapatite and other bioglass materials are also used as an injectable bone filler. There is cross-over with tissue engineering as osteoinductive surface coatings are being designed. Impregnation with growth factors, bone morphogenetic proteins (BMPs) and antimicrobial agents is in development.

Biomaterials in tissue engineering

There are numerous biomaterials including polymers, ceramics and metals in use and under development for tissue engineering scaffolds. Specific details are beyond the scope of this chapter but it is important to understand the requirements of a scaffold:

- Biocompatible and non-toxic degradation products.
- Biodegradeable resorption at the same rate as tissue repairs.
- Tissue ingrowth, vascularization and nutrient delivery by porous network of interconnected macro- and micro-pores.
- Mechanical properties comparable to, and maintenance of structural integrity of, replaced load-bearing tissue.

Materials testing

In light of well-publicized implant failures, it is important to be aware of the standards and tests related to biomaterial testing in orthopaedics. The International Standards Organization (ISO) and American Standard Testing and Materials (ASTM) Committee guide biocompatibility testing. The tests include mechanical testing of endurance and wear testing in load simulators with a minimal number of cycles of force and displacement, depending on the implant. Animal testing assesses the response of the tissue to the material and tests the material to implantation.

European conformity (CE) marking and/or USA Food and Drug Administration (FDA) approval provide regulation of the end product prior to being launched on the market. Orthopaedic implants are FDA class III devices requiring extensive pre-market approval. However, if the manufacturer can demonstrate 'substantial equivalence' of all or pieces of the device to previously cleared devices, approval can be given without specifically demonstrating safety or effectiveness with clinical studies. For example, different surface coatings, bearing surface and head size could be equivalent to a previously approved device; however the combination may be untested. Novel devices require a full clinical trial for approval for use in patients.

Viva questions

1. Discuss the advantages and disadvantages of bone cement in hip arthroplasty.
2. Explain what forging is and how the material properties are affected.
3. Discuss the available femoral stem materials and the relevance of surface coating to implant fixation.
4. Describe the processing of highly cross-linked UHMWPE and its advantages and disadvantages.
5. Explain the testing and approval process prior to implant marketing.
6. Explain your choice of material for an intramedullary device.

Further reading

Böstman O, Pihlajamäki H. Clinical biocompatibility of biodegradable orthopaedic implants for internal fixation: a review. *Biomaterials* 2000;**21**(24):2615–21.

Gravius S, et al. Mechanical in vitro testing of fifteen commercial bone cements based on polymethylmethacrylate. *Z Orthop Unfall* 2007;**145**(5):579–85.

Kurtz SM. UHMWPE *Biomaterials Handbook: Ultra High Molecular Weight Polyethylene in Total Joint Replacement and Medical Devices*. Academic Press, Oxford, 2009.

Williams DF. *The Williams Dictionary of Biomaterials*. Liverpool: Liverpool University Press, 1999.

19 Biomechanics and Joint Replacement of the Hip

Mark Mullins, Thomas Youm and John Skinner

Introduction

The hip joint is the most common site for arthroplasty, with around 70,000 hip replacements performed annually in the UK. The success or failure of management of hip problems is dependent on a sound understanding of the biomechanics of the hip joint and how the various components of this may be modified. In addition, it is important to appreciate the factors that affect implant survival in order to be optimally informed when selecting an implant for a particular patient.

Biomechanical factors in hip pathology

The basis of **free-body analysis** is covered in Chapter 16. The hip effectively functions as a multi-axial ball-and-socket joint upon which the upper body is balanced during stance and gait. Having a stable hip joint is critical to all motion, while supporting the forces encountered during daily activity. The dynamic forces on the hip joint are enormous. Normal walking exerts a force of three times the body weight through the hip joint, increasing to seven times the body weight in fast walking. Even the seemingly innocuous activity of straight-leg raising puts a force in excess of twice the body weight across the joint.

The **joint reaction force** (JRF) is the compressive force at the femoroacetabular articulation. The JRF results from the need to balance the moment arms of the body weight with the pull of the hip abductors in order to maintain a level pelvis. The primary contributors to the JRF are the muscular forces generated to level the pelvis during standing and gait, with a smaller contribution from body weight.

Free-body analysis of the hip joint makes certain assumptions. These include a single-leg stance and that the weight of the leg is one-sixth of the total body weight. **Figure 19.2** shows the free-body analysis for the hip joint.

It is important to note the direction of action of the abductor muscle force (F_{ab}), as the primary role of this group of muscles is to stabilize the pelvis in single-leg stance. Resolving the moments:

$$F_{ab} \times A = B \times 5/6\, F_{bw}$$

$$F_{ab} \times 0.05 = 0.15 \times 500$$

$$F_{ab} = 1500\ \text{N}$$

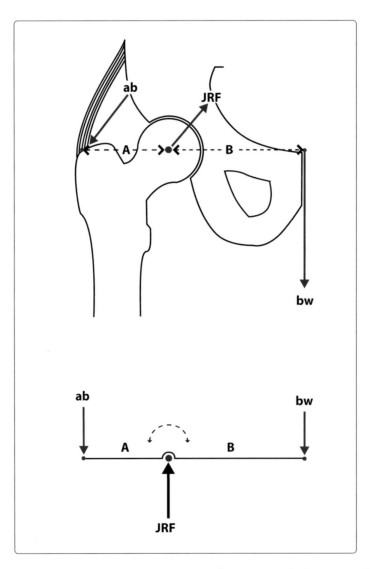

Figure. 19.1 Factors affecting the joint reaction force (JRF) on the hip. W: weight.

The hip JRF, as represented in **Figure 19.1**, is calculated by resolving the vector triangle shown in **Figure 19.3**.

The major determinant of joint pathology is the JRF, which is the resultant of the abductor force F_{ab} and 5/6 body weight F_{bw}. Of these two factors, the abductor force predominates, but a reduction in either will reduce the JRF and, thus, symptoms at the hip joint. In osteoarthritis, the near-frictionless articular cartilage is worn away and the resultant increased frictional forces exert a resistant moment. To overcome this, an increased abductor force is required.

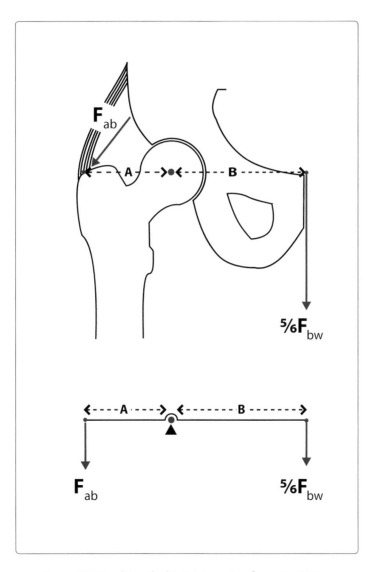

Figure 19.2 Resolving the hip joint reaction force. A = 0.05 m; B = 0.15 m; body weight (bw) = 600 N F_{ab}: abductor force.

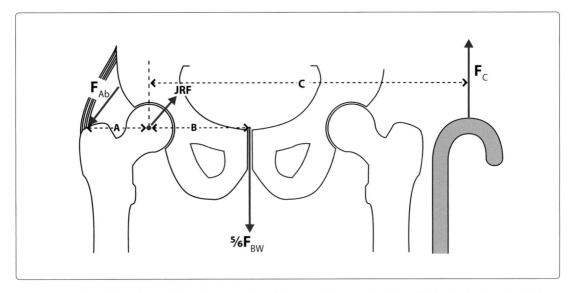

Figure 19.3 Effect of a walking stick in the contralateral hand on joint reaction force (JRF). A = 0.05 m; B = 0.15 m; C = 0.50 m; body weight (bw) = 600 N; Fc = 100 N ; F$_{ab}$: abductor force.

Strategies to reduce joint reaction force

- **Reduce body-weight moment**:
  - reduce body weight;
  - decrease lever arm:
  - medialize the axis of rotation;
  - Trendelenburg gait.
- **Help the abductors**:
  - provide additional moments:
    - walking stick in opposite hand;
    - suitcase in ipsilateral hand.
  - increase abductor lever arm:
    - increase offset;
    - osteotomy;
    - lateral transfer of greater trochanter;
    - varus angulation of stem of total hip replacement (THR).
  - improve abductor line of function.

In a **Trendelenburg gait**, the patient sways the body weight over, towards the affected side. This lateral motion decreases the body-weight moment arm and, hence, the JRF. The effect of using a walking stick in the contralateral hand is shown in **Figure 19.3**. Resolving the moments clockwise:

$$500 \times 0.15 = (F_{ab} \times 0.05) + (100 \times 0.5)$$

Therefore, F_{ab} is 500 N, a reduction of 67% when using a walking stick.

Carrying a suitcase in the ipsilateral hand provides another anticlockwise moment, thereby reducing the abductor force.

Acetabular and femoral osteotomies

The inherent osseous stability of the hip can have significant consequences on the forces and contact areas experienced at the joint surface. This is clearly demonstrated in the evaluation of the force transfer across the hip in the setting of hip dysplasia, coxa vara and coxa valga. In dysplastic conditions there is insufficient coverage of the femoral head by the acetabulum, and articular surface contact is concentrated on a small area of cartilage on the lateral aspect of the acetabulum. These contact pressures can be as high as two and a half times body weight during a single-leg stance. **Periacetabular osteotomies** improve the anterior, lateral and superior coverage of the femoral head and have been shown to significantly decrease the contact force across the articular cartilage. This is accomplished by increasing the joint surface area across which the contact force is distributed, while optimizing the mechanical advantage of the abductor musculature and decreasing the force necessary to maintain pelvic balance.

Intertrochanteric osteotomy is another powerful procedure that can be used to redirect the femoral head into the acetabulum. The goals of the osteotomy are to optimize the contact surfaces between the joint, to centre the vertical JRF well within the dome of the acetabulum and to redirect the muscular balance of the gluteus medius and minimus muscle. The **varus osteotomy** has obvious advantages in **increasing the abductor lever arm** as well as providing a more horizontal line of action of the abductors. It may also increase congruency and displace the JRF medially. In a **valgus osteotomy**, the main effect is to make the capital drop osteophyte weight bearing, thus increasing the size and quality of the surface available for weight bearing. Other effects are possible, depending on the precise pattern of abnormality in the proximal femur; these effects may include **lengthening the abductor lever arm** and making the abductor action **more horizontal**.

Total hip arthroplasty

The aims of hip replacement are to relieve pain by excising the painful joint and to improve function by increasing the offset and lever arm of the hip, which will consequently improve the line of abductor action as well as correcting any limb length discrepancy. Sir John Charnley applied the basic principles listed above to his low-friction arthroplasty. He advocated routine lateralization of the abductors and medialization of the centre of rotation by deepening the socket and using a small head size. Although these principles are well founded in biomechanical terms, they are not universally applied today, for the reasons discussed in this section.

Frictional torque of hip arthroplasty depends on:

- Materials bearing surface made from (ceramics, cobalt chrome, steel).
- Femoral head size.
- Polyethylene (if used) thickness.
- Peripheral or equatorial versus polar contact.

Greater force is required to initiate than to maintain movement. At low speed and with poor lubrication, **stick-slip** movement (also known as **stiction-friction**) may occur. This produces torques some 40 times higher than in unaffected arthroplasties and may cause acetabular loosening.

In addition, the combination of thick polyethylene and small head size diffuses load more than thin polyethylene, leading to lower frictional torque and decreased stress at the cup interface, with widening of stress dissipation within the bone (and therefore less loosening) (**Figure 19.4**).

Acetabular component

Deepening the socket by removing the subchondral bone plate results in plastic deformation of the softer cancellous bone, which undergoes necrosis, with formation of a fibrous membrane. There is subsequent bone resorption, leading to decreased stiffness and, ultimately, failure of the construct. Because of this and in order to preserve bone, sockets are no longer routinely medialized but are placed in the correct **anatomical location**, with a smaller head size effectively medializing the centre of rotation.

Laboratory tests have demonstrated that the acetabular preparation that gives the strongest fixation in cemented cups is the use of **three large keyholes** with preservation of the subchondral plate. However, even the weakest combinations have a lowest turning moment to failure some four times higher than the greatest frictional moments.

Modern cemented acetabular cups often have **flanges** to compress the cement, **grooves** to increase the surface area and improve bonding and **pods** to prevent bottoming out. However, deep grooves reduce polyethylene thickness, which may result in stress risers predisposing to creep, fatigue and failure.

Uncemented cups rely on an initial press-fit or screw fixation before bone on-growth. As yet, there are no long-term data to support their increased popularity.

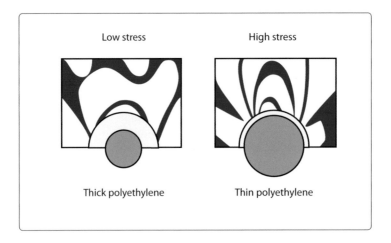

Figure 19.4 Effect of polyethylene thickness and femoral head size on dissipation of stress within bone.

Femoral component

A stylized femoral component is shown in **Figure 19.5**. As discussed above, increasing the offset of a hip joint – in this case, using a stem design with a large medial offset – results in an increased abductor lever arm. Although this may be advantageous with weakened post-operative abductor function, if it is achieved by increasing the neck length this leads to an increase in stress transfer at the tip of the component and an increase in strain on the medial cement mantle, which can lead to implant failure.

There are three commonly used modes of femoral stem fixation:

- **Cementless** fixation.
- **Cemented** – all interfaces fixed (**composite beam**).
- **Cemented** – bone interface fixed, stem cement interface free to slip (**taper slip**).

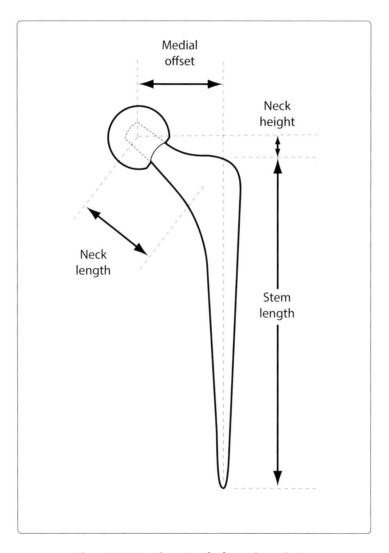

Figure 19.5 Key elements of a femoral prosthesis.

A well-bonded cementless implant and a cemented implant with all interfaces fixed produce similar stresses at the interface between the implant (including cement) and bone. These are high shear stresses, low compressive stresses and medium tensile stresses.

By contrast, implants using cemented taper fit exhibit low shear stresses, high compressive stresses and almost no tensile stresses. The ability of bone cement to undergo creep and stress relaxation is primarily responsible for the conversion of tensile stress to compressive stress at the cement–bone interface.

A constant source of interest in hip arthroplasty is the optimal bearing surface for young high-demand patients. The place of metal/polyethylene bearing surface is well established in lower-demand patients, but in more challenging cases the option of hard-on-hard bearing surfaces such as ceramics now exists. As yet, although there are attractive possible benefits in terms of wear debris and its nature, there are few long-term clinical studies to support its use. In addition, ceramic bearings have the additional potential complication of head or liner fracture, which presents extreme difficulties in revision surgery due to third-body particles. At present, the surgeon should have good reasons for departing from well-proven technology.

Hip resurfacing with metal-on-metal bearings is an attractive concept, as it is bone-conserving, allows normal femoral loading, avoids stress shielding, improves functional results, restores anatomy (although it may not restore offset as well as once thought) and reduces the risk of dislocation. In addition, lubrication at the interface is likely to be fluid-film in nature. However, the surgery is not conservative on the acetabulum, and the long-term effect of raised plasma metal ion levels is concerning (possible risks of sensitivity, teratogenicity, carcinogenicity and lymphocyte activation) (see Chapter 25).

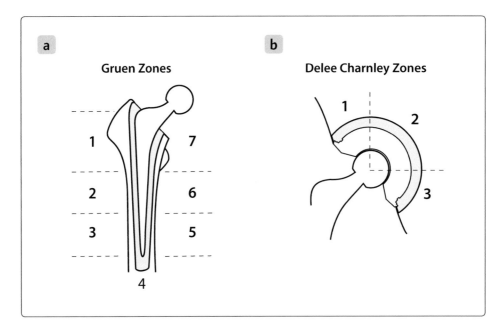

Figure 19.6 Radiolucent zones of the femur (a) and the acetabulum (b).

Osteolysis and wear in hip arthroplasty

The most common mode of failure for established implants is osteolysis from wear debris. This debris is generated from all surfaces where contact and movement occur, and it is important to consider that this may arise from modular components, at the prosthesis–cement and cement–bone interfaces and at bearing surfaces.

Radiolucent zones have been characterized in the femur by Gruen *et al.* (1979) and in the acetabulum by Delee and Charnley (1976) (**Figure 19.6**). The subsequent **modes of femoral component failure** have also been characterized by Gruen *et al.* (1979) (**Figure 19.7**).

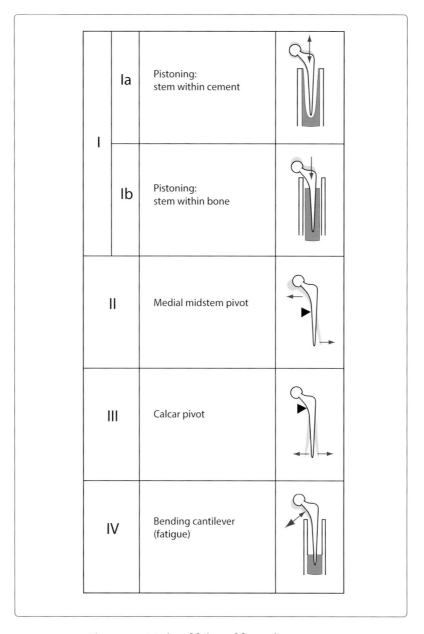

Figure 19.7 Modes of failure of femoral components.

Since the turn of the twenty-first century, there has become a vogue for 'mini-incision' THR. The exact definition of this term is unclear, with wound sizes of less than 10 cm or 12 cm being suggested, as well as the use of alternative approaches such as the two-incision technique. Some of the factors driving this change have undoubtedly been the potential commercial gains together with the goal of shorter inpatient stay. As yet, only the proponents of these techniques have demonstrated markedly improved results in terms of inpatient stay; how much of this has been due to improved anaesthesia, rehabilitation programmes and social support is unclear. It is vital to stress that any decrease in inpatient stay should not be at the expense of the long-term survivorship of the prosthesis. These moves have, however, encouraged all arthroplasty surgeons to consider ways of optimizing the surgical procedure and associated patient care.

Summary

In conclusion, knowledge of the biomechanics of the hip is essential in order for informed decisions about patient management and implant design to be undertaken. Published long-term data on differing implants must also be considered in the light of previous experiences, such as the Capital hip replacement; meta-analyses such as the **Swedish Hip Register** are particularly valuable.

Viva questions

1. Which total hip prosthesis would you use, and what is the evidence to support this choice?
2. Describe the modes of failure of different types of total hip replacement (THR).
3. When planning a THR, which are the important factors to consider?
4. When reviewing a THR in a follow-up clinic, what clinical symptoms and radiological signs are of particular concern?
5. Which approach do you prefer for THR, and what are its relative merits and weaknesses?

Further reading

Barrack RL, Mulroy RD, Jr, Harris WH. Improved cementing techniques and femoral component loosening in young patients with hip arthroplasty: a 12-year radiographic review. *J Bone Joint Surg Br* 1992;**74**:385–9.

DeLee JG, Charnley J. Radiological demarcation of cemented sockets in total hip replacement. *Clin Orthop Relat Res* 1976;**121**:20–32.

Gruen TA, McNiece GM, Amstutz HC. Modes of failure of cemented stem-type femoral components: a radiographic analysis of loosening. *Clin Orthop Relat Res* 1979;**141**:17–27.

Murray DW, Carr AJ, Bulstrode C. Survival analysis of joint replacements. *J Bone Joint Surg Br* 1993;**75**:697–704.

Murray DW, Carr AJ, Bulstrode C. Which primary total hip replacement? *J Bone Joint Surg Br* 1995;**77**:520–27.

Ong KL, Manley MT, Nevelos J, Greene K. Review: biomechanical issues in total hip replacement. *Surg Technol Int* 2012;**22**:222–8.

20 Biomechanics and Joint Replacement of the Knee

Alister Hart, Joshua Lee, Richard Carrington and Paul Allen

Biomechanics of the normal knee

Relevant bone geometry

Femur

The **medial femoral condyle** is larger and extends more distally in comparison to the lateral condyle.

Tibia

There is **asymmetry** of the **tibial plateaus**. In the sagittal plane, the medial tibial plateau is slightly concave with a sloped anterior surface and a horizontal posterior surface. The lateral tibial plateau is slightly convex, with a flat horizontal articular surface; anterior and posterior to this the surface slopes downwards accommodating the anterior and posterior horns of the lateral meniscus. The tibial plateaus are made more congruent to the femoral condyle by the presence of the menisci. The asymmetry of the femoral condyles and tibial plateaus allows for rotation of the tibia about its anatomical long axis during knee flexion.

Tibiofemoral alignment and malalignment

Normal alignment is described in the frontal and lateral planes. The normal frontal alignment is described by the **weight-bearing axis** (from the centre of the hip to the centre of the ankle) of the limb passing through the centre of the knee (**Figure 20.1**). In **varus malalignment**, the centre of the knee is lateral to the weight-bearing axis; in **valgus malalignment**, the centre of the knee is medial to the weight-bearing axis.

The centre of the knee lying just posterior to the weight-bearing axis describes normal lateral alignment. The result of this is an extension force, requiring passive resistance of the posterior capsule and ligaments with minimal muscular action. If the centre of the knee is located well

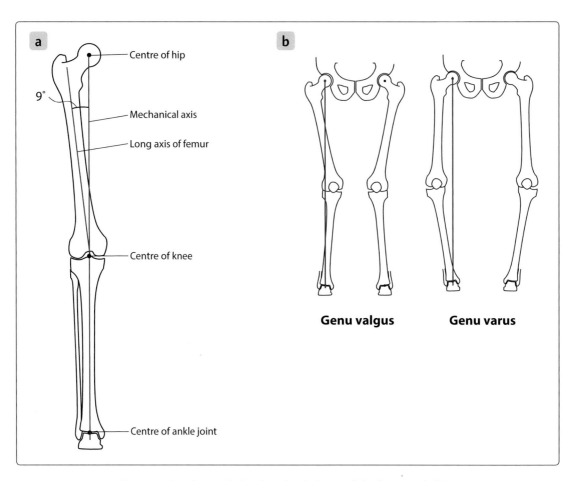

Figure 20.1 a: Anatomical and mechanical axes of the femur and tibia;
b: abnormalities of coronal mechanical axis alignment.

behind the weight-bearing axis, then there will be hyperextension malalignment. If the centre of the knee is located in front of the weight-bearing axis, then flexion malalignment exists.

Knee joint motion

Flexion–extension and femoral rollback

It was thought that the femur rolled across the tibia with flexion because the cruciate ligaments, in conjunction with the femur and tibia, provided a rigid four-bar linkage. This mechanism produces a mixture of femoral **rollback and slide**, which allows the high degree of flexion seen in the normal knee (**Figure 20.2**). This simplistic mechanism has been used to design successful knee replacements.

Studies using magnetic resonance imaging (MRI) of cadaveric and living knees has revealed that during flexion the lateral femoral condyle does rollback across the tibia, with relatively little rollback of the medial femoral condyle. This difference in the amount of rollback leads to internal rotation of the tibia in relation to the femur with **flexion**.

The **biomechanical functions** of femoral rollback are two-fold: to **increase the lever arm** of the quadriceps and to allow **clearance** of the femur from the tibia in deep flexion (see **Figure 20.2**). During knee extension, the femur rolls forwards, increasing the lever arm of the hamstrings to act as a brake on hyperextension.

The rigid four-bar linkage mechanism is disputed. Anatomically, one visualizes the four linked bars of two cruciate ligaments and the two areas of bone that lie between the insertions of the cruciates, but in practice the ligaments are not rigid and do not have a single isometric point at all positions of flexion. The result is variable tension in different bundles of fibres of the same ligament at different degrees of flexion.

The **flexion–extension axis** for the knee is reasonably approximated to the **trans-epicondylar line** (TEL). A lateral view of the femur reveals that the posterior projections of the condyles are defined by two concentric circles centred on the TEL.

Rotation during flexion–extension

The **medial compartment** is deeply dished due to the concave tibial plateau and a relatively fixed meniscus. The result is an **anteroposterior excursion** of the tibiofemoral contact point of less than 1 cm. The **lateral compartment**, with its convex tibial plateau and much more mobile lateral meniscus, has a much greater excursion (2 cm) of the tibiofemoral contact point; in full flexion the contact point is shared between the tibia and posterior horn of the meniscus. This asymmetry in movement leads to axial rotation of the lateral compartment around the medial compartment by up to 30° over the whole of flexion range.

From extension to full flexion, the tibia internally rotates with respect to the femur. From full flexion to extension, the tibia externally rotates with respect to the femur. The external rotation of the tibia on the femur that occurs during the terminal degrees of knee extension is termed the **screw-home mechanism** and results in tightening of both the cruciate ligaments, locking

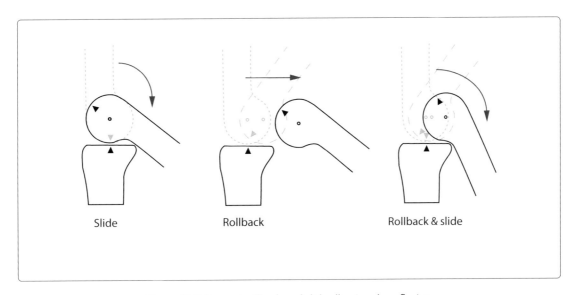

Figure 20.2 Femoral rollback and slide allowing deep flexion.

the knee such that the tibia is in the position of maximal stability with respect to the femur. Contraction of the popliteus, causing internal rotation of the tibia, is responsible for the unlocking of the knee when the knee moves from full extension to initiation of flexion.

The geometry and alignment of the bony anatomy creates articular surfaces with a constant flexion–extension gap, so that the tension is maintained in the supporting ligaments throughout flexion and extension.

The patellofemoral joint

The biomechanical function of the patella is to act as a pulley for the quadriceps and increase the power of the quadriceps by increasing the moment arm. Patellectomy reduces quadriceps strength by at least 20%.

Patellofemoral joint alignment

The **Q angle** is defined by the intersection of lines joining the centre of the patella with the anterior superior iliac spine and the tibial tubercle. The normal Q angle varies between 5 and 20°. Women have an increased Q angle compared with men. Angles greater than 20° are associated with patellofemoral instability and pain.

Patella and trochlear geometry

Patella geometry is variable and can be grouped into three types according to **Wiberg** (**Figure 20.3a**). Type 1 has equal medial and lateral facets, which are both concave. Type 2 has a concave lateral facet and a smaller concave medial facet. Type 3 has an even smaller medial facet, which is convex. Wiberg proposed that the patella with a deficient medial facet is more likely to develop patellofemoral osteoarthritis (OA).

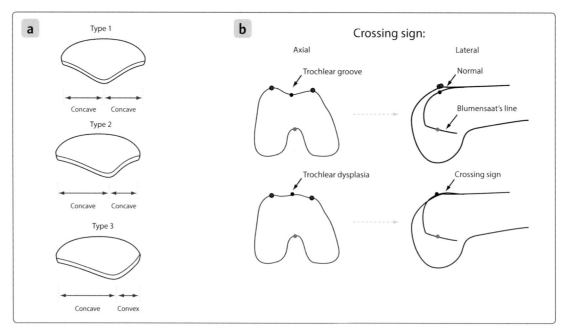

Figure 20.3 a. Wiberg classification of patellar geometry b. Crossing sign in Dejour's classification of trochlear dysplasia (Grade A).

The patella sits in the trochlea, providing the bony restraint of the patellofemoral joint. In the normal trochlea, the sulcus angle (the angle formed between the highest point of the medial femoral condyle to the sulcus and lateral femoral condyle) is on average $137° ± 8°$. The highest point of the lateral femoral condyle is more anterior than the medial and the sulcus deepens more distally. Trochlea geometry is also very variable and Dejours has classified the degree of trochlea dysplasia into four types based on the lateral radiograph and axial (computed tomography[CT]/MRI) imaging:

- **Grade A**, crossing sign (on true lateral radiograph of the knee the line of the trochlea groove crosses the anterior border of either of the femoral condyles) and relatively shallow trochlea.
- **Grade B**, crossing sign and flat or concave trochlea.
- **Grade C**, crossing sign and double contour (line seen on lateral radiograph due to hypoplastic medial femoral condyle).
- **Grade D**, features of grade C plus vertical join between facets or cliff pattern (seen on axial imaging).

The variables that determine patella tracking are patella geometry (Wiberg type 3 patella tracking laterally due to its deficient medial facet), dysplasia of the trochlea and a laterally placed tibial tubercle (increase in the Q angle). Measurement of the tibial tuberosity–trochlear groove (TT–TG) distance by superimposing two CT images (through TT and through trochlear sulcus) indicates laterally placed TT when the TT–TG is greater than 20 mm. In such cases a medial transfer of the TT may be indicated.

In addition to the bony contours, soft tissues provide additional static restraints to the patella. Of particular interest in recent years is the function of the **medial patellofemoral ligament** (MPFL). It is a distinct condensation of capsular fibres within layer 2 of the medial structures of the knee, originating from the medial femoral epicondyle and part of the superficial medial collateral ligament, inserting into the superomedial aspect of the patella. It provides a medial check-rein to the patella and is commonly disrupted in acute patella dislocations. In recurrent dislocation of the patella, if the bony anatomy is within normal limits, then it may be appropriate to reconstruct the MPFL.

Patellofemoral joint motion

The patella first engages the femoral sulcus at 20° of knee flexion and tracks along a conforming groove. At 20° of flexion, the distal part of the patella makes contact first. As the knee flexes, the contact area of the patella shifts proximally. Beyond 90° the patella rotates externally, and only the medial facet articulates. At extreme flexion, the patella lies in the intercondylar groove.

Patellofemoral contact pressure is 0.5 times body weight during walking, increasing to between 2.5 and 3.3 times body weight when ascending and descending stairs.

Functional biomechanics

There are **static** and **dynamic** elements to the biomechanics of the knee. The static elements include the **alignment** of the articulating bones, the **geometry** of their weight-bearing surfaces, and the **laxity** of the connecting ligaments. The dynamic elements are the **coordinated activity** of the muscles. Proprioception helps to optimize knee function within the static limits.

How is stable movement of the knee achieved?

There are **primary and secondary restraints** to all degrees of freedom of movement of the knee. Sectioning studies have quantified the contribution of the secondary restraints. Individual ligaments have primary and secondary functions.

Anterior translation

The **primary restraint** to anterior translation of the tibia on the femur is the **anterior cruciate ligament** (ACL). The ACL is composed of two bundles – the anteromedial (tight in flexion) and the posterolateral (tight in extension). When the knee is flexed to 30°, the ACL provides 87% of the restraint against anterior translation.

The **secondary restraints** to anterior translation are as follows:

- Iliotibial band: 24%
- Mid-medial capsule: 22%.
- Mid-lateral capsule: 20%.
- Medial collateral ligament (MCL): 16%.
- Lateral collateral ligament (LCL): 12%.
- Menisci.

In addition, the hamstrings are dynamic stabilizers of anterior translation.

The ACL is important in controlling the anteroposterior tibiofemoral contact point at all positions of flexion. The function of the ACL, to resist varus, valgus and rotational forces, is most relevant in combined ligament injuries.

Posterior translation

The **primary restraint** to posterior translation of the tibia is the **posterior cruciate ligament** (PCL). The **secondary restraint** is the LCL.

The primary function of the PCL is to resist posterior tibial translation on the fixed femur. The PCL is also a secondary restraint to external rotation, varus and valgus joint space opening, and hyperextension. The PCL contributes 95% of the restraining force to posterior translation at 90° of knee flexion. The posterolateral corner (LCL, arcuate ligament, popliteal muscle/tendon complex, posterolateral capsule, fabellofibular ligament) provides 59% of additional restraining force after the PCL has been sectioned, and the MCL supplies an additional 16% restraint.

Internal rotation

The **primary restraint** is the **ACL**. The **secondary restraints** are the popliteal oblique ligaments (POL) and posteromedial complex (PMC).

External rotation

The **primary restraints** to external rotation are the **popliteofibular ligament**, and the LCL and the posterolateral complex at 30 degrees of flexion. The MCL is important also at all degrees of flexion.

Valgus

The **superficial MCL is the primary restraint** to valgus stress at all angles, with its least effect at full extension. The PMC is tight at full extension but slackens with flexion greater than 30°. The deep MCL has little resistance to valgus load. The ACL acts as a secondary restraint to valgus force.

Varus

The **LCL is the primary restraint** to varus stress in all positions of flexion. Its greatest effect is at 30°, and its least effect is at full extension. The ACL and posterolateral structures are the secondary restraints to varus stress.

The posterolateral structures

The posterolateral corner of the knee is composed of the iliotibial band, biceps femoris tendon, LCL, popliteus tendon, fabellofibular ligament, popliteofibular ligament (PFL), arcuate ligament, coronary ligament, posterior horn of the lateral meniscus, middle third of the lateral capsular ligament and posterolateral joint capsule.

There are three distinct layers within the lateral structures of the knee:

- **Superficial layer**: iliotibial tract and biceps.
- **Middle layer**: quadriceps retinaculum anteriorly and the two patellofemoral ligaments posteriorly.
- **Deep layer**: superficial and deep capsular lamina. The superficial lamina includes the LCL and the fabellofibular ligament. The deep lamina consists of the coronary ligament, popliteus hiatus, arcuate ligament and PFL.

The LCL is a primary restraint to varus rotation at 30° of knee flexion and a secondary restraint against external rotation and posterior displacement. The PFL prevents excessive posterior translation and varus angulation, and restricts excessive primary and coupled external rotation (greater effect at 30° than at 90°).

Isolated PCL sectioning results in increased posterior translation that is maximal at 70–90° of knee flexion. Combined sectioning of the LCL and PFL results in increased varus rotation, external rotation and posterior translation that is maximal at 30° of flexion. Combined LCL, PFL and PCL injury results in increased varus rotation, external rotation and posterior translation at all angles of knee flexion. Additionally, isolated sectioning of the popliteus muscle belly does not cause significant posterolateral instability of the knee.

Biomechanics of knee arthroplasty

Introduction

Before the modern designs of condylar total knee replacement (TKR), TKR was performed using fixed hinges with poor medium- and long-term survival. Condylar TKRs were conceived by three groups (Insall *et al.*, Freeman and Samuelson, and Walker and Sledge) between 1969 and 1974. This enabled resurfacing of the distal femur and proximal tibia with implants whose shape resembled the natural knee.

TKRs can be classified according to their degree of constraint, whether the PCL is retained or sacrificed or whether they are mobile or fixed-bearing. **Figure 20.4** shows the range of TKR designs available on the market.

Natural knee motion is complex, involving six degrees of freedom (translation and rotation about each of the axes x, y and z). Rigid-hinge TKR allows only one degree of freedom (rotation about the x axis), resulting in flexion and extension. This provides a stable articulation, but it also increases the force transmitted to the implant–cement–bone interface and thus increases the risk of loosening. Modern hinge designs use **sloppy hinges**, by incorporating metal on polyethylene bushings and rotating platforms. The development of the non-hinged TKR reflects the evolution of the understanding of knee kinematics, stability, constraint and conformity.

The first **condylar TKRs** were cruciate-sacrificing. Stability in the sagittal plane (resisting anteroposterior translation) was achieved by a curved tibial articulating surface. The surface is therefore **conforming** because the radii of the tibial and femoral surfaces are similar. Importantly, this does not imply that the knee is constrained, since constraint is a function of the surface contours together with the peri-articular soft tissues. Stability in the coronal plane (resisting varus/valgus forces) was achieved with the median intercondylar eminence. To reiterate, **conformity** is a purely **static mechanical** concept, whereas **constraint** is a **dynamic kinematic** concept.

The **PCL-retaining TKR** is thought to replicate knee kinematics more closely because the native PCL causes femoral rollback and increased stability. This is controversial. These implants have low conformity with a **round-on-flat design** to allow femoral rollback. In the coronal plane, the disadvantage of a round-on-flat design is that **lift-off** can occur, followed by **slam-down** and **edge-loading** of the polyethylene, resulting in increased contact stress and wear.

The **PCL-substituting** (or **posterior-stabilized**) TKRs have increased tibial contouring (conformity) in both the sagittal and the coronal planes. Sagittal plane stability is achieved with the femoral cam and tibial post. Coronal plane stability is achieved with the conforming surfaces and collateral ligaments.

The most **constrained condylar TKR** are **revision TKR designs** such as the Total Condylar III (TC3)™ prosthesis with an intimately fitting cam and spine mechanism

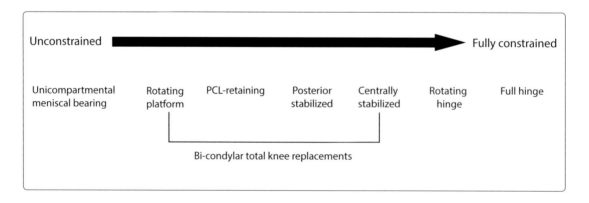

Figure 20.4 The spectrum of constraint in knee arthroplasty. PCL: posterior cruciate ligament.

that is broader and more elevated than the posterior stabilized TKR. The TC3 allows 2° of internal and external rotation and 1.25° of varus and valgus motion. Its use is restricted to partial collateral ligament insufficiency or bone loss requiring augments to recreate an equal flexion–extension gap. The greater constraint of such devices increases the forces transmitted to the implant–cement–bone interface and therefore, intramedullary stems are used to distribute the forces over a larger area.

Condylar TKR design

A successful TKR is well fixed to the supporting bone, is durable and allows good knee function with near-normal knee kinematics. This requires a compromise of competing objectives. For example, replication of the sliding and rolling back of the normal femur during deep flexion requires low conformity, such as that seen with a flat polyethylene tibial tray in the sagittal plane. The disadvantage is reduced contact area and high contact stress, resulting in increased wear. Higher conformity increases contact area, but higher constraint transmits greater force to the bone–cement–implant interface to increase the risk of loosening.

Kinematics of TKR

Flexion–extension is controlled by the geometry of the femoral condyles and the polyethylene insert. The natural femoral condyles have two radii of curvature – a large **anterior radius** in contact with the tibia during extension and a small **posterior radius** in contact during flexion. Most condylar TKRs approximate this natural geometry. However, some, such as the Triathlon TKR ™, have a single femoral radius. Most TKRs have matched medial and lateral condylar geometry. An exception is seen with the medial pivot knee design, which has a more conforming medial compartment and a less conforming lateral compartment capable of sliding, in an attempt to replicate the internal/external rotation in flexion/extension of the normal knee as described earlier in this chapter.

Condylar design compromise

The ideal TKR minimizes contact stress but allows near normal knee kinematics and provides sufficient constraint to ensure stability throughout functional use. Unfortunately, constraint is defined by its limitation of degrees of freedom.

If a TKR is designed such that it is completely conforming in the coronal and sagittal planes, then contact stress would be low but kinematics would be similar to a simple hinge with virtually only one degree of freedom, i.e. flexion and extension. This would increase the torsional stress across the joint, causing loosening (unless the stress was dissipated through a rotating platform).

The condylar compromise

- Contact stress inversely proportional to constraint.
- Normal kinematics inversely proportional to constraint.
- High contact stress causes loosening.
- Increased constraint increases loosening.

Solution: compromise constraint to allow low contact stress and reduce loosening.

Thus, the femoral and polyethylene radii determine both the rotation and the flexion–extension constraint. In terms of **coronal plane geometry**, a relatively **flat-on-flat** design can result in edge-loading and consequent slam-down during varus–valgus loading, whereas a **curved-on-curved** design reduces edge-loading, spreading the load over a wider area during varus–valgus loading (**Figure 20.5**).

Polyethylene thickness

Polyethylene inserts with a thickness greater than 8 mm reduce the variability in contact stress, resulting in less polyethylene wear. However, the manufacture, sterilization and storage of polyethylene are also important in reducing wear. For more detail, see Chapter 25.

Biomechanical goals of TKR

From a purely anatomical perspective, the following goals allow optimal biomechanical performance of a condylar TKR:

- Restore the mechanical axis so that it passes through the centres of the hip, knee and ankle.
- Make the bone cuts perpendicular to the mechanical axis.
- Preserve the level of the joint line.
- Balance the ligaments.
- Ensure rigid durable fixation.

These goals are achieved through design and surgical technique.

Mechanical alignment

Restoring the mechanical alignment prevents a net varus or valgus force, which causes uneven contact pressure on the polyethylene and early failure. It also prevents instability and pain through unbalanced ligaments. In the case of incompletely correctable deformities, additional soft-tissue releases are required for ligament balance.

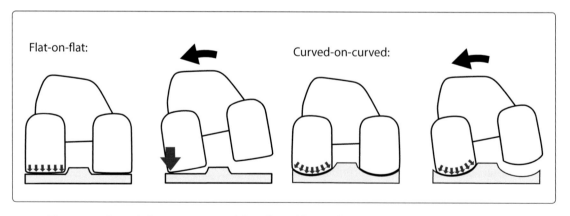

Figure 20.5 Coronal plane geometry and the effect of flat-on-flat' versus 'curved-on-curved' designs.

Mechanical alignment is determined by the femoral and tibial bone cuts. The femur and tibia are cut in order to allow the thickness of the prosthesis to recreate the original thickness of the bone and cartilage in both flexion and extension and with joint line height preserved.

Tibial bone cuts

The natural tibial plateau is 3° varus to the mechanical axis; however, it is recommended that the tibia is cut perpendicular to the mechanical axis because this is more easily reproduced in the surgical setting as well as even loading of the medial and lateral sides of the tibia. Tibial component rotation is a critical variable, and malrotation can lead to poor patella tracking including dislocation, anterior knee pain and stiffness. The tibial tubercle is slightly externally rotated in the natural knee; one surgical technique is to align the rotation of the tibial component using a line connecting the centre of the tibial tray to the medial third of the tibial tubercle.

Femoral bone cuts

The valgus cut angle is the angle between the femoral anatomical axis and the mechanical axis. It is between 5 and 7° and should be calculated with full-length lower-limb X-rays in certain patients, e.g. very tall/very small patients, history of previous trauma or congenital deformity.

The valgus cut angle aims to cut the femur perpendicular to the mechanical axis. The femoral component is 3° externally rotated with respect to the femoral neutral axis, in order to create a rectangular flexion gap with the tibia. The natural tibia is in 3° of varus, but the recommended tibial cut is perpendicular to the mechanical axis, therefore placing the tibial component in 3° of valgus with reference to the natural tibia. To create a rectangular flexion gap in this situation, the femur must be cut with 3° of external rotation. If, after the femoral and tibial cuts, the flexion gap is not equal, then the tight ligaments on the concave side of the deformity usually require release.

There are several methods used to judge femoral component rotation (**Figure 20.6**). The **epicondylar axis** is actually 1–3° externally rotated to the neutral axis, and therefore a femoral component that is parallel to this axis is in optimum position. Note that this line is almost universally present at revision surgery. **Whiteside's line** is a vertical line joining the roof of the notch with the deepest point of the trochlear. A line perpendicular to Whiteside's line is the epicondylar axis. The **posterior condylar axis** is parallel to the neutral axis and 3° internally rotated in relation to the epicondylar axis, when the posterior condyles are not worn or hypoplastic.

Ligament balancing

Ligament balancing in both the coronal and the sagittal planes is essential in order to create a stable knee, reduce wear and maintain function. The degenerate knee has either contracted or stretched ligaments. A degenerate knee with a **pre-operative varus deformity** that has non-parallel flexion or extension gaps usually has a contracted MCL, which must be released. A degenerate knee with a **pre-operative valgus deformity** that has non-parallel flexion or extension gaps usually has contracted lateral structures (popliteus, LCL, iliotibial band). A degenerate knee with a pre-operative **fixed flexion deformity** that is tighter posteriorly after

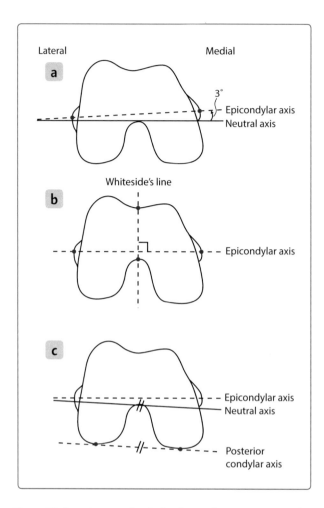

Figure 20.6a–c Axes used to judge femoral component rotation.

bone cuts are made has tight posterior structures (capsule and PCL).The release is therefore performed on the concave side of the deformity. A pre-operative correctable deformity is likely to be balanced after the bone cuts have been made.

The order of structures to be released for a **varus** knee is as follows: osteophytes, deep MCL, posteromedial corner with attachment of semimembranosus, superficial MCL and PCL.

The order of structures to be released for a **valgus** knee is as follows: osteophytes, lateral capsule, iliotibial band (tight in extension), popliteus (tight in flexion), LCL, intermuscular septum and lateral head of gastrocnemius.

PCL and TKR function

The normal PCL is taut in knee flexion, preventing posterior translation of the tibia and allowing femoral rollback to occur in deep flexion, enabling a greater degree of flexion by preventing impingement. There are two schools of thought in regards whether to preserve or excise the PCL.

In an unconstrained TKR sacrificing the ACL and PCL risks flexion instability and, without femoral rollback, may limit flexion to 95°. Preserving the PCL should reduce flexion instability and allow femoral rollback. Conversely, in a degenerate knee, the PCL is contracted and unlikely to function normally.

PCL resection combined with a cam-and-post mechanism to mimic the femoral rollback was developed in the 1970s as the solution to this problem. Modern designs of PCL-sacrificing TKR use, first, a relatively **high tibiofemoral congruency** to reduce contact stress and increase anteroposterior stability and, second, a **cam-and-post mechanism** to control femoral rollback. Some surgeons cite biomechanical reasons for choosing a posterior-stabilized TKR, such as previous patellectomy (weakens the extensor mechanism, which increases anteroposterior instability), inflammatory arthritis (which can cause late rupture of the PCL) and previous trauma to the PCL. Advocates of PCL retention note that use of a PCL-sacrificing TKR requires the removal of a significantly large bone block to accommodate the cam mechanism. This can lead to fracture of one of the condyles intraoperatively; if the implant needs to be revised in the future, retention of bone stock is important and at the original surgery significantly more bone has been removed than in a PCL-retaining design.

Patellofemoral joint in TKR

There are three design solutions for patellar implants: **dome** (eliminates rotational alignment problems), **anatomical** (increases conformity but requires accurate alignment of components and soft-tissue balancing) and **mobile bearing** (the need for metal backing here reduces the thickness of the polyethylene and early loosening and has largely been discontinued).

Optimizing patella tracking in TKR

The Q angle (defined earlier) is formed between the intersection of the line describing the direction of pull of the quadriceps superior to the patella and the line describing the direction of the patella tendon. Increasing the Q angle increases the force acting in a lateral direction at the patellofemoral joint, which causes patella maltracking and subluxation.

The key to optimal patellar tracking is correct rotational alignment of the femoral and tibial components. Internally rotating the tibial component effectively externally rotates the tibial tubercle, increasing the Q angle. Tracking can be improved further by aligning the femoral component with the lateral cortex of the lateral femoral condyle and by slight medialization of the patella component.

Patella height in TKR

A short patella tendon causes patella baja. If the patient has patella baja preoperatively, then one should consider recreating the correct patellar height by lowering the joint line by under-resecting the distal femur, over-resecting the tibia, or upsizing the femur to balance the flexion gap and placing the patella dome superiorly.

If the joint line is inadvertently raised as a consequence of TKR, then the patella tendon becomes functionally short. This can result in impingement of the inferior patella pole on the polyethylene insert during flexion.

Biomechanics of TKR failure

Factors that cause polyethylene wear in TKR

- **Thickness of polyethylene**: if the polyethylene used is less than 8 mm thick, then the contact stress is greater than the yield strength of the polyethylene. Note that polyethylene insert thickness is usually expressed as the thickness of the tibial base plate and polyethylene together, so that an 8 mm insert may be approximately 6 mm thick at its lowest point.
- **Articular geometry**: flat polyethylene reduces the contact surface area and increases the contact load. Conforming polyethylene has the opposite effect.

Other factors include the method of **polyethylene sterilization**, **increased conformity** leading to increased backside wear and the use of **all polyethylene components** (see Chapter 25).

Backside wear

Backside wear is wear of the non-articulating surface of the tibial insert. This has been observed in all designs of knee prostheses, independent of the capture mechanism of the polyethylene insert. There is no effective way to eliminate backside wear in modular tibial components, though some designs of locking mechanism are better than others in reducing micro-motion. In addition, the top surface of tibial trays in nearly all TKR designs is highly polished in an attempt to reduce the amount of wear.

What factors in TKR design increase the probability of loosening?

Factors that affect load transfer and increase the probability of implant loosening include:

- Flexible implant (low thickness/length ratio).
- Small contact area.
- Load transfer at the edges of contact (e.g. caused by a large varus–valgus movement, or anteroposterior or medial-lateral instability) in an unbalanced knee.
- Features that concentrate stress, e.g. peripheral tibial tray pegs.

Viva questions

1. Which total knee replacement (TKR) would you use, and what is the evidence to support this choice?
2. When planning a TKR, which are the important factors to consider?
3. When reviewing a TKR in a follow-up clinic, what clinical symptoms and radiological signs are of particular concern?
4. How would you correct a varus/valgus/fixed-flexion knee deformity during TKR?
5. What factors contribute to failure of TKRs?

Further reading

Alpert JM, McCarty LP, Bach BR Jr. The posterolateral corner of the knee: anatomic dissection and surgical approach. *J Knee Surg* 2008;**21**(1):50–4.

Conditt MA, Stein JA, Noble PC. Factors affecting the severity of backside wear of modular tibial inserts. *J Bone Joint Surg Am* 2004;**86**:305–11.

Freeman MA, Pinskerova V. The movement of the normal tibio-femoral joint. J Biomech 2005;**38**:197–208.

Morgan H, Battista V, Leopold SS. Constraint in primary total knee arthroplasty. *J Am Acad Orthop Surg* 2005;**13**:515–24.

Sharkey PF, Hozack WJ, Rothman RH, Shastri S, Jacoby, SM. Insall Award paper. Why are total knee arthroplasties failing today? *Clin Orthop Relat Res* 2002;**404**:7–13.

21 Biomechanics of the Spine

Amir Ali Narvani, Arun Ranganathan, Brian Hsu and Lester Wilson

Introduction

Interest in biomechanics of the spine developed in the latter half of the twentieth century. Sir Frank Holdsworth proposed the two-column model of the spine in 1963. Most of our current understanding of spinal biomechanics dates back to the work conducted by White and Panjabi, who published their work for the first time in 1978. Denis proposed the three-column model of the lumbar spine to explain spinal instability following fractures. The basic element of spinal biomechanics is the functional spinal unit.

Functional spinal unit

The functional spinal unit is the **smallest physiological unit of the spine that exhibits biomechanical properties similar to that of the entire spine** (White and Panjabi). This includes two adjacent vertebral bodies, the intervertebral disc, facet joints and all adjoining ligaments, but excludes muscles (**Figure 21.1**). It is also called a **spinal motion segment** or an **articular triad**.

It is also important to define the **neutral zone** and the **elastic zone**. The neutral zone is the motion region of the joint **which functions independent of the osseoligamentous complex and a relatively small load produces a large displacement** on the **load displacement curve** (**Figure 21.2**). On the other hand, the elastic zone is the remaining area of the joint, which produces **maximum resistance to displacement by a load**. The neutral zone and the elastic zone put together constitute the total range of motion present in a joint.

Definition of spinal stability

White and Panjabi defined spinal stability as the ability of the spine under **physiological loads** to **limit patterns of displacement that can damage or irritate the spinal cord or nerve roots** and, in addition, to **prevent incapacitating deformity or pain caused by structural changes**.

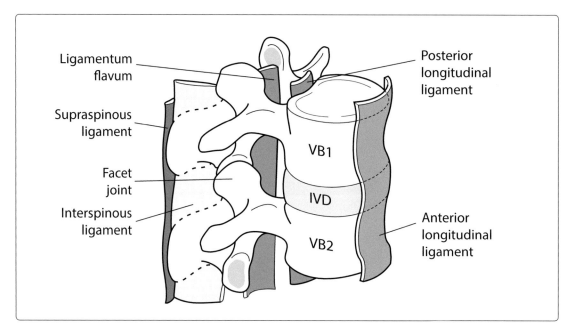

Figure 21.1 Components of a functional spinal unit.

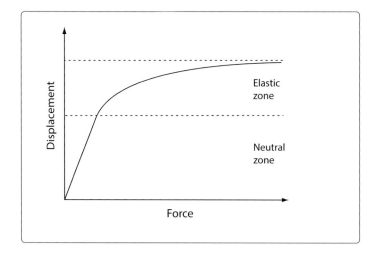

Figure 21.2 Force–displacement curve for spine demonstrating the neutral and elastic zones. The complete range of movement is the neutral zone and the elastic zone.

Concepts in developing a force-body diagram of the lumbar spine

Forces acting on the spine include:

- Body weight.
- Tension in the spinal ligaments.
- Tension in the surrounding muscles.
- Intra-abdominal pressure.

With the patient in an upright posture, the total body centre of gravity is **always anterior to the spinal column** and hence the spine is always subject to a **constant forward bending moment**. The perpendicular distance between the spinal muscles and the joints is relatively small and hence large forces are generated to resist the torque produced by the weight of the body during movements and while lifting weights. **Figure 21.3** illustrates these large forces, chiefly compression, tension and shear.

A complete free-body diagram of the lumbar spine should include the individual weights of the head, trunk, upper limb and the weight lifted, along with their respective distances from the centre of spinal motion. This becomes more complicated if the angular inclination at every level of the vertebral column is included and if segmental trunk weight is considered, depending on the level of the spine that is being considered for the free-body diagram. **Figure 21.4** illustrates a simplified force-body diagram to show the torque experienced by the erector spinae muscles to counteract forces at the L5–S1 level while lifting a weight.

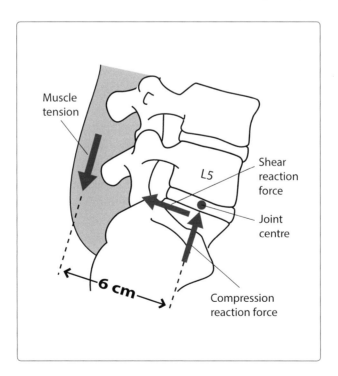

Figure 21.3 Forces generated within a segment of the lumbar spine.

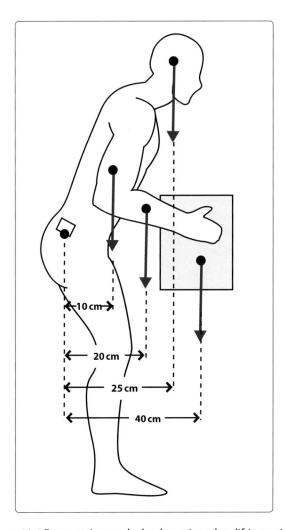

Figure 21.4 Forces acting on the lumbar spine when lifting weights.

During stance phase, postural muscles are consistently firing and active. Normal positioning of vertebral segments and with adequate sagittal alignment ensures that the energy expenditure and activity in the postural muscles is minimal. If the line of centre of gravity is displaced forwards (usually the case but can be rarely backwards), the muscles have to counteract by increased activity and energy expenditure. Factors influencing the load on the spine during activities such as lifting weights include the size, shape, weight and density of the object, the relative displacement of the object from the centre of motion in the spine, the degree of spinal flexion and the rate of loading.

If the weight of the head and upper limb is neglected in order to understand the effect of posture on spinal loading, the free-body diagram can be further simplified. **Figure 21.5** demonstrates the increased load experienced by the spine when loads are lifted with the spine in forward flexion.

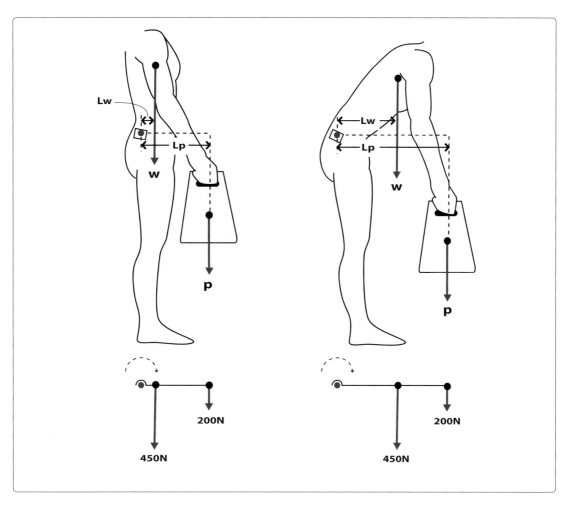

Figure 21.5 Free-body diagram of the lumbar spine when lifting a weight with the spine straight and in flexion, the latter increasing the load on the spine. Lw: Lever arm for body weight. Lp: Lever arm for weight carried in hand.

The spine comprises a long column with important anatomical units that can function independently and also in unification with each other, to produce synchronous motion. In order to understand the biomechanical concepts for the different parts of the spine, they have been divided into three functional and anatomical units, the **cervical spine** including the upper cervical spine and the occipitocervical junction, the **thoracic spine** and the **lumbar spine** including the lumbosacral junction.

Biomechanics of the cervical spine

The head houses five specialized sensory functions and the cervical spine helps to scan the surroundings in three-dimensional planes. The cervical spine subserves the **largest range of motion** yet protects the spinal cord throughout the full range of motion. Functionally the cervical spine can be divided into **four subunits** – the **occipitocervical joint**, the **atlantoaxial joint**, the **C2–3 joint** and the **subaxial cervical spine**.

Nodding (flexion and extension) is the chief motion occurring in the **atlanto-occipital (O–C1) joint**, and in all other planes of motion the O–C1 joint articulates and functions as a fixed segment. The occipital condyles are convex and the atlantal sockets are concave; the condyles move forward and backward in flexion and extension. Extremely strong ligaments stabilize the O–C1 joint. Softer constraints to this motion are provided by the structures in the throat impacting against each other and the posterior neck muscles. The firm endpoint to this rolling motion is the abutment of the rim of the socket against the base of the skull. Similarly the cranial vault impinging against the posterior cervical musculature limits extension.

The **atlantoaxial (AA) joint** permits a large degree of rotation. The AA joint can be divided into a median AA joint and a lateral AA joint constituted by the lateral masses. The arch of atlas pivots around the odontoid peg during axial rotation by a rotatory motion at the median AA joint and forward–backward coupling of the two lateral AA joints. The joint has an interesting architecture. It is biconvex and the atlas and axis rest on the tips of the convexity during static positioning. Intra-articular meniscoids render stability and determine the extent of joint contact during various degrees of motion. During rotation, the atlas slides down the anterior slope of the axis on one side and down the posterior slope on the contralateral side, thereby causing a decreased relative height between the atlas and axis. The strong capsule of the AA joint, transverse ligaments and the alar ligaments act as restraints to this motion. Bony endpoint to backward motion is provided by abutment of the atlantial arch against the odontoid peg; however, there is no bony anatomical constraint to forward sliding. Integrity of the odontoid peg and the ligaments prevent AA dislocations.

The **C2–3 joint** was always regarded as a part of the subaxial spine until recently when important anatomical differences were noticed. The superior articular process of C3 faces superiorly, posteriorly and is medially inclined at 40°. It forms a socket for the base of the C2 vertebra. It has also been noticed that the direction of coupling in lateral flexion is opposite to the remaining subaxial vertebrae. C2 rotates away from the axis of rotation of the rest of the subaxial cervical vertebrae in lateral flexion.

The **subaxial cervical vertebrae** articulate with each other through the intervertebral discs in front and the facet joints posteriorly. The end plates of subjacent vertebrae are angled forwards and downwards favouring flexion–extension in this region of the cervical spine. The posterior ends of the vertebral bodies form an ellipsoid joint between the convexity of the vertebral body above and the concavity of the posterior end of the body below; this culminates in the uncinate processes bilaterally. The intervertebral joints constitute a saddle joint that permits flexion–extension in the sagittal plane, and facetal sliding facilitates side-to-side rocking motion in the transverse plane. Rotation is possible in a plane perpendicular to the axis of the facet joints and the cervical facets are normally oriented 45° to the transverse plane of the vertebral bodies. Any horizontal rotation leads to lateral flexion of the vertebral body towards the side of rotation. The structure of the intervertebral disc also varies in the cervical spine, in that it lacks a posterior annulus except for a few longitudinal fibres in the median plane. Transverse fissures are a normal feature in cervical discs, which also assist axial rotation.

This wide range of motion is chiefly brought about by various groups of muscles acting in co-ordination. The chief anterior muscle is the sternocleidomastoid, which is a primary flexor and rotator. The muscles responsible for lateral bending are the scalenei. The most superficial of the posterior muscles are the trapezei, beneath which lie the primary extensors of the cervical spine. They fall into two groups, those that connect the cervical spine to the occiput (splenius capitis, semispinalis capitis and longissimus capitis) and those that connect the cervical spine to the cervical spine (splenius cervicis, semispinalis cervicis and longissimus cervicis). The suboccipital muscles (rectus capitis posterior minor and major, and obliquus capitis superior and inferior) stabilize the occiput, C1 and C2 articulations.

Biomechanics of the thoracic spine

The thoracic spine is unique in being the **least mobile segment of the spine** and having additional **stability and stiffness as a result of its articulation with the rib cage**. The thoracic spine is the largest segment of the spine and consists of 12 vertebrae. The thoracic spine is normally **kyphotic**, placing the vertebral bodies anteriorly under compression and the posterior arches in tension. The kyphosis is brought about predominantly due to the fact that the anterior height of the vertebral body is less than the posterior in the thoracic spine. The antero-posterior (AP) diameter increases from T1 to T12, whereas the medio-lateral diameter decreases from T1 to T3 and then increases to T12. The laminae overlap significantly compared to other regions of the spine. The spinal canal is narrowest in the thoracic spine making the spinal cord very vulnerable to stenosing conditions. The range of motion being very restricted in this region acts as a protective mechanism, making it less prone to degenerative conditions. The facets being coronally orientated resists any degree of translation. At T11 and T12, the orientation of the facets becomes transitional and the oblique sagittal orientation at this level is a direct reflection of this. The thoracic facets have a coronal angulation of 20° and a sagittal angulation of 55°. Demifacets superior and inferior to the disc articulate with rib heads as a synovial joint. Resection of the laminae and interspinous ligaments in cadaveric thoracic spines produced a large increase in the range of flexion–extension. The 11th and 12th ribs differ from the rest of the ribs and articulate with the side of the facets. The rib cage increases the stiffness of the thoracic spine especially in extension and rotation, and to a lesser degree in flexion. The ribs and sternum increase the moment of inertia in rotation and also the compressive tolerance of the spine by a factor of 4.

The thoracic discs are shorter and the annulus is much thicker giving greater resistance to rotation. The range of motion in the upper thoracic spine is 4°, 6° in the mid-thoracic region and 12° in the lower thoracic segments. Lateral flexion is 6° in the upper thoracic spine and 8–9° in the lower thoracic spine. Rotation in the upper thoracic spine is 9°.

Biomechanics of the lumbar spine

The **vertebral bodies in the lumbar spine are the largest in the spinal column** and they can sustain large loads. The lumbar intervertebral discs are large and they have a tough outer fibrocartilage with criss-crossed collagen fibres in the annulus fibrosus. The nucleus pulposus in the lumbar spine is slightly posteriorly disposed compared to the other regions of the spine. A combination of these factors helps the lumbar discs to counter large degrees of compression, tension and shear stresses. Further details on the intervertebral disc are in Chapter 15.

In the lumbar region, the facets are oriented at right angles to the transverse plane and at 45° to the frontal plane. This permits flexion, extension and lateral flexion but no rotation. The facets and the discs have a coupled function in load bearing. The disc is loaded in flexion and the facets take more than 30% of the load in hyperextension. Spinal ligaments are static stabilizers of the spine. All spinal ligaments except the ligamentum flavum have high collagen content, and this limits their extensibility during spinal motion. The ligamentum flavum primarily attaches to the posterior arches of adjacent vertebrae. It is rich in elastin content and hence contracts in extension and expands in flexion. This also helps maintain spinal canal dimensions during motion. The ligaments farthest away from the centre of rotation bear the maximum stress and maximally limit the motion. Thus the **anterior longitudinal ligament is maximally stressed in extension**, the **interspinous and supraspinous ligaments in forward flexion** and the **transverse ligaments in lateral flexion**. The range of flexion gradually increases in the lumbar motion segments and reaches 20° at L5–S1. Lateral flexion is limited to about 30° in the lumbar spine. Lateral rotation is 20° in the upper lumbar spine and increases to 50° in the lumbosacral junction.

The main extensors are erector spinae, multifidus and intertransversarii muscles. The main flexors are psoas, rectus abdominis, internal and external oblique and the transverse abdominal muscles. The first 50–60° of spinal flexion occurs in the lumbar spine, with the maximum percentage occurring in the L5–S1 region. Further flexion is caused by tilting of the pelvis, which is controlled by the posterior hip muscles. In complete flexion, the erector spinae become inactive due to the flexion–relaxation phenomenon. There is residual activity in the quadratus lumborum and lateral lumbar erector muscles when the superficial erector spinae are inactivated. The sequence of muscular activity is reversed in extension, with posterior rotation of the pelvis being caused by the gluteus maximus and the hamstrings.

Normal sagittal plane alignment of the spine

In neonates, the spine normally has a gentle convex curve posteriorly along its entire length. As head control is developed, a secondary lordotic curve develops in the cervical spine. Once the child starts to ambulate and develops, the upright posture lordotic curvature of the lumbar spine develops. Hence, the only fixed curves are the thoracic and sacral curves. Wedging of bones causes the thoracic and sacral curves and wedging of discs causes the cervical and lumbar curves. The formation of sagittal curves is thought to be a mechanism for force dissipation and injury prevention. It is also thought that the kyphosis in the sacral region and the thoracic region is to allow adequate volume to accommodate the thoracic and pelvic cavity. The spine is normally straight in the coronal plane except when a person has scoliosis. The normal range of cervical lordosis is 20–40°, the average thoracic kyphosis is 35° (range 20–50°) and the average lumbar lordosis is 60° (20–80°). Interestingly, 75% of the lumbar lordosis occurs between L4 and S1, of which 47 % is at L5–S1.

Normal sagittal alignment assists postural muscles to work efficiently and economizes energy in gait and ambulation. A plumb line dropped in the lateral position from the C2 dens passes near the body of C7 anterior to the thoracic spine, posterior to the lumbar spine and through the posterosuperior corner of the S1 vertebral body. Any displacement of this line anteriorly is taken as positive and posteriorly is taken as negative. Thoracic kyphosis is usually directly proportional to the lumbar lordosis.

It is important to know the definition of certain parameters that are important determinants of spinal sagittal balance (**Figure 21.6**).

- **Sacral inclination** (SI) or **sacral slope** is the angle between the line of the posterior S1 vertebral body and the horizontal axis (mean, 50°, range 43–58°).
- **Lumbar lordosis** (LL) is the angle between L1 and S1 and measures 60° (range 30–80°).
- **Pelvic incidence** (PI) is the angle formed by drawing a perpendicular line starting from the mid-point of the sacral end plate and a line connecting this point to the centre of the femoral head. PI is fixed for a person after growth and is not affected by posture or pelvis position.
- **Pelvic tilt** is the angle between the line connecting the mid-point of the sacral plate to the bi-coxo-femoral axis and the vertical plane.

The relationship between these parameters is given by the formula:

SI + pelvic tilt = PI

PI should normally be within 10° of LL and this rule is useful in osteotomy planning for spinal sagittal plane imbalance.

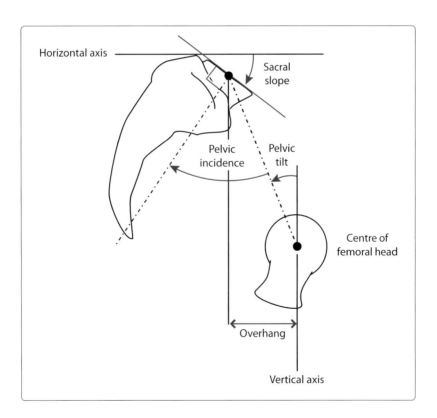

Figure 21.6 Important parameters for spinal sagittal balance.

Viva questions

1. What is spinal stability?
2. What unique features of the spine contribute to stability?
3. What do you know about the subsystems of the spine?
4. What is a functional spinal unit?
5. How does vertebral anatomy change as one proceeds caudally in the spine?

Further reading

Mercer S, Bogduk N. The ligaments and annulus fibrosus of human adult cervical intervertebral discs. *Spine* 1999;**24**:619–26.

Panjabi MM. The stabilizing system of the spine: part I. Function, dysfunction, adaptation and enhancement. *J Spin Disord* 1992;**5**:383–9.

Panjabi MM. The stabilizing system of the spine: part II. Neutral zone and instability hypothesis. *J Spin Disord* 1992;**5**:390–6.

Resnick DK, Weller SJ, Benzel EC. Biomechanics of the thoracolumbar spine. *Neurosurg Clin North Am* 1997;**8**:455–69.

White AA, Panjabi MM. *Clinical Biomechanics of the Spine.* Philadelphia, PA: J B Lippincott, 1990.

22 | Biomechanics and Joint Replacement of the Shoulder and Elbow

Mark Falworth, Prakash Jayakumar and Simon Lambert

SHOULDER

The shoulder demonstrates the greatest range of motion of any joint in the body. Complex biomechanical principles control its multiplanar range of movement. The resultant high degree of freedom and lower level of constraint may lead to an increase in the development of pathological conditions. A balance is required between mobility and range of motion versus stability required to generate power within the joint and stabilize the arm in space. Understanding the biomechanics is essential in order to contend with the treatment of these conditions and the challenge of design and development of joint replacement prostheses.

Anatomy

The shoulder is a complex of three articular joints and two physiological joints. The articular joints include the **glenohumeral** (GHJ), **acromioclavicular** and **sternoclavicular joints**. The physiological joints include the **scapulothoracic joint** and **subacromial joint** (between the rotator cuff and inferior surface of the acromion). The individual osseous components have specific anatomical configurations and soft-tissue attachments to optimize function.

Humerus

The humerus is composed of the head, neck (surgical and anatomical) and the shaft. The head is **superiorly inclined** and **eccentrically placed in relation to the shaft**, with a neck–shaft angle of around 130–140° and positioned 9 mm posterior to the central shaft axis, respectively. It is **retroverted** by around 30° in relation to the trans-epicondylar axis. The angle of inclination, posterior offset and version must be replicated during prosthetic replacement to achieve optimal biomechanics and limit early failure.

Scapula and glenoid

The **scapula** is **anteverted** 30–40° in relation to the coronal plane. The **glenoid** is around 7° **retroverted** from the plane perpendicular to the scapular plane, and demonstrates around 3–5° of **superior tilt** in relation to the vertical plane (**Figure 22.1**). The surface area

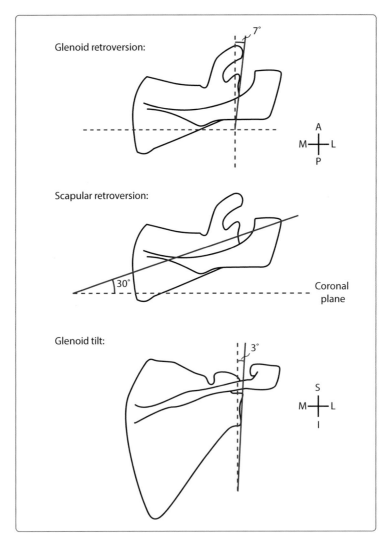

Figure 22.1 Glenoid and scapular orientation.

of the glenoid is only approximately one-third that of the humeral head. Joint congruency and thus stability is increased by the distribution of cartilage of the glenoid fossa and the presence of the glenoid labrum.

Clavicle

The clavicle functions as a strut suspending the GHJ, maintaining the lateral position of the shoulder and providing important muscular attachments.

During shoulder movements, the clavicle circumducts around the sternoclavicular joint medially and laterally, and the articulation with the acromion is maintained by the coracoclavicular and acromioclavicular ligaments. Disruption of these structures leads to destabilization of the scapula, protraction of the shoulder and scapulothoracic dyskinesia.

Joint movement

Normal shoulder function is reliant on coordinated glenohumeral and scapulothoracic movement. Failure of normal movement of either joint and/or malcoordination leads to abnormal kinetics and potential increase in the risk of pathology, such as impingement or instability.

A range of muscles are involved in movements on the shoulder and their action is dependent upon the position of the arm in space at the point of movement. Muscles controlling movements can be classified into **glenohumeral**, **scapulothoracic** and **thoracohumeral** (*Table 22.1*).

Glenohumeral motion

The rotator cuff muscles force the humeral head firmly into the glenoid fossa and minimize humeral head translation. A cuff deficient shoulder has a significant impact on the glenohumeral

Table 22.1 Muscles controlling shoulder movement

Glenohumeral movement	Scapulothoracic movement	Thoracohumeral movement
Deltoid	Trapezius	Pectoralis major
Supraspinatus	Levator scapulae	Latissimus dorsi
Infraspinatus	Rhomboid major	
Subscapularis	Rhomboid minor	
Teres minor	Serratus anterior	
Teres major	Pectoralis minor	
Biceps brachii		
Coracobrachialis		
Triceps		

articulation. Forward elevation in the scapular plane involves combined activity of deltoid and supraspinatus creating a vertical shear force, which in the presence of cuff deficiency leads to **superior migration** of the humeral head (**Figure 22.2**).

Deltoid and supraspinatus are also active during shoulder abduction. Supraspinatus plays a more dominant role in the initiation of abduction whilst deltoid activity increases with elevation of the arm. The vectors of both muscles equalize at around 90° of abduction (**Figure 22.2**). Thus, patients with a supraspinatus tear may experience pain and weakness around 30° of elevation compared with 90°, where there is greater power, compensation and recruitment of deltoid.

Scapulothoracic motion

Scapular rotation on the thorax confers important roles: the glenoid functions as a **stable base** during arm elevation; it **minimizes the risk of mechanical impingement of the rotator cuff**; it **preserves the deltoid muscle fibre length**; it **limits the degree of humeral head translation**; it **maximizes the range of shoulder movement** and **enables concavity compression** of the humeral head into the glenoid throughout the range, allowing optimal transfer of net joint reaction forces through the glenoid fossa. The humeral head rolls and translates during shoulder movements, up to 11 mm inferiorly during high elevation. Thus, a fixed, rigid glenoid would fail to prevent increasing translation and minimize the range of motion. Moreover, a malpositioned glenoid may cause instability and impingement.

Scapulothoracic dynamics are important factors in assessing a painful shoulder and it is important to define the relationship between glenohumeral and scapulothoracic movements, and identify any scapulothoracic dyskinesia. The coordination of glenohumeral and scapulothoracic movements are variable and dependent on the degree of arm elevation. Zero to 30° of abduction and 60° of forward flexion primarily involves glenohumeral movement. Beyond 30° the ratio of scapulothoracic to glenohumeral movement is 2:1 and beyond 120° the ratio is around 1:1.

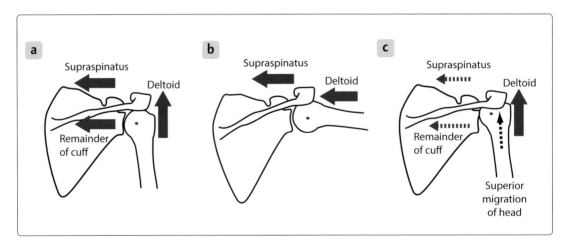

Figure 22.2 a) Muscle forces across the glenohumeral joint at initiation of abduction; b) muscle forces in 90 degrees of abduction; c) muscle forces in presence of weak/deficient cuff

Glenohumeral stability

The GHJ is reliant on the synchronous function of both static and dynamic stabilizing factors. A combination of structural and functional features provides joint stability at various stages throughout the range of motion (*Table 22.2*).

Static factors

Humeral head and glenoid version

Reduced retroversion and abnormal offset of the humeral head and **excessive retroversion of the glenoid** may have significant impact on the stability of the shoulder and should be factored into surgical treatment for instability. Less than 30° of humeral head retroversion may lead to anterior instability and be an indication for a humeral shaft rotation osteotomy.

Glenoid version plays an important role in the osseous stability of the shoulder. Normal scapular anteversion in relation to the coronal plane counters retroversion of the glenoid and prevents posterior instability. Cases involving glenoid dysplasia may be associated with posterior instability. Excessive retroversion of the glenoid may be an indication for a scapular neck osteotomy.

Glenoid arc

The articulating area of the glenoid and humeral head is essential for maintaining osseous stability. The **effective glenoid arc** is defined as the area of the glenoid articular surface available

Table 22.2 Static and dynamic factors affecting glenohumeral joint stability

Static factors	Dynamic factors
Structural features	Structural features
Humeral head and glenoid version	Scapular rotators
Glenoid arc	Rotator cuff
Labrum	Biceps
Glenohumeral ligament and capsule	Deltoid
Coracohumeral ligament	
Functional features	Functional features
Conformity	Proprioception
Vacuum effect	
- Intra-articular pressure	
- Suction effect	
- Adhesion–cohesion	
Surface area	

for humeral head compression. The **balance stability angle** is defined as the angle between the centre of the glenoid and the limit of the effective glenoid arc in any direction. Bony loss of the glenoid may reduce the glenoid arc and balance stability angle, leading to instability.

Labrum

The glenoid labrum is a fibrocartilaginous ridge-shaped structure that increases GHJ congruency, humeral head coverage and contact surface area by deepening the glenoid fossa. It provides **20% of stability to the shoulder**. The combined depth of the labrum–glenoid concavity is 9 mm in the superior–inferior axis and 5 mm in the anteroposterior (AP) axis. The labrum increases glenoid depth by 50%, acting as a type of '**chuck-block**' preventing abnormal translation. It provides an attachment for glenohumeral ligaments and the long head of biceps superiorly. Superiorly, it is triangular in cross-section, meniscal in appearance and relatively mobile. Inferiorly it is rounded in cross-section and more firmly attached. This limits translation of the GHJ. The **weakest parts of the capsule and labral complex are anteroinferior and posterosuperior**, which are the classic zones of injury in **Bankart lesions** and **superior labrum anterior and posterior (SLAP) tears**, respectively.

Glenohumeral ligament and capsule

The glenohumeral capsuloligamentous complex is composed of the glenohumeral ligaments (superior, middle and inferior) blended into the joint capsule. These ligaments become taut at varying degrees of humeral head rotation and elevation.

The **inferior glenohumeral ligament** (IGHL) is the primary stabilizer of the abducted GHJ and the most frequently injured portion of the capsule resulting in instability. The IGHL originates either directly from the labrum (85%) or the glenoid rim (15%) and inserts just inferior to the greater and lesser tuberosities. It is composed of anterior and posterior bands with a zone inbetween, formed by a portion of ligament known as the axillary pouch, which extends from the inferior two-thirds of the glenoid rim to the inferior one-third of the humeral head, supporting the humeral head like a hammock. The anterior band tightens at 90° abduction and external rotation, spanning the mid-zone of the GHJ and preventing anterior and inferior translation of the humeral head. The posterior band tightens and increases flexibility in flexion and internal rotation. Insertion and orientation of the IGHL is more consistent when compared with the other glenohumeral ligaments.

The **middle glenohumeral ligament** (MGHL) originates from the supraglenoid tubercle and the anterosuperior labrum between the 1 o'clock and 3 o'clock positions, and blends in with subscapularis as it inserts into the lesser tuberosity. The MGHL provides anterior stability between 0 and 90° of abduction. Maximal restraint to anterior displacement is provided by the MGHL between 45 and 60° of abduction and the IGHL beyond 60°.

The **superior glenohumeral ligament** (SGHL) originates from the supraglenoid tubercle just anterior to the long head of biceps that it covers, and inserts into the humerus near the lesser tuberosity. The **rotator interval** is formed by the SGHL and the coracohumeral ligament. It has an important role in shoulder stability and functions as an inferior stabilizer and limiter of internal rotation of the adducted arm.

Coracohumeral ligament

The coracohumeral capsuloligamentous complex is a key component of the rotator interval. It is composed of a thickening of the anterosuperior capsule with a lateral extension that blends in with the superficial fibres of supraspinatus and subscapularis. The ligament inserts into the dorsolateral coracoid and contains anterior and posterior bands that insert into the lesser and greater tuberosities, respectively. The anterior band becomes taut with the arm in external rotation and the posterior band becomes taut in internal rotation, resulting in resistance to anterior-inferior translation during these movements.

Rotator interval lesions may increase humeral head translation and should be factored into the surgical treatment strategy when managing atraumatic types of shoulder instability.

Conformity

Greater congruency of the articulating joint confers greater stability. Conversely, reduced congruency risks increased translation and instability. Conformity is optimized by three features: the glenoid radius is around 2 mm greater than that of the humeral head; the glenoid concavity is increased by gradual increase in thickness of the cartilage layer away from the central zone of the glenoid fossa toward the periphery; joint loading and impact causes cartilage deformation and greater conformity.

Vacuum effect

A vacuum effect is caused by three different mechanisms:

- Intra-articular pressure: **negative intra-articular pressure** within the GHJ provides a suction-type effect, centring and drawing the humeral head into the glenoid. Joint penetration disrupts the pressure differential and allows easier translation of the humeral head.
- Suction effect: the glenoid labrum provides a suction effect on the humeral head, acting like a plunger.
- Adhesion–cohesion: two wet surfaces, such as the humeral head and glenoid, create an adhesion–cohesion bond when coming into contact with each other and provide increased GHJ stability.

Surface area

The force transmitted through the humeral head onto the glenoid fossa is dependent on the surface area of the interface. The glenoid fossa is one-third the size of the humeral head. This is a relatively small surface area and the size differential generates high forces across the joint interface augmenting glenohumeral stability.

Dynamic factors

Dynamic stabilizers of the shoulder during active movement enable glenohumeral rotation with minimal translation, where the centre of rotation of the humeral head is closely related to the centre of rotation of the glenoid. In the anaesthetized patient, the effects of dynamic stabilizers are minimized and the cuff is defunctioned allowing increased translation of the humeral head.

Ultimately, forces act across the GHJ and cause a **concavity compression force** that maintains stability. Concavity compression relies on three factors: **integrity of the muscles** compressing the humeral head into the glenoid fossa; the **structural relationship between the glenoid fossa and the humeral head**; and the **glenohumeral ligaments** at the limits of motion.

Scapular rotators

Scapular muscles are a key link in the **kinetic chain** where they transfer energy from the lower limbs and trunk to the kinetic energy of the shoulder and upper limb, whilst providing a stable base for shoulder movements. The position of the scapula influences glenoid version and the degree of superior angulation. Chronic or repetitive scapular protraction may lead to excessive strain and insufficiency in the anterior band of the IGHL. Normal scapulothoracic dynamics and coordinated scapulohumeral rhythm are dependent upon normal function of the **rotatory force couple** and **pectoral girdle musculature**. The rotatory force couple consists of an **upper component** (levator scapulae, upper trapezius and upper fibres of serratus anterior) and a **lower component** (lower trapezius and lower fibres of serratus anterior). Disruption of one or more of these components may lead to increased risk of shoulder instability.

Rotator cuff

The rotator cuff maintains the centre of rotation of the humeral head and provides significant stability to the shoulder. Rotator cuff contraction causes a **compressive force** driving and stabilizing the humeral head within the glenoid fossa (**Figure 22.3**). This action maximally contributes to joint stability at the mid-range of shoulder motion whilst the glenohumeral and coracohumeral ligaments are most effective at the limits of motion.

Subscapularis provides anterior stability when the arm is in neutral and has a decreasing effect when the arm is placed in abduction. Infraspinatus and teres minor act in combination, reducing the strain on the antero-inferior glenohumeral ligament in abduction and external rotation.

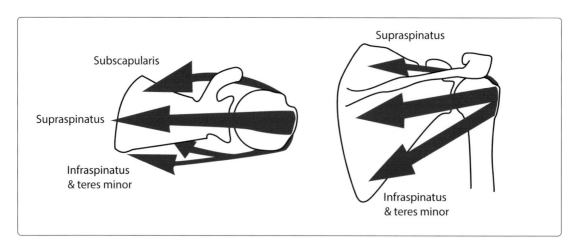

Figure 22.3 Rotator cuff direction of action maintaining centre of rotation and humeral head compression.

A 50% decrease in rotator cuff muscle forces causes around a 50% increase in anterior displacement of the humeral head. Large rotator cuff tears or those that involve supraspinatus extending into infraspinatus and disrupting the transverse force couple may cause superior migration of the humeral head. Isolated cuff tears do not usually result in significant migration.

Biceps

The biceps tendon originates from the superior labrum in a Y-shaped fashion. The tendon reduces both anteroposterior and superior–inferior translations and its role may become more prominent in cases with concurrent rotator cuff tears or labral deficiencies.

Deltoid

The deltoid provides superiorly directed shear force to the humeral head with the arm in adduction, whilst at 90° of abduction its line of action works synergistically with the rotator cuff to increase concavity compression forces. In a cuff deficient shoulder, overriding action of the deltoid leads to superior translation of the humeral head and destabilization of the GHJ.

Proprioception

Proprioception plays an important role in shoulder stability. The GHJ capsule, particularly anteriorly and inferiorly, contains numerous mechanoreceptors. In a normal shoulder, dynamic proprioception improves hand position sense following the initiation of movement. Abduction and external rotation of the shoulder involves the humeral head making contact with the capsule, which may trigger a signal via these receptors to the stabilizing muscles of the shoulder. Progressive instability leads to increased capsular stretch and greater proprioceptive disorganization leading to muscle patterning instability, dislocations and/or subluxation and progression to GHJ wear and reduced core stability. In multidirectional or muscle patterning instability, there is a reduced capacity to recruit proprioceptors which may lead to a disruption in motor control of the upper limb. Thus, treatment should commence early on in the pathological process.

Prosthetic replacement

Prosthetic replacement of a shoulder joint with an **intact rotator cuff and deltoid muscle** requires an **unconstrained prosthesis** positioned in-line with normal glenohumeral anatomy.

The aim of prosthetic replacement of the **humeral component** is to select an implant that **matches the size of the humeral head** and to position it in order to **restore the normal centre of rotation**. This involves surgical replication of anatomical factors including the **angle of stem insertion**, maintaining the **natural neck–shaft angle**, correct **version of the humeral head**, matching and **dialling in both the AP and medial–lateral humeral offset** and ensuring correct cuff tension. Mismatch of these anatomical parameters can alter the centre of rotation of the humeral head and result in abnormal humeral head translation, decreased range of motion, instability, dysfunction, abnormal wear pattern at the glenohumeral interface and ultimately, failure of the implant.

Prosthetic options include **thin-stem cemented**, **press-fit uncemented** and **surface replacement arthroplasty**. Thin-stem cemented prostheses can be optimally positioned within the humeral shaft in order to replicate the normal centre of rotation of the humeral head. However, the risk of cement complications and accurate first time placement must be considered. Press-fit uncemented stem designs involve a fixed stem position within the shaft and thus require an adjustable component between the stem and the head, plus or minus an eccentric Morse taper, in order to adjust the centre of rotation and 'dial in' AP and medial–lateral offset. Surface replacement arthroplasty is a less complex implant that avoids the potential pitfalls of stem insertion. This concept aims to replicate normal humeral head anatomy. This implant requires adequate humeral head bone stock, a factor that may prevent adequate exposure of the glenoid and thus positioning and placement of the glenoid component when total shoulder arthroplasty is performed.

The aim of prosthetic replacement of the **glenoid component** is to position the implant with the correct degree of version and inclination. Prosthetic options include **flat back** or **spherical back** designs. Spherical back implants may decrease lift-off, loosening and slippage of the component at the bone–cement interface.

Prosthetic replacement of a shoulder joint with **rotator cuff deficiency** requires a **constrained prosthesis**. The lack of cuff to constrain the prosthetic humeral head causes superior migration during the initiation of abduction resulting in an abnormal centre of humeral head rotation and abnormal articular contact pressures, which ultimately lead to poor function and instability. Unconstrained total shoulder arthroplasty in these cases results in excessive shear forces, causing superior eccentric loading of the glenoid component, glenoid loosening and the **rocking horse phenomenon** and ultimately failure.

Fixed fulcrum implants were developed to contend with this musculotendinous deficiency. First generation designs included reverse ball-and-socket type devices that often failed due to loosening of the glenoid component due to excessive torque. Next generation **reverse shoulder prostheses** (e.g. Delta reverse prosthesis, DePuy International Ltd, Leeds, UK) include a large glenoid hemisphere without a neck, and a humeral cup orientated in a horizontal position (**Figure 22.4**). This implant configuration **medializes the centre of rotation**, **increases recruitment of the anterior and posterior fibres of deltoid as abductors**, and **increases the tension in deltoid** due to the lowered position of the humerus. The action of deltoid is optimized in the presence of a deficient rotator cuff. This restores some movement, but rotation, especially external rotation, is rarely restored. Ultimately this reduces the torque on the glenoid component, providing greater stability to the humeral head.

A major issue with this implant design is notching of the scapular neck. This may be due to inferior impingement or formation of polyethylene granuloma causing bony lysis.

ELBOW

The principal role of the elbow is to provide a functional link between the shoulder and the hand in order to place the hand in space. The elbow also provides a stable axis for forearm motion and acts as a weight-bearing joint. Complex joint biomechanics are involved in maintaining stability and function.

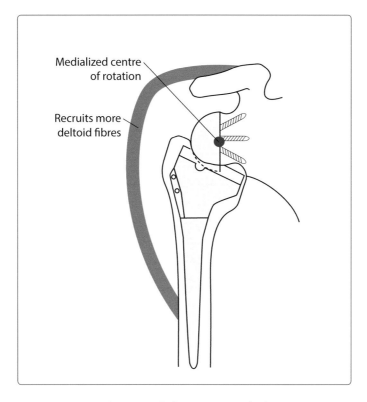

Figure 22.4 Delta reverse prosthesis.

Anatomy

The elbow joint is composed of three articulations: the **ulnohumeral**, **radiohumeral** and **proximal radioulnar joint**.

The **ulnohumeral (ulnotrochlear) joint** consists of the ulnar trochlear notch articulating with the trochlea of the distal humerus and forming a simple hinge joint. The distal humerus is angled anteriorly by 40° in relation to the humeral shaft, and recessed anteriorly and posteriorly to accommodate the coronoid and olecranon processes, respectively. This adaptation improves congruity, stability and optimizes range of movement, allowing a flexion–extension range of around 140°.

The **radiohumeral (radiocapitellar) joint** consists of the radial head articulating with the capitellum. The capitellum has a much smaller radius than the radial head, making this joint less congruent than the ulnohumeral joint. This configuration enables rotational movement at the elbow irrespective of the degree of elbow flexion.

The **proximal radioulnar joint** consists of the articulation between the side of the radial head and the radial notch of the ulna. The joint is stabilized by the annular ligament and the normal range of movement includes 85° of supination to 75° of pronation from neutral. The axis of forearm rotation runs through the centre of the radial head and the capitellum.

The **carrying angle** is a valgus angulation of the forearm at the elbow ranging from 11° in males to 14° in females, measured in extension. This is caused by the trochlear axis, passing through the trochlea and capitellum, which lies around 6° off the perpendicular axis to the humeral shaft.

Four distinct muscle groups control elbow movement: **flexion** (biceps brachii, brachialis and brachioradialis), **extension** (triceps and anconeus), **pronation** (pronator teres and pronator quadratus) and **supination** (biceps brachii and supinator). Flexion–extension involves muscle groups matched and providing antagonistic stabilizing action. Pronation–supination involves muscle groups matched and acting in opposite directions.

Free-body diagram

Forces acting across the elbow are variable. A free-body diagram can be used to illustrate the forces acting across the elbow flexed to 90° whilst carrying a mass held in the hand. Joint reaction force can be calculated by resolving clockwise versus anticlockwise moments and assuming forces about the elbow maintain equilibrium (**Figure 22.5**).

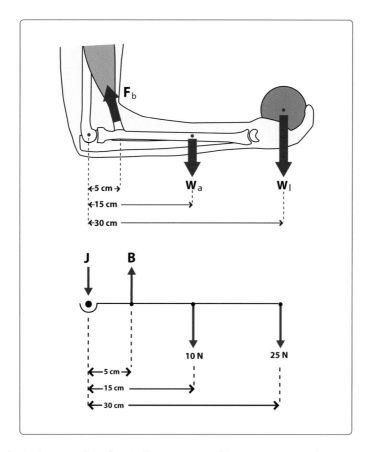

Figure 22.5 Free-body diagram of the flexed elbow. B: Force of biceps; J: resultant force; F_b: Force of Biceps; W_a: Weight of arm; W_l: Weight of load.

Clockwise (extension) moment = anticlockwise (flexion) moment

$(25\text{ N} \times 0.3) + (10\text{ N} \times 0.15) = (B \times 0.05)$

$7.5 + 1.5 = 0.05B$

$9/0.05 = B$

$180\text{ N} = B$

Joint reaction force $+ 25 + 10 = 180$

Joint reaction force $= 180 - 35$

Joint reaction force $= 145\text{ N}$

Elbow stability

Elbow stability is achieved by static and dynamic components. Static stabilizers include osseous stabilizers and soft-tissue stabilizers (*Table 22.3*). Dynamic stabilizers include muscles crossing the elbow joint. Different primary and secondary stabilizers are effective depending on the instability forces applied (*Table 22.4*).

Table 22.3 Static and dynamic factors affecting elbow joint stability

Static factors	Dynamic factors
Osseous stabilizers	*Muscles crossing elbow joint*
Radiohumeral joint	Biceps brachii
Ulnohumeral joint	Triceps
Coronoid process	
Soft tissue stabilizers	
Medial collateral ligament	
Lateral collateral ligament	
Anterior capsule	

Table 22.4 Stabilizers of the elbow

Instability	Primary stabilizer	Secondary stabilizer
Valgus stress	Anterior oblique ligament (medial collateral ligament)	Radiocapitellar joint Ulnohumeral joint
Varus stress	Ulnohumeral joint	Anterior capsule in extension Lateral collateral ligament in flexion
Posterolateral rotatory instability	Lateral ulnar collateral ligament	

Osseous constraints

The ulnohumeral joint is a primary stabilizer during application of varus stress. The olecranon forms the ulnohumeral articulation and significant bone loss can occur before overall stability is affected.

The largest joint reaction forces in the elbow are due to posteriorly directed forces caused by extensor and flexor musculature at the distal humerus. The major osseous constraint and articular contribution to elbow stability **resisting posterior displacement is the coronoid process**. A minimum of 50% of the coronoid process is required to maintain ulnohumeral stability. Bony deficiency of 50% will lead to a significant loss of stability, especially in full extension. An intact radial head enhances resistance to posterior displacement in the presence of a deficient coronoid.

The radiohumeral joint is a secondary stabilizer during application of valgus stress. As a secondary stabilizer, its role is maximally effective when the medial collateral ligament (MCL) is disrupted and conversely, the radial head plays a minimal role when the MCL is intact. The **radial head** is a key stabilizer that tensions the MCL. It is **essential for maintaining stability if the MCL and/or lateral collateral ligament (LCL) are disrupted or the distal radioulnar joint is injured**. Radial head excisions in the presence of an intact and functioning MCL may lead to proximal migration of the radius, causing pain and instability at the distal radioulnar joint.

Soft-tissue stabilizers

The main soft tissue stabilizers of the elbow are the **MCL, LCL** and **anterior capsule**. The **MCL** is composed of three components: the **anterior oblique ligament** (AOL), the **posterior oblique ligament** (POL), and the **transverse ligament** (TL) (**Figure 22.6**). The MCL, particularly the AOL, is the primary restraint and stabilizer of the elbow in valgus stress. It is tight in extension and loose in flexion. The POL is tight in flexion and loose in extension. The TL (Cooper's ligament) connects the coronoid to the tip of the olecranon. Its role in stabilizing the elbow is unclear.

In radial head fractures, the radial head can be excised if the MCL is intact. Cases with concurrent attenuation or disruption of the MCL may lead to progressive valgus deformity unless the lateral column is maintained by a radial head replacement.

The **LCL** is composed of four components: the **radial collateral ligament** (RCL), **annular ligament** (AL), **lateral ulnar collateral ligament** (LUCL) and **accessory lateral collateral ligament** (ALCL). The LUCL may have a role in posterolateral instability. Other factors, including increased elbow flexion, may also increase the degree of rotatory instability (*Table 22.4*).

The **anterior capsule** is a secondary stabilizer during varus stress (in extension), and also plays a role in stability during valgus stress, distraction and hyperextension forces.

Muscles crossing the elbow joint also play a role in maintaining elbow stability and their action is dependent on the joint position.

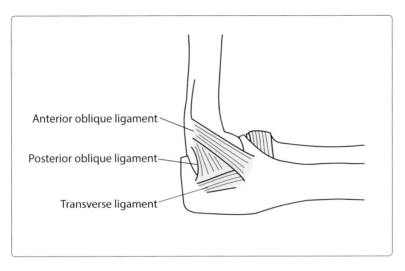

Figure 22.6 Medial collateral ligament.

Prosthetic replacement

Total elbow arthroplasty may be indicated in the management of elbows affected by rheumatoid arthritis, osteoarthritis and post-traumatic arthritis. Prostheses are mainly classified into **linked** and **unlinked** implants. Implant choice is dictated by the integrity of the osseous and ligamentous structures, as well as surgeon preference.

Linked (semiconstrained or sloppy hinge) prostheses allow some varus–valgus laxity and thus enable reduction of force transmission at the bone–cement–implant interface. Laxity is variable, ranging from 7° to 10°, and is dependent on the implant. This can be increased further by performing releases of the collateral ligaments at the time of surgery.

Unlinked prostheses are dependent on constraint gained from the articulating geometry of the implant as well as the inherent stability from surrounding bone, ligaments and muscles. Stability is further enhanced in some implant systems that include radial head components to act as a further stabilizing factor. This reduces varus–valgus laxity and enhances stress distribution at the bone–cement–implant interface. Ultimately, implants must be placed accurately in order to avoid abnormal wear patterns and failure.

Viva questions

1. What anatomical factors are involved in maintaining shoulder stability?
2. How do the muscles of the shoulder girdle control arm elevation and abduction?
3. Discuss the principles in the design of a total shoulder arthroplasty in the cuff deficient shoulder.
4. Discuss the management of a comminuted fracture of the radial head with respect to maintaining elbow stability.
5. Draw a free-body diagram of an arm held in 90° of elbow flexion and carrying a mass in the hand. Resolve the forces through the elbow and calculate the joint reaction force.

Further reading

Boileau P, Watkinson DJ, Hatzidakis AM, Balg F. Grammont reverse prosthesis: design, rationale, and biomechanics. *J Shoulder Elbow Surg* 2005;**1S**:147–61S.

Burkart AC, Debski RE. Anatomy and function of the glenohumeral ligaments in anterior shoulder stability. *Clin Orthop* 2002;**400**:32–9.

Lippitt SB, Vanderhooft JE, Harris SL, et al. Glenohumeral stability from concavity compression: a quantitative analysis. *J Shoulder Elbow Surg* 1993;**11**:27–35.

Morrey BF, An KN. Stability of the elbow: osseous constraint. *J Shoulder Elbow Surg* 2005; **1S**:174–8S.

Mura N, O'Driscoll SW, Zobitz ME, et al. The effect of infraspinatus disruption on glenohumeral torque and superior migration of the humeral head: a biomechanical study. *J Shoulder Elbow Surg* 2003;**2**:179–84.

23 Biomechanics of the Hand and Wrist

Nicholas Saw, Livio Di Mascio and David Evans

Introduction

The biomechanics of the hand and wrist represent a subject of immense complexity, and a thorough understanding is difficult because of:

- The series of joints involved, many of which move together to produce composite movements.
- The muscles that power movement often cross more than one joint and contraction produces functional movement in concert.
- The role of ligamentous restraints in the wrist and distal radioulnar joint.
- Carpal and distal radioulnar joint (DRUJ) kinematics not being understood fully.

Nonetheless, some principles can be considered to help us in our appreciation of the hand. This chapter is divided into the hand, the carpus, the DRUJ and the paralyzed hand.

The hand
Joints and movement

For each axis of movement, there should be two motors acting perpendicular to the axis, as seen with flexor digitorum profundus (FDP) and the lateral bands of the extensors at the distal interphalangeal (DIP) joints of the fingers. For three axes of movement – **flexion/extension** (F/E), **abduction/adduction** (A/A) and **rotation** – six motors are required. This makes for a bulky mass of muscle, which would interfere with prehension and increases the complexity of coordination. To simplify matters, no joints rotate in the hand; joints with two axes of movement allow perceived rotation. This perceived rotation is achieved by circumduction about joints with non-parallel and offset axes.

Planes of movement

In the anatomical position, the forearm is supinated, with the palm facing forward. Description of finger and wrist movement is straightforward. The thumb's resting position is out of the plane of the palm. For this reason, description of thumb movements can be more confusing. Flexion and extension of the thumb occur parallel to the plane of the palm, abduction and adduction occur perpendicular to the palm. Opposition represents a combination of these movements that brings the thumb pulp to face the little finger pulp.

Interphalangeal joints

The interphalangeal (IP) joints are simple single-axis hinge joints. They allow **flexion** and **extension** and are powered by two motors. The axis of movement is just anterior to the origin of the collateral ligaments. There is a small trochlea and groove to provide some rotational stability. This is enhanced in most functional positions, as the joint reaction force creates compression of the joint. The **collateral** and **accessory collateral ligaments** and **volar plates** provide further static stability. The collateral ligaments are taught in extension and the volar plate aids static stability of the joint in this position.

Metacarpophalangeal (MCP) joints

These ellipsoid joints have two axes of movement: **F/E** and **A/A**. The F/E axis is transverse about the metacarpal head. The A/A axis, however, is flexed 30° from the metacarpal shaft and is cone shaped. Therefore, abduction and adduction can occur in the true sense in the anatomical plane relative to the middle finger, but can also occur allowing for a cone-shaped range of movement when combined with F/E with the apex of the cone at the metacarpal head. This movement is perceived clinically as circumduction.

This circumduction at the MCP joint aids opposition and precision pinch grip. Due to the cam shape of the metacarpal head, the collateral liagments are lax between full extension and 30° of flexion and are taught in flexion. This allows for dexterity in extension and stability in power grip. The compressive joint reaction force and the collaterals and volar plate again provide static stability. The ulna collateral ligament of the thumb in particular acts as a passive restrictor of abduction at the MCP joint in pinch.

Passive immobilization of the small joints of the hand should be performed with the IP joints in extension and the MCP joints in flexion. In this position the collateral liagments are taut and therefore will be less prone to creating joint stiffness due to loss of tissue compliance.

Carpometacarpal joints

Movement at the carpometacarpal (CMC) joints of the fingers is limited, especially in the index and middle fingers. These two metacarpals are bound rigidly to the distal carpal row and transmit the forces from hand to wrist. The **middle finger metacarpal** acts as a cantilever from which a strong fibrous framework extends, attaching to and holding in place the **flexor sheaths**. This framework, mediated through the collateral ligaments to the deep transverse metacarpal ligament, suspends the flexor mechanisms from the metacarpal heads and transverse arch. In rheumatoid arthritis, the synovitis weakens the radial collateral ligaments in particular and disrupts the attachments to the arch, with secondary consequences such as extensor tendon subluxation, MCP joint subluxation, ulnar drift and loss of flexion power.

The CMC joint of the ring and little finger metacarpals do allow for a degree of F/E. This range of movement is minor but allows for better opposition of the little finger when combined with circumduction and also allows for grip accomodation, particularly with power grip.

The CMC joint of the thumb is vital to the prehensile hand, and the remainder of this section discusses this joint alone. The **thumb CMC joint** is a saddle joint and so has two axes of movement: **F/E** and **A/A**. There is no axis of rotation. These two axes are not perpendicular but are skewed relative to each other and to the anatomical plane. The radii of the joint surfaces of the trapezium and metacarpal are also different. The result is a F/E axis across the trapezium that is designed for flexion towards the hypothenar eminence: a functional movement for any grip. The A/A axis is through the metacarpal, but, like the MCP joint described earlier in the shape of a shallow cone, apex volar and ulnar, allows circumduction.

The result is that the thumb metacarpal can **abduct**, **extend** and **pronate** (because of the offset axis and differential radii) to increase the span to grasp an object and oppose the thumb. Flexion and adduction then allow for grip: pulp-to-pulp pinch, key pinch and power grip.

The thumb CMC and MCP joints almost always work in unison, as the motors cross both joints. Therefore, the metacarpal and phalanges usually describe the same movements in different arcs. For example, to flex the metacarpal and extend the phalanges is of little functional use; it is better to extend and then flex both together in order to grasp an object.

Stability of the CMC joint is due to a combination of muscles holding the joint and strong ligaments with thickened capsule. The thumb CMC joint is congruent only at extremes of movement: there is often a degree of translation with focal point loading. In adduction and flexion, the most useful movement for any grip, only the volar surfaces of the CMC joint are under load – up to 120 kg in a power grip. The large contact pressures on the volar surface can contribute to degenerative change. The **volar oblique** or **beak ligament** between the ulna side of the metacarpal and tubercle of the trapezium is a major restraint to dorsal translation in combination with the **dorso-radial capsule**. The latter should be repaired carefully after trapeziectomy.

Motors that power movement

The motors can be divided into **extensors** (supplied by the radial and posterior interosseous nerves), **flexors** (supplied by the median and anterior interosseous nerves) and **intrinsics** (supplied by the median and ulnar nerves). The long flexors and extensors cross many joints and so have the greatest excursions to deal with the range of positions of the hand.

Amplitude of tendon excursion (3–5–7)

- Wrist flexors and extensors: 30 mm.
- Finger extensors and extensor pollicis longus (EPL)/flexor pollicis longus (FPL): 50 mm.
- Finger flexors: 70 mm.

Extensor mechanism

The origins of the extensors are the common extensor origin, radius, ulna and interosseous membrane. Brachioradialis (BR) crosses the elbow and acts as an elbow flexor as well as a midpronator or midsupinator, depending on forearm rotation. Extensor carpi radialis longus (ECRL) acts as a wrist extensor and radial deviator as well as a weak elbow flexor. Both BR and ECRL are innervated by the radial nerve and allow the above movements in posterior interosseous nerve (PIN) palsy, whereas extensor carpi radialis brevis (ECRB) and the rest of the extensors are innervated by the PIN.

The extensor mechanism over the dorsum of the digits represents a complex interplay of extensor and intrinsic function contributing to the accurate positioning of each joint in space (**Figure 23.1**).

The **long extensors** receive contributions from the **lumbricals** (radial side) and **interossei** to form the **extensor hood** over the **proximal phalanx**, with a complex pattern of interweaving fibres that allow for the formation of a differential pulley system. The **intrinsics** and **extrinsics** work in concert to control the tension in the whole system, effecting IP joint extension via the central slip to the middle phalanx and lateral bands to the distal phalanx to allow coordinated positioning. In essence, the long flexors and extensors may be thought to provide the power and the intrinsics the fine control for hand function.

Flexor mechanism

The **FDP** inserts onto the distal phalanx after traversing through the chiasma of the **flexor digitorum superficialis** (FDS) as FDS divides and rotates around FDP to attach to the middle phalanx. FDP is a mass action muscle, although FDP to the index has some independent action. For this reason, if one tendon of FDP is tethered or shortened, the DIP joints of the other fingers will exhibit a degree of flexor lag once the tethered tendon reaches maximum flexion: the **quadriga effect** (analogous to a Roman chariot with four parallel horses controlled by the charioteer via a single rein).

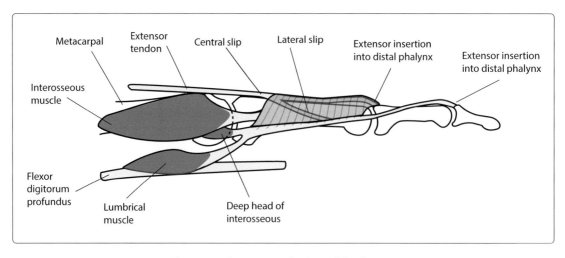

Figure 23.1 Extensor mechanism of the fingers.

The tension generated by the muscle fibres is equal throughout the tendon to its insertion, but the torque generated is dependent on the moment arm. The flexors work with an increasing torque proximally as the moment arm about the axis of rotation increases (**Figure 23.2**).

Pulleys

A system of thickenings within the fibro-osseous sheaths of the flexor tendons are known as the flexor pulleys. These pulleys keep the flexor tendons closely apposed to the bones, counteracting the large torque forces generated from muscle contraction. Without this pulley system, the flexor tendons would tend to 'bowstring' and thus create an even greater torque force at each joint and subsequent fixed flexion contractures (**Figure 23.3**).

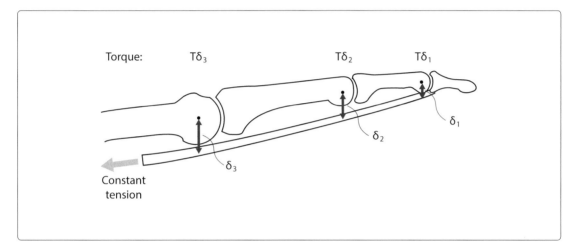

Figure 23.2 Increasing torque of the finger flexors proximally.

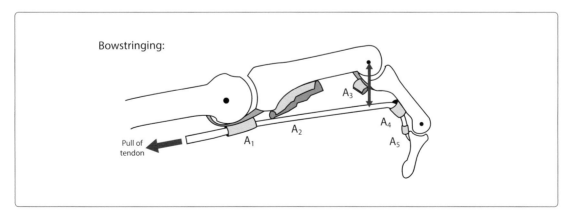

Figure 23.3 Incompetence of the annular pulleys, especially that of the A_2 or A_4, leads to dysfunction of the flexor apparatus and subsequent fixed flexion deformity.

This pulley system is well described, with these thickenings of the flexor sheath creating the annular **A1–A5 pulleys**. The flexor retinaculum also functions as a pulley across the wrist. The **cruciate pulleys (C1–C3)** sit between the A pulleys and provide support to the flexor sheath. The **A2 and A4 pulleys** are the most important, in that order, and should be preserved or, if damaged, reconstructed.

Intrinsics

Finger intrinsics

The **lumbricals** are unique in that their origin is from a tendon (FDP) and their insertion into the extensor hood (another tendon) on the radial side. They act as **guy ropes** between the flexors and extensors to allow correct adjustment of tension for finger balance. The interossei arise from the metacarpal shafts and are responsible for abduction (mnemonic for dorsal interossei: **DAB**) and adduction (mnemonic for palmar interossei: **PAD**), also contributing to the extensor hood. Both lumbricals and interossei allow for the flexion of the MCP joints and extension of the IP joints on their own (therefore in radial nerve palsy, IP joint extension but not MCP joint extension is still possible) and they coordinate the positioning of the fingers for function. The lumbricals are the more effective MCP joint flexors because they have a greater mechanical advantage, being further from the axis of flexion. MCP joint stability is further improved by contraction of the interossei.

The intrinsics allow finger flexion without curling. The MCP joints flex first, followed by the IP joints. This lets the hand describe a large round shape for grasping. With intrinsic paralysis, attempts to hold an object result in the rolling up of the fingers from distal to proximal (FDP and FDS alone), hyperextension at the MCP joints as a result of unopposed extrinsic extensors, and failure to grasp, i.e. the **intrinsic minus hand**. Intrinsic tightness results in MCP joint flexion and proximal interphalangeal (PIP) joint extension, i.e. the **intrinsic plus position** (the **Bunnell test** can be used to differentiate intrinsic from extrinsic tightness clinically, a positive test being when PIP joint flexion is less than MCP joint extension than with MCP joint flexion).

With the lumbricals bridging flexors and extensors, paradoxical extension of the IP joint can occur with attempted flexion. This can be seen when an FDP tendon has been divided distal to the origin of the lubrical. As this FDP contracts to flex the finger, the force from the FDP passes through the lumbrical to the extensor mechanism to act as an extensor of the IP joint, i.e. the **lumbrical plus** finger.

Another structure that links the flexor and extensor apparatus is the **spiral oblique retinacular ligament of Landsmeer (SORL)**. It arises from the proximal phalanx and A2 pulley, passes anterior to the F/E axis of the PIP joint and inserts on to the lateral slips of the extensor tendon on to the distal phalanx, dorsal to the F/E axis of the DIP joint. As the PIP joint extends, the SORL becomes tighter and tends to passively extend the DIP joint. Therefore, IP joint extension is linked in a controlled way.

Thenar muscles

The **thumb intrinsics** have dual innervation from the ulnar (terminal motor) and median (recurrent motor) nerves. The adductor pollicis (AP) is generally under ulnar control, the abductor pollicis brevis (APB) median, and the flexor pollicis brevis (FPB) and opponens pollicis (OP) variable. The latter three arise from the flexor retinaculum and scaphoid or trapezium. OP acts to pronate and flex the metacarpal at the CMC joint. APB and FPB cross both the CMC and MCP joints and therefore act to position the whole thumb in abduction and flexion. APB is unique in being able to abduct the thumb for opposition, and its loss may cause a significant functional loss (e.g. in severe carpal tunnel syndrome).

The importance of thumb adduction by AP is not so much the action itself but rather the role of resisting abduction, especially working in concert with FPB. In pinch grip, AP generates the large moment arm required to provide a stable post across the CMC and MCP joints to resist the large forces applied at the thumb tip. It is possible to pinch quite well without an FPL to flex the IP joint, as the volar plate and collaterals provide a stable extended IP joint to pinch against, at least initially. FPL however, cannot compensate for the loss of AP. In an ulna nerve palsy, the AP is denervated, therefore, in an attempt to hold a sheet of paper between the adducted thumb and index finger, a trick manoeuvre is used. The thumb is pronated sufficiently for FPL (anterior interosseous nerve) to perform a lateral pinch, and there may be some flexion of the index MCP joint to facilitate this. This is the basis for **Froment's test**.

As **EPL** crosses the wrist, it acts as a radial deviator. In addition, EPL is also a powerful adductor of the thumb at the CMC and MCP joints and may trick the orthopaedic surgeon in an intrinsic palsy. When EPL and FPL contract together, FPL tensions the EPL, which can then provide lateral pinch. The resulting posture of the thumb in this situation is characteristic: there is flexion across the IP and MCP joints (stronger FPL moment arm) and extension at the CMC joint (stronger EPL moment arm). The EPL alone is able to lift the thumb off a flat surface (retropulsion). From its origin, EPL angles around Lister's tubercle in the third dorsal compartment to insert on to the distal phalanx that it extends.

Abductor pollicis longus (APL) and **extensor pollicis longus** and **brevis** (EPB) also aid in positioning the thumb, although supplied by the PIN. APL and EPB are extensors and abductors of the thumb and, acting with AP, stabilize the thumb metacarpal for independent MCP joint flexion. However, they also cross the wrist anterior to the axis of F/E and are weak abductors and flexors of the wrist.

Hypothenar muscles

These muscles essentially mirror the thenar muscles, and their significance should not be underestimated. They allow the little finger to oppose the thumb and thereby cup the hand. This allows water to be held, which is a vital act. They also contribute to grip by providing a cushioning mass of muscle and by increasing the breadth of the hand for stability. Try gripping a racquet without the little finger to see their contribution.

The wrist

The biomechanics of the carpus and DRUJ are horrendously complicated, and their instabilities are beloved of examiners. Fortunately, a complete understanding is unnecessary for examinations and is indeed mostly beyond many surgeons. It is, however, important to understand the general principles involved.

Some general observations first:

- The wrist and hand are **suspended off the ulna**, not the other way round.
- The wrist is **inherently unstable**, with the ligaments providing static and the muscles dynamic stability.
- The bones of the proximal carpal row form an **intercalated segment**.

The carpus

The carpus may be divided into the **distal** and **proximal carpal rows**. The distal row comprises the trapezium, trapezoid, capitate and hamate. The proximal row comprises the scaphoid, lunate and triquetrum. The pisiform may be considered as the sesamoid of the flexor carpi ulnaris (FCU) tendon and as such is an important stabilizer of the wrist.

The distal row is bound together tightly by interosseous ligaments and functions as a single unit. The proximal row, however, has no tendons attached and functions as an intercalated segment between the radius and ulna and the distal carpal row. Their movement is therefore dependent on the geometry of the bones and the forces applied against the restraining ligaments. These need to be considered.

The radiocarpal joint consists of the articular surface of the radius, with its scaphoid and lunate facets, and the triangular fibrocartilage complex (TFCC). These articulate primarily with the scaphoid and lunate, as the triquetrum is held within the insertions of the TFCC and its contact with the ulna disc is limited. The forces generated across the neutral wrist are transmitted primarily through the capitate/scapholunate articulation at the mid-carpal joint, and the radioscaphoid and radiolunate articulations at the radiocarpal joint. The lunate can be considered the key to proximal row movement. It is wedge shaped, being wider volarly and radially, and this shape tends to tilt the lunate dorsally when it is under load from the capitate.

The ligaments of the wrist may be classified as **extrinsic** or **intrinsic**. The extrinsic ligaments are arranged in two V-shapes. The **volar extrinsic ligaments** are strongest and arise from the radius and ulna with their apex on the lunate and capitate. The **dorsal extrinsic ligaments** run in a distal/ulnar direction and resist translation of the carpus down the sloping radius in a volar and ulnar direction (**Figure 23.4**).

Their names describe the bones to which they attach, such as the radioscaphocapitate (volar) and radiotriquetral (dorsal), these two being the most important. The **intrinsic ligaments** run between the carpal bones, binding tightly to fix the bones (distal row) or somewhat more loosely to allow some intercarpal movement (proximal row). The scapholunate and lunotriquetral ligaments are two such intrinsic interosseous ligaments that allow limited motion.

Carpal kinetics

Conceptually, one of the easiest ways to consider carpal kinetics is to remember two points. First, the **scaphoid flexes in radial deviation** to get out of the way so the trapezium can approach the radial styloid, and **extends in ulna deviation** to fill the space vacated by the trapezium. Second, the **lunate** can be thought of as a torque lever suspended between the opposing moments of the **scaphoid (flexion)** and **triquetrum (extension)**. The whole system is under constant and changing tension; therefore, if any part is disrupted, then abnormal and unlinked rotation will

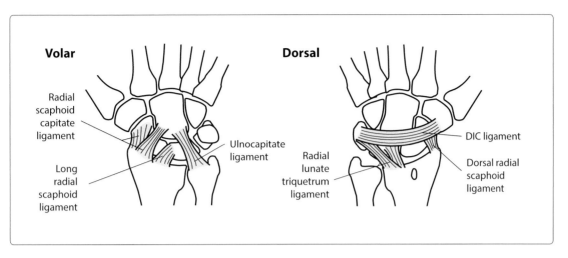

Figure 23.4 Extrinsic ligaments of the wrist. DIC: dorsal intercarpal.

occur. The lunate will then tilt with the intact part within the chain. It is the direction of tilt of the lunate that is described in the instability.

The F/E axis of the wrist is just distal to the radial and ulnar styloids, and the radioulnar axis passes through the capitate. The axis of pronation/supination passes from the radial head to the tip of the ulna styloid and occurs through the radioulnar articulation.

A combination of mid-carpal and radiocarpal movement is responsible for flexion (45° mid-carpal, 40° radiocarpal) and extension (25° mid-carpal, 35° radiocarpal). Abduction of 60° and adduction of 20° occurs around the axis of the capitate.

Normal wrist movement

In radial deviation, the scaphoid flexes to allow the trapezium to approach the radius. The flexion torque is transmitted to the lunate by the scapholunate ligament (SLL), augmented by the capitate pressing on the volar lip of the lunate. The triquetrum is pulled along with the hamate to a non-articulating position relative to the ulna.

On ulnar deviation, the scaphoid extends to fill the space vacated by the trapezium, passing an extension moment to the lunate via the SLL. The capitate presses on the dorsal lip of the lunate to tilt it dorsally. The hamate now engages the triquetrum, and the helical shape of the triquetrohamate joint causes triquetral extension, in addition to the torque from the lunotriquetral ligament (LTL).

With axial loading, the greatest force is transmitted across the mid-carpal joint at the capitoscapholunate articulation. The proximal row then changes shape to adapt to the forces. The extensors tend to exert a dorsal force on the capitate, which then tends to tilt the lunate and triquetrum dorsally. The volar facing radial articulation accentuates this. The scaphoid, however, tends to flex with axial loading due to the tension in the volar extrinsic ligaments, so the lunate is under two opposing moments. The stability of the whole construct is dependent on the integrity of the scapholunate and lunotriquetral interosseous ligaments. Disruption allows for independent movement, leading to carpal instability.

The action of radial deviation and extension followed by ulnar deviation and flexion is functionally important. For this reason, ECRL and FCU, the muscles that produce this movement, are among the most powerful. During this functional 'dart throwing motion', the scaphoid is effectively locked in flexion within the proximal row. Thus, this motion is essentially a mid-carpal movement. In the less common action of moving from ulnar extension to radial flexion, the scaphoid is free to move, and so this is a radiocarpal movement.

Abnormal carpal movement

As described earlier, the carpal bones are held together with intrinsic ligamentous restraints under constant tension. Disruption may occur by failure of the ligamentous restraints or by fractures uncoupling the bony architecture. This may lead to carpal instability. Carpal instability is difficult to describe and understand, but bearing in mind the normal carpal interaction, its classification can be explained.

There are many classifications described, including the **Mayo** and that used by the **International Wrist Investigators Workshop**. The mechanics behind the Mayo classification are described; its two main subtypes being **carpal instability dissociative (CID)** and **carpal instability non-dissociative (CIND)**.

Carpal instability dissociative

This is instability, **ligamentous** or **osseous**, within a **carpal row**. It may be visible without loading (**static**) or only under load or movement (**dynamic**). CID includes disruptions of the SLL or LTL so the proximal carpal dynamics are affected. Initially, the injury may not be seen on plain radiographs but may be seen only under stress views or under screening (dynamic instability). If untreated, the disruption may become more permanent and visible on plain radiographs (static). The normal scapholunate gap can be variable, especially in children, so never forget to compare with the contralateral wrist.

Note that the scaphoid tends to flex and the lunate and triquetrum extend. The SLL and LTL hold this proximal row under balanced tension. If the SLL is disrupted, the scaphoid flexes, the lunate extends with the triquetrum via the intact LTL and a **dorsal intercalated segmental instability (DISI)** pattern occurs.

If the LTL fails, then the triquetrum extends and the lunate tilts volarly with the flexing scaphoid, as the flexed scaphoid transmits its torque via the intact SLL to the lunate. This results in a **volar intercalated segmental instability (VISI)** pattern. The pattern of instability is named after the direction in which the lunate tends to abnormally tilt (**Figure 23.5**).

There may be nothing to see on plain radiographs, or there may be a visible gap between the bones, flexion of the scaphoid (ring sign of seeing the flexed scaphoid end on) and reduction of the carpal height ratio as the capitate slides dorsally or volarly shortening the carpus (**Figure 23.6**). Abnormal measurements on radiographs indicative of carpal instability are shown in *Table 23.1*.

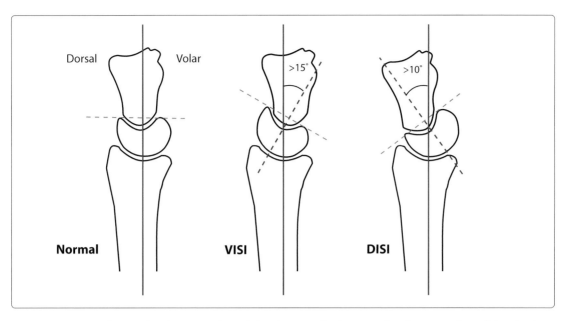

Figure 23.5 Dorsal intercalated segmental instability (DISI) and volar intercalated segmental instability (VISI).

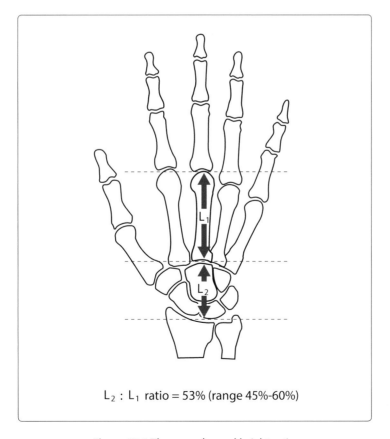

$L_2 : L_1$ ratio = 53% (range 45%-60%)

Figure 23.6 The normal carpal height ratio.

Table 23.1 Abnormal measurements on radiographs in DISI and VISI

	DISI	VISI	Normal
Scapholunate angle	>70°	<30°	30°–60°
Capitolunate angle	>-30°	>30°	-20°–10°
Radiolunate angle	>-15°	>20°	-20°–10°
Carpal height ratio	<0.54	<0.54	0.54 ± 0.03
Scapholunate distance	3 mm+	<2 mm	<2 mm

DISI: dorsal intercalated segmental instability; VISI: volar intercalated segmental instability.

Carpal instability non-dissociative

This describes carpal instability **between** the **distal and proximal rows** (mid-carpal instability, MCI), at the radiocarpal joint, or both. The rows themselves are intact. This pattern is less common than CID and results from significant **disruption** of the **extrinsic ligaments** that uncouple the dynamics of the carpus. The patient often describes a 'clunk', as occurs in MCI when the distal row suddenly reduces on to the proximal row in ulnar deviation. In individuals with ligamentous laxity, such as gymnasts, there may be MCI without significant trauma.

If the very strong radiocarpal ligaments are disrupted, then the carpus may slide down the ulna inclination of the radius, uncoupling the radiocarpal articulation. Ulnar translocation of the carpus is seen on radiographs when more than 50% of the lunate projects beyond the ulnar edge of the radius. The whole carpus may slide (**type I ulnar translocation**) towards the ulna, increasing the gap between the radial styloid and the scaphoid. In **type II ulnar translocation**, the distance between the radial styloid and the scaphoid remains normal and the scopholunate space is widened. It is important to distinguish between the two types of ulnar translocation since the appearance of a wide scapholunate gap may lead to the erroneous diagnosis of scapholunate dissociation.

Depending on the direction in which the lunate is tilted, a DISI or VISI deformity may be seen. However, as the proximal row is intact, the scapholunate angle is normal. As the lunate is tilted, the capitolunate angle is abnormal and the carpal height ratio may be reduced.

Carpal instability complex

Carpal instability complex (CIC) results when instability **within and between rows** is combined. CIC results from significant disruption of intrinsic and extrinsic soft tissues, or fractures, and the movement of the carpal bones reflects the disruptions.

It is simplest to describe the CIC by the individual components. For example, if the SLL is disrupted, then the end result may be a CID with a DISI deformity. If the radiocarpal ligaments are disrupted, then the result may be a CIND in isolation with translation of the whole carpus. However, if both the SLL and the extrinsic ligaments are disrupted, except for the radioscaphoid ligament, then the scaphoid would remain in position while the lunate slides ulnar-wards, and a **type II ulnar translocation** is seen. The combination of the SLL and extrinsic ligamentous injury creates a CIC.

Combined LTL and SLL injuries may result in CIC. This is seen most commonly in traumatic perilunate injuries. As described by Mayfield, the stages of perilunar injury progress in a stepwise manner from SLL to capitolunate to LTL to radiolunate disruption. The reverse Mayfield pattern may also be seen, usually in association with TFCC or DRUJ injuries, starting with the LTL. These injuries probably do not happen in a precise sequence, but they show how a CIC can develop with combinations of ligamentous injuries.

Time plays a factor in the evolution of the CIC patterns, as untreated CID increases the strain on the extrinsic ligaments that may well have been damaged in the initial injury. These extrinsic ligaments may then become gradually attenuated and dysfunctional, resulting in a CIC pattern.

Adaptive carpus and scaphoid fractures

The alignment of the carpus is dependent on the geometry of the bones and the soft tissues. It follows that if these are altered, then the carpus will adapt in order to compensate for these changes. In situations where there is a malunion of the distal radius, most commonly seen following a Colles' type fracture, the radial articulation may lose its normal volar anatomical tilt. The carpus will adapt to this new alignment, usually with the proximal row translating and tilting dorsally. The distal row exhibits a compensatory flexion, and an adaptive DISI deformity may be seen (**carpal instability adaptive, CIA**).

The scaphoid itself is under two opposite moments. There is a flexion moment exerted on the distal pole (as described earlier) and an extension moment exerted proximally by the triquetrum and lunate via the LTL and SLL. The radioscaphocapitate ligament acts as the fulcrum for scaphoid movement. If the scaphoid fractures across the waist, these moments are uncoupled and the classic humpback deformity of the flexed distal pole is seen. There may also be a DISI deformity as the lunate and the proximal scaphoid tilt dorsally. The situation is the same in tran-scaphoid perilunate injuries, with the additional ligamentous disruption causing a combined instability, i.e. CIC.

Axial instability

This pattern of instability results from longitudinal or crushing forces disrupting the carpus and the CMC joints. The line of the force disrupts the wrist axially and may affect the radial or ulnar side, or both.

Implications of carpal instability

The carpus is designed to function as a whole. Uncoupling of the normal intercarpal and radiocarpal movement affects the axis of movement, causing restriction, and affects joint loading, leading to a predictable pattern of arthritic collapse. Both cause pain. The most commonly examined patterns of degenerative change are the **scapholunate advanced collapse (SLAC)** and **scaphoid non-union advanced collapse (SNAC)**. Although the pathogenesis is complex, the progression of degenerative change can be simplified and understood from the biomechanics, most of which have already been covered in this chapter.

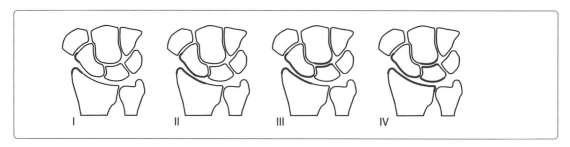

Figure 23.7 Scapholunate advanced collapse (SLAC). With chronic scapholunate ligament injury, a progressive and predictable pattern of arthritic collapse ensues. Stage I, affecting the radial styloid–scaphoid junction; stage II, affecting the entire radioscaphoid joint; stage III, affecting the entire radioscaphoid joint and the capitolunate articulation; stage IV, osteoarthritis affects both the radiocarpal and intercarpal joints and may involve the distal radioulnar joint.

SLL disruption uncouples the flexing scaphoid from the extending lunate, initially causing a dynamic instability. The capitate is still under the axial loading forces pulling it proximally and may widen the gap on stress radiographs. The carpal height may therefore be shortened. Left untreated, a static DISI deformity develops. The scaphoid tends to stay flexed and impacts on the dorsal rim of the radius, causing abnormal loading of the radiocarpal joint in addition to any chondral damage from the initial injury. This degenerate change progresses between the radial styloid initially and scaphoid (**SLAC stage I**). Once the arthritic disease has encompassed the entire scaphoid facet articulation it has entered **SLAC stage II**. The capitate continues to push down on the widened scapholunate interval, and degenerate change occurs at the lunocapitate articulation (**SLAC stage III**) (**Figure 23.7**).

The SNAC wrist is similar, except that the uncoupling of the forces occurs across the fractured scaphoid rather than through the scapholunate joint. The pattern of forces across the wrist is similar, with scaphostyloid arthrosis occurring initially (**SNAC stage I**). The proximal pole of the scaphoid extends with the lunate, so the capitate impinges on the proximal scaphoid, leading to scaphocapitate arthrosis (**SNAC stage II**). Unchecked, the lunocapitate articulation becomes affected (**SNAC stage III**). Ultimately, the carpus is shortened and collapses, and degenerative change progresses to affect the radiocarpal articulation.

The distal radioulnar joint complex

Pronation and **supination** of the wrist involve the proximal and distal radioulnar joints and the interosseous membrane. Whilst bearing in mind that proximal disruption will affect wrist movement, only the DRUJ will be considered here.

The **ulna** is the fixed structure around which the radius rotates. The axis of rotation has been described. The extent of the ulnar articular surface (130°) is greater and the radius of the curvature smaller than the shallow sigmoid notch of the radius, so the contact areas vary in rotation. There is about 60% joint contact with the wrist in the neutral position, and this decreases to 10% in full pronation or supination. Relative to the ulna, there are also volar translation and proximal migration of the radius in pronation and dorsal translation and distal migration in supination (the radius slides forwards or back on the ulna). There is also a normal proximal migration of the radius – up to 7 mm – with axial loading resisted by the interosseous membrane and proximal radiocapitellar joint. Like all joints, the stability of the DRUJ is dependent on static and dynamic stabilizers. The TFCC is also discussed here.

The **TFCC** describes a complex structure linking the DRUJ to the ulnar carpus and consists of the **articular disc and meniscal homologue,** the **volar and dorsal radioulnar ligaments,** the **ulnocarpal ligaments** and the **extensor carpi ulnaris sheath.** The TFCC binds the radius, ulna and carpus to form a stable platform for movement. In addition, the extensor carpi ulnaris (ECU) and pronator quadratus (PQ) contribute to dynamic stability and the articular shape itself, and the relationship of the radius and ulna with the interosseous membrane are important static stabilizers, which should not be underestimated in providing DRUJ stability.

The volar and dorsal radioulnar ligaments arise from the edges of the radial notch and attach to the fovea and base of the ulna styloid. There is debate as to the specific contribution of each ligament to the stability of the DRUJ, but in essence they bind the radius to the ulna through the whole arc of movement, each becoming tight at full pronation or supination. The ulnocarpal ligaments comprise the ulnolunate, ulnocapitate and ulnotriquetral. These ligaments link the carpus to the ulna and so help to stabilize the DRUJ. The axis of pronation and supination can be thought to pass along the ulnotriquetral ligament.

The ECU is bound to the distal ulna by its own sheath, and so its relationship to the ulna is fixed. The sheath itself provides stability, but the ECU also has a major dynamic role dependent on its position relative to the radius. When the wrist is loaded in pronation, e.g. when holding a pen, the ECU acts to compress the DRUJ by squeezing it together. In supination, the carpus tends to sublux dorsally, and the contraction of the ECU exerts a counterforce to prevent this. If the ECU is displaced from its normal position, as in rheumatoid arthritis, then subluxation of the ulna head (or in fact the radius from the ulna) becomes more pronounced. The contraction of PQ compresses the DRUJ, particularly in supination, to prevent subluxation.

As mentioned it is worth pointing out that although by convention we normally describe dorsal or volar subluxation of the ulna head, what in fact occurs is subluxation of the radius and carpus relative to the ulna, with supination of the carpus.

Wrist motors

The wrist motors are all the muscles that cross the wrist, including long flexors and extensors. The dedicated wrist motors, ECU and FCU, and flexor carpi radialis (FCR) and extensor carpi radialis longus/brevis (ECRL/B), often work in controlled antagonism to provide a stable platform for hand movement. Interestingly the antagonism is actually most pertinent between ECRL/B and FCU, which allows for the functional 'dart throwing motion' of the carpus on the wrist. As previously described, the proximal carpal row is near stationary during this motion, which is believed to provide a stable platform for the generation of force and accuracy during certain power and precision grip activities. For power grip, wrist extension is necessary, and this synergism of movement is of use in tendon transfers.

The paralyzed hand

This section describes the tendon transfers that may be used to restore function following nerve injury or tendon rupture. Before contemplating a transfer, several principles need to be considered:

- The joint must be **passively mobile**.
- The **gain in function** must be greater than the potential loss.
- The **motor** must be of sufficient power (generally one MRC grade will be lost) and excursion.
- Ideally there should also be:
  - **one motor per joint** to be moved;
  - a **straight line of pull**;
  - **synergistic transfers**;
  - **sensibility** of the recipient part.

The number of motors available also affects what can be achieved. In severe neurological loss, as in brachial plexus injuries, the role of tenodesis and fusion (simplify the machine) cannot be forgotten. Below is a list, though by no means exhaustive, of transfers. When there is a selection, those in italics are suggested.

Radial nerve

- **Loss**: wrist and MCP joint extension.
- **Transfer**:
  - pronator teres (PT) to ECRB (less radial deviation than ECRL);
  - *palmaris longus (PL) to EPL*; or
  - FDS IV to EPL;
  - FCR (better) or extensor digitorum communis (FCU) to EDC.

Low ulnar nerve

- **Loss**: intrinsics.
- **Transfer**:
  - to prevent clawing:
    - FDS tenodesis;
    - MCP joint capsulodesis;
    - *FDS to lateral band*;
    - ECRL plus graft to lateral band.
  - thumb adduction:
    - ECRB plus graft;
    - EIP through second metacarpal space;
    - FDS IV rerouted through fascial pulley.
  - first dorsal interosseous (DIO):
    - *often not needed*: flex all fingers to form post for pinch;
    - ECRL or APL to first DIO.

High ulnar nerve

- **Loss**: the above plus FCU and FDP.
- **Transfer**:
  - suture FDPs together;
  - ?FCR to FCU (remaining radial flexors: PL and APL).

Low median nerve

- **Loss**: thumb opposition.
- **Transfer**:
  - PL to APB;
  - *extensor indicis (EIP) to APB*;
  - *FDS IV to APB*;
  - abductor digiti minimi (AbDM) to APB.

High median nerve

- **Loss**: the above plus PT, finger and thumb flexors (except ulnar FDP).
- **Transfer**:
  - AbDM or EIP to APB;
  - suture FDPs together;
  - reroute biceps or ECU to radius for pronation;
  - *ECRL to FPL*;
  - BR plus graft to FPL.

Viva questions

1. What is an intrinsic plus/intrinsic minus/lumbrical plus hand?
2. What is Froment's test? What is its anatomical basis?
3. What is carpal instability? What are the common types seen clinically?
4. What are the principles of tendon transfer?
5. What tendon transfers are suitable for a median/ulnar/radial nerve palsy?

Further reading

Brand PW, Hollister AM. *Clinical Mechanics of the Hand*. London: Mosby, 1999.

Buchler U (ed). *Wrist Instability*. London: Taylor and Francis, 1996.

Cassidy C, Ruby LK. Carpal instability. *Instr Course Lect* 2003;**52**:209–20.

Gilula LA, Mann F, Dobyns JH, Yin Y. Wrist terminology as defined by the International Wrist Investigators' Workshop (IWIW). *J Bone Joint Surg Am* 2002;**84**:1–66.

Goodman HJ, Choueka J. Biomechanics of the flexor tendons. *Hand Clin* 2005;**21**:129–49.

24 Biomechanics and Joint Replacement of the Foot and Ankle

Rohit Madhav, Amit Amin, Deborah Eastwood and Dishan Singh

Introduction

The foot and ankle consist of a complex arrangement of joints and soft-tissue units that work together to allow efficient bipedal ambulation. As the foot projects forward from the ankle, it provides stability during stance and assists with overall body balance. It is required to be flexible to accommodate uneven ground, but also to convert to a rigid lever for stability during heel strike and push-off.

The ankle and subtalar joint complex work in tandem, forming a functional unit that dissipates axial, bending and torsional forces encountered during weight bearing. In walking and running, the muscles and tendons controlling the position of the foot successively absorb and release energy in a way that assists the body to move in its path so that the centre of gravity is not subjected to rapid acceleration and deceleration forces and the eye level undergoes minimal movement.

The inherent stability and congruity provided by the static and dynamic structures in this region is reflected in the low incidence of primary foot and ankle osteoarthritis.

Nomenclature

Embryologically, the foot is initially aligned with the leg but then rotates through 90° during development. Therefore, hindfoot movements are described in the axis of the leg, while forefoot movements are described at 90° to this. There is no general agreement regarding the terms used to describe foot movements, and there is particular disagreement between the definitions used by paediatric orthopaedic surgeons and those preferred by adult foot and ankle surgeons. The terms described here are based on those of the American Orthopaedic Foot and Ankle Society (AOFAS) (*Table 24.1*).

Table 24.1 AOFAS definitions of foot and ankle movements

Dorsiflexion/plantarflexion	Sagittal plane movements up and down (e.g. ankle)
Varus/valgus	Coronal (frontal) plane angulation towards or away from midline (e.g. hindfoot)
Adduction/abduction	Transverse plane movements towards and away from midline (e.g. midfoot)
Pronation/supination	Describes movement in three planes and three joints, i.e. supination is ankle plantarflexion, hindfoot varus, and midfoot adduction
Inversion/eversion	Specific to the subtalar joint, as one axis of rotation produces movement in two planes (hindfoot varus, forefoot supination/hindfoot valgus, forefoot pronation)
Concentric contraction:	Musculotendinous unit shortening whilst muscle contracting
Eccentric contraction	Musculotendinous unit lengthening whilst muscle contracting

Body motion during gait

The centre of gravity displaces in vertical, horizontal and lateral directions during the gait cycle. The coordinated actions of the hip, knee, foot and ankle convert individual series of motion arcs into a smooth sinusoidal curve in each of the planes. Vertical and lateral displacements average 4–5 cm and require controlled acceleration and deceleration. Horizontal movement (propulsion) occurs with each rotatory movement of the pelvis, resulting in torques of approximately 7–8 Nm in the tibia, with an average rotation of 19°. During the first third of the

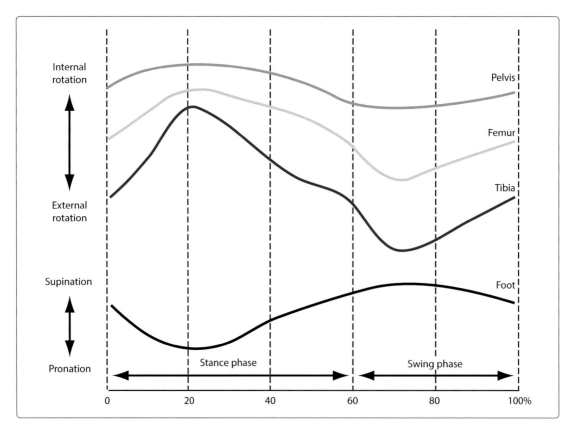

Figure 24.1 Rotation of the pelvis, femur and tibia in the transverse plane during walking.

stance phase of gait, the lower leg undergoes internal rotation. External rotation occurs during the subsequent two-thirds of stance (**Figure 24.1**).

Biomechanics of the ankle

Anatomy and kinematics

The talar dome is wider anteriorly (mean difference 2.4 ± 1.3 mm) than posteriorly. Its medial side has a narrower radius of curvature and a smaller articular facet compared with its lateral side. Anatomically, the shapes and articular surfaces of the talus and mortise represent a section of a **frustum of a cone** (**Figure 24.2**), with its apex medial (mean conical angle 24 ± 6°). The apex coincides with the deltoid ligament. The axis of rotation of this diverging cone is the same as that of the ankle joint.

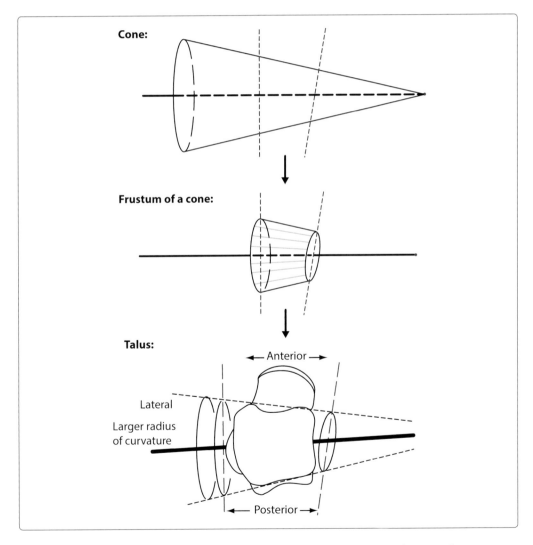

Figure 24.2 The talus and ankle mortise fit geometrically as a section of a frustum of a cone.

The ankle joint can be simplified into a **uniplanar hinge joint** with motion occurring about a transverse axis joining the tips of the malleoli. The axis is oblique by 10° (82 ± 3.6), and the talus in its mortise rotates a few degrees around a sagittal axis centred at the apex of the cone, helped by the larger radius of curvature of its lateral edge. Thus, plantarflexion results in forefoot adduction and hindfoot inversion and dorsiflexion leads to forefoot abduction and hindfoot eversion (**Figure 24.3**). Put another way, with ankle movement, the foot goes from 'down and in' to 'up and out'. Therefore, whilst considered a uniplanar hinge, ankle joint motion is described as triplanar.

The distal tibiofibular syndesmosis is held together by the anterior inferior tibiofibular ligament, the posterior inferior tibiofibular ligament, the interosseus ligament and transverse tibiofibular ligaments. With ankle dorsiflexion, the wider anterior talus engages within the mortise, relying on some opening within the syndesmosis, typically about 2 mm. Isolated syndesmotic sprains (high ankle sprains) and a variety of ankle fractures can result in syndesmotic injury. Malreduction of the syndesmosis and instability have been shown to increase ankle joint contact pressures and may result in long-term predisposition to osteoarthritis.

Symptomatic osteoarthritis of the ankle is **nine times less prevalent than that of the hip and knee**. Factors include the **highly congruent nature of the articulation**, a **uniform cartilage mantle** that better resists compressive forces, and the **biomechanical make-up of the cartilage** that is more resistant to indentation.

Minor deviations of the inclination of the axes of the ankle due to epiphyseal injury, ligamentous injury or malunion of a fracture can result in severe pathological alterations in the joint, although symptomatic degenerative change remains relatively uncommon.

The total range of motion of the ankle joint in the sagittal plane is approximately 10–20° of dorsiflexion to 25–30° of plantarflexion. Even with the most oblique axis, a normal ankle provides only 11° of tibial rotation. An average of 19° is required for propulsion, and thus the subtalar joint needs to be a significant contributor to rotational movement.

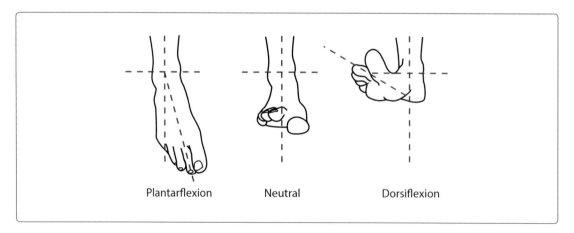

Plantarflexion   Neutral   Dorsiflexion

Figure 24.3 The effect of the oblique orientation of the ankle joint on forefoot position with dorsiflexion and plantarflexion.

The normal pattern of ankle joint motion during gait has been studied extensively. At **initial contact** (heel strike in normal gait), the ankle is in **neutral to slight plantarflexion**. The ground reaction causes immediate **plantar flexion** (at 7% of the gait cycle), but the motion rapidly reverses to **dorsiflexion** during mid-stance as the body passes over the supporting foot (at 35% of the cycle). The motion then returns to **plantarflexion** with heel-rise during the late stance phase (40–62% of the cycle). At lift-off at the beginning of the swing phase, the ankle is in **plantarflexion**. The motion reverses towards **dorsiflexion** in the middle of the swing phase (foot clearance) and changes again to slight **plantarflexion** and **pre-positioning** for initial contact (**Figure 24.4**).

At normal walking speed (about 6 km/h), an individual averages 60 cycles per minute and spends 60% of each cycle in stance phase on each leg. The first 10% of the gait cycle after heel-strike is a period of double stance, i.e. both feet are in contact with the ground. As the individual walks faster, the period of double stance becomes reduced, until eventually, as the individual begins to jog or run, double stance disappears altogether and is replaced by periods when neither foot is on the ground. In sprinting, heel-strike is replaced by forefoot strike.

Kinetics of the ankle

Owing to the smaller load-bearing surface of the ankle, higher stresses are generated across this joint compared with the knee and hip. At 500 N of load, the ankle has a contact area of 350

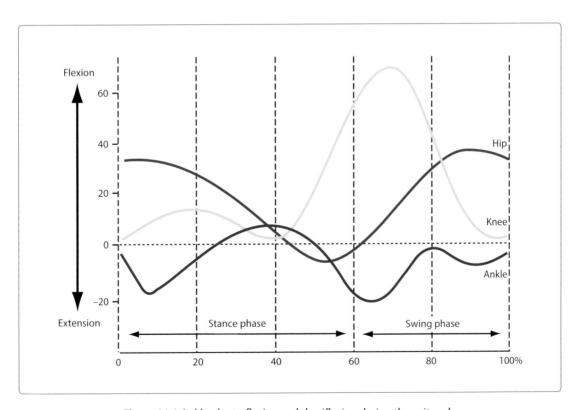

Figure 24.4 Ankle plantarflexion and dorsiflexion during the gait cycle.

mm^2 as compared with 1100 and 1120 mm^2 for the hip and knee, respectively. Changes in the tibiotalar contact area are produced by lateral talar shift, a frequent sequelae of major sprains and fractures of the ankle. If talar shift is not corrected, it can lead to significant biomechanical alterations in the joint. One mm of talar shift has been shown to reduce the ankle joint surface contact area by 42%, leading to a significant rise in joint contact stress and, hence, early degenerative changes. Recent studies using unconstrained models have replicated and validated this original work.

When an individual stands on both feet, each ankle supports approximately one-half of the body weight. The line of gravity of the body passes a few centimetres anterior to the transverse axis of the ankle joint, and hence the body weight produces a dorsiflexing torque on the joint that varies between 3 Nm and 24 Nm as a result of body oscillations. Therefore, standing with the body weight distributed evenly on both feet requires some activity in the plantar flexor muscles. The main **compressive force** in the ankle during gait is produced by contraction of the **gastrocnemius** and **soleus muscles** and is transmitted through the Achilles tendon. When these and other muscles in the lower leg are involved in balancing the body, the joint reaction force at the ankle increases in proportion to the amount of muscle force used for these balancing activities. For an individual standing on tiptoe, the joint reaction force is about 2.1 times the body weight and the **Achilles tendon** force reaches about 1.0 times the body weight (a total of three times the body weight). This explains why a patient with degenerative arthritis has pain when rising up on tiptoes.

Anatomy of the Achilles tendon

The tendo Achilles is the largest and strongest tendon in the body and is formed by the conjoined tendons of gastrocnemius and soleus. It has a **spiral arrangement**, with its medial fibres inserting posteriorly and the lateral fibres inserting anteriorly on to the **calcaneal tuberosity**. Thus, when performing a percutaneous lengthening via two incisions, the cuts must be made perpendicular to the fibres, i.e. distal-anterior and medial proximal (**DAMP technique**) in order to cut the correct bundles and achieve a slide. Another popular method, popularized by paediatric orthopaedic surgeons, is the **triple cut or Hoke technique**, with incisions approximately 3 cm apart in one plane (medial, lateral, medial), dividing 50% of the tendon each time.

Biomechanics of the subtalar joint and the foot

As discussed earlier, the unique qualities of the foot allow it to be flexible when necessary, as in when walking barefoot, and yet suitably rigid, converting the 26 bones (28 with the sesamoids) and 57 joints into a solid unit, as required for ballet dancing *en pointe*.

Anatomy and kinematics of the subtalar joint

Sometimes the foot functions as a single unit, and at other times it functions as a subtle grasping appendage. The potential of the normal foot to be a prehensile limb has been well demonstrated by patients with complete amelia of the upper extremities and who dress themselves, feed themselves and even write with their feet and toes.

The **talus** is a bone with **no muscle attachments**. It sits atop the calcaneum stabilized only by the ligaments and cradled by all the tendons passing from the leg to the foot. The subtalar joint is commonly referred to as a **torque converter**, and it has been modelled as a **mitred hinge**, transforming tibial rotation into forefoot pronation and supination via inversion and eversion (**Figure 24.5**).

On average, the subtalar joint can be inverted 20° and everted about 5°. Throughout the stance phase of gait, the average range of motion of the subtalar joint is only 6° in normal feet and 12° in flat feet, a so-called **functional range of motion**. The foot rests in slight supination during the swing phase; at heel-strike, it rotates into slight pronation as the lower limb is internally rotated in the first 15% of the stance phase and the heel strikes the ground slightly lateral to the longitudinal axis of the leg (**Figure 24.6**).

One degree of tibial rotation would yield 1° of foot motion if the axis was at 45°. The flat-footed individual has a more horizontal subtalar axis, and thus the same tibial torsion has greater rotatory effect on the foot; the opposite occurs for the cavus foot. If movements at the subtalar joint are congenitally blocked, as in tarsal coalition, then the ankle joint remodels into a ball-and-socket joint to allow inversion and eversion.

The subtalar joint also demonstrates **linear motion**, i.e. anteroposterior movement. This is likened to the **Archimedes spiral screw** (mean helix angle 12°), where rotational movements are converted to linear motion. The calcaneum moves forwards in inversion and backwards in

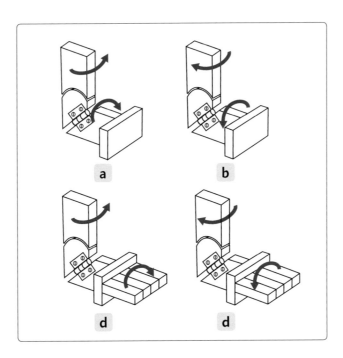

Figure 24.5 In the mitered hinge model of the subtalar joint, tibial rotation causes subtalar joint (a) inversion and (b) eversion and forefoot (c) supination and (d) pronation.

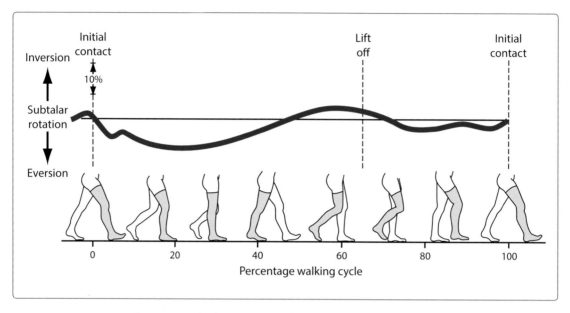

Figure 24.6 Subtalar inversion and eversion during the gait cycle.

eversion. For practical purposes, foot motion can be considered to be of two distinct types – non-weight bearing and weight bearing. Active weight-bearing motion of the foot differs from passive motion because of forces produced by the body weight and by muscle contractions that act to stabilize the joints. When an individual stands on the ball of the foot, the hindfoot inverts slightly and the midfoot is in plantarflexion and the forefoot exhibits some pronation, creating an arch. Standing flatfooted on an externally rotating leg also raises the arch by moving the heel into slight inversion and causing the forefoot to twist into pronation. Rotating the leg internally has the opposite effect: it lowers the arch.

Mid-tarsal/transverse tarsal joint motion

The transverse tarsal joints (**Chopart's joints**) lie just anterior to the talus and calcaneum and are associated closely with the subtalar joint. They represent motion between the **talus** and **navicular** and between the **calcaneum** and **cuboid**. The talonavicular joint is key to understanding hindfoot kinematics. If the talus is considered to sit relatively free in the ankle mortise, held by ligaments from the tibia and fibula, the foot essentially moves around an instant centre of rotation at the talonavicular joint. If an isolated talonavicular fusion is performed, 80% of hindfoot motion is eliminated, in contrast to 60% if an isolated subtalar joint fusion is performed.

Motion at the **talonavicular joint** is aided by its ball-and-socket type geometry, whereas the **calcaneocuboid joint** is saddle shaped. The axes of these two joints are positioned in a frontal plane; the superior axis passes through the talar neck and the inferior axis passes through the calcaneal body. When the foot is in **eversion** (i.e. with the arch flat or foot pronated), these two axes fall into parallel alignment in the same plane and the midfoot is able to flex and extend with ease in relation to the hindfoot. However, when the heel is **inverted** (i.e. with the arch elevated or foot supinated), the axes diverge, and flexion and extension movements of the midfoot, with respect to the hindfoot, are significantly restricted. During the mid-stance phase, the pronated 'flat' foot is mobile and can adapt to the uneven ground. In the late stance phase, with heel inversion and forefoot supination, the locked Chopart's joints turn the foot into a stiff lever arm to push off with. This mechanism may be why patients are able to tolerate a pronated foot or flat foot more easily than they tolerate a varus or supinated foot, as in club foot.

Intertarsal and tarsometatarsal joint motion

Motion of the surfaces of the intertarsal and tarsometatarsal joints is restricted by the shapes of the bones, the many restrictive ligaments, and surrounding muscles. **Gliding motion** occurs between the **cuneiform** and **cuboid** and also within the tarsometatarsal joints during gait. Since the total extension of any two bones of the intertarsal joints is small, for practical purposes motion may be considered as translation of power into motion (gliding) of one surface across another. Total midfoot motion ranges from just a few degrees of dorsiflexion to about 15° of plantarflexion and is distributed through all the tarsal bones.

Tendons, ligaments and plantar fascia support the bony arch and its shape is affected by the tarsometatarsal joints (known together as **Lisfranc's joint**). In essence, the **dorsum** of the arch is subjected to **compressive stresses** across the articular surfaces, while the **plantar muscles**, **ligaments** and in particular the **plantar fascia** are under **tensile stress** (like a bow and a bow string). The arch may be raised by passive means through external rotation of the tibia during standing and also through extension of the toes and tightening of the plantar fascia.

The midfoot functions as a rigid lever converting hindfoot forces into forefoot propulsive forces during the gait cycle, and therefore stability is essential in this region. Following a Lisfranc injury that is missed or not reduced, a flat-foot deformity results with or without instability.

Metatarsal break

In the latter part of stance phase, as the weight is transferred to the forefoot, there is an axis through which all the toes extend at the **metatarsophalangeal joints**. This oblique axis, which overlies the metatarsophalangeal joints, is called the **metatarsal break**. It varies considerably among individuals in its orientation to the long axis of the foot, from 50 to 70°. It is a generalization of the instant centres of rotation of all five metatarsophalangeal joints. The obliquity of this break conforms to the transverse crease formed in shoes.

Function of the plantar fascia

The function of the plantar fascia is complex. From its attachment to the calcaneum, the plantar fascia extends forwards to span all the tarsal and metatarsophalangeal joints and to attach to the plantar aspect of the proximal phalanges. The result is a **truss-like** structure whose links are the tarsal bones and ligaments of the foot, which is held at its base by a tether, the plantar fascia. The **windlass mechanism** is formed at the metatarsophalangeal attachment of the fascia. As the metatarsophalangeal joints are extended passively when one stands on the ball of the foot, the plantar fascia is pulled distally across them, shortening the distance from the calcaneum to the metatarsal heads. This process makes the base of the truss shorter. The tarsal joints are locked into a forced flexed position and the height of the longitudinal arch of the foot is increased. Thus, extension of the toes helps to turn the foot into a rigid lever before push-off (**Figure 24.7**).

Kinetics of the foot

During normal stance, approximately 50% of the load is borne by the heel and 50% is transmitted across the metatarsal heads, predominantly the first and between the second and third heads. A slight change in the foot structure alters the load distribution. At heel-strike, the ground reaction force is slightly medial to the centre of the heel pad. When the foot rolls into slight valgus shortly thereafter during the flat-foot portion of stance, the ground reaction force progresses slightly laterally to lie beneath the cuboid and then forwards towards the base of the first metatarsal. Towards the end of the stance phase, the ground reaction force courses medially to reach beneath the second metatarsal head and then proceeds to the hallux at toe-off. Thus, during the stance phase of gait, the centre of the load progresses forwards rapidly, from the heel to the great toe (**Figure 24.8**).

The extrinsic muscles provide active control of the foot. The **anterior leg muscles** are active at **heel-strike**, while **posterior calf muscles propel the foot forwards to toe-off**. The soft tissues of the sole are especially adapted to absorb shock at heel-strike and to protect the bony structures through the stance phase of gait and push-off.

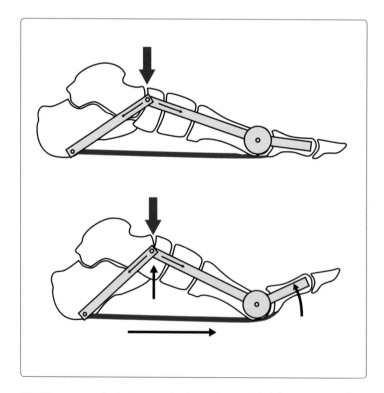

Figure 24.7 The truss and windlass mechanism raises arch height, increasing foot stability.

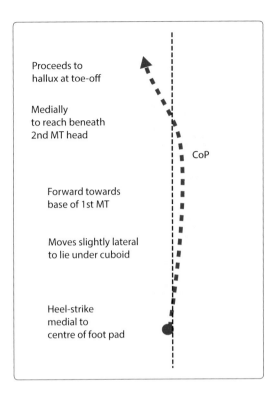

Figure 24.8 Path of the centre of pressure during normal gait. CoP: centre of pressure; MT: metatarsal.

Total ankle replacement (TAR)

Summary of biomechanical considerations

The ankle is not a simple single-axis hinge, and its axis of rotation changes with loading and rotation. The ankle transmits large axial (four to seven times body weight) loads and large shear forces (80% of body weight). The ligaments contribute significantly to stability in all positions of the joint. The challenge therefore, with ankle arthroplasty design, is to replicate these complex biomechanics, to optimize function and enhance prosthesis longevity.

Surgical considerations

Current research supports TAR as a **viable option for patients with ankle osteoarthritis**, with the **ideal** patient being **low-demand**. Those with concomitant subtalar osteoarthritis often benefit from motion preservation at the ankle joint, as a tibiotalocalcaneal fusion has been shown in gait studies to produce significant functional deficit. Gait analysis has also shown **TAR to be superior to ankle fusion with respect to gait symmetry and timing**, although stride length was found to be inferior to normal controls.

Absolute contraindications include **infection, talar avascular necrosis and neuromuscular disease**. With respect to **relative contraindications, coronal plane deformity of >10° has been**

shown to be associated with higher revision rates, and careful attention should be directed to ligament balance and ancillary bony and soft-tissue procedures in these cases.

Prosthesis longevity remains undetermined and salvage of a failed TAR often requires a complex and difficult fusion.

Early designs

Introduced in the 1970s, the **first-generation implants** consisted of **two-part constrained** or **unconstrained cemented components**. The **constrained-hinge types** had **high failure rates**, predominantly at the implant–bone interface, due to large load transmission. The **unconstrained designs** relied on malleolar and ligamentocapsular elements for stability. Their **positioning** was therefore **critical**, relying heavily on **accurate soft-tissue balancing**. These failed due to instability in inversion/eversion and internal/external rotation. **Cemented implants** required considerable bony resection, leaving soft cancellous bone for support, which led to **migration and subsidence** of components.

Second generation two-component implants were designed to be **uncemented and semiconstrained**, such as the Agility total ankle prosthesis. This design incorporated a wide tibial component and an inferior tibiofibular fusion to allow more even, lower pressure distribution. Problems with this implant included **inferior tibiofibular non-union** and **talar component loosening**.

Modern designs

Third generation designs incorporate **mobile-bearing technology** with improved prosthesis surface biology and design, allowing improved bonding with host bone. These designs aim to **reduce stress at the bone–implant interface**, and **improve congruity in all joint positions**, minimizing polyethylene wear and potentially aseptic loosening. Initial designs like the Scandinavian Total Ankle Replacement (STAR) have shown promising mid- to long-term results. However, with medially-based pain commonly seen after TAR and often attributed to overtensioning of the deltoid ligament, the design of the talar component has been called into question.

Thus, with a view to increasing congruity and reducing ligament imbalance **newer designs**, like the SALTO and Hintegra prostheses, employ **anatomical talar components**, and early reports are encouraging although long-term follow-up is awaited from independent series.

Viva questions

1. What is the ideal position in which to fuse an ankle joint?
2. What is the mechanism by which eccentric contraction of muscle is achieved?
3. Describe the windlass mechanism and its role in gait.
4. Describe changes in the gait cycle with:
   (a) gastrosoleus weakness
   (b) tibialis anterior weakness.
5. What do you know about ankle joint replacements?

Further reading

Inman VT, Ralston HJ, Todd F. *Human Walking.* Baltimore, MD: Williams & Wilkins, 1981.

Jackson MP, Singh D. Total ankle replacement. *Curr Orthop* 2003;**17**:292–8.

Mann R, Coughlin M. *Surgery of the Foot and Ankle,* 7th edn. London: Mosby, 1999.

Ramsey PL, Hamilton W. Changes in tibiotalar area of contact caused by lateral talar shift. *J Bone Joint Surg Br* 1976;**58**:356–7.

Singh AK, Starkweather KD, Hollister AM, Jatana S, Lupichuk AG. Kinematics of the ankle: a hinge axis model. *Foot Ankle* 1992;**13**:439–46.

25 Friction, Lubrication, Wear and Corrosion

Gurdeep Biring, Iain McNamara, Marcus Bankes, Jay Meswania and Gordon Blunn

Introduction

Tribology is defined as the science that deals with the interaction between surfaces in motion and consequences of that interaction, i.e. **friction, lubrication and wear**. Sir William Hunter described the tribological features of synovial joints succinctly in 1743: "Both are covered with a smooth crust, to prevent natural abrasion; connected with strong ligaments to prevent dislocation; and enclosed in a bag that contains a proper fluid deposited there, for lubricating the two contiguous surfaces".

Natural synovial joints are subjected to an enormous range of loading conditions; for example, approximately five to ten times the body weight passes through the hip and knee at heel-strike. Articular cartilage has limited ability to repair and therefore, efficient lubrication is necessary in order to minimize friction and prevent cartilage wear.

This chapter aims to define tribology in normal synovial joints and in joint replacements, with reference to corrosion in the latter.

Friction

Friction is defined as the resistance to sliding motion between two bodies in contact. Surface friction comes from the adherence of one surface to another or the viscosity of the sheared lubricant film between the two surfaces. The force required to overcome the fluid's viscosity is much less than the surface adhesion.

For dry friction, three laws of friction have been defined:

- Frictional force (F) is directly proportional to the applied load (W). i.e. $F = \mu f \times W$ where μf is the coefficient of friction.
- F is independent of the apparent area of contact.
- Kinetic (sliding) friction is independent of sliding velocity (V).

In a rotational system, such as a hip replacement, it is important to describe torque rather than force:

Frictional torque = frictional force (F) × radius (r) = $\mu_f \times W \times r$

Even the smoothest polished surfaces appear rough when viewed at high enough magnification. The projections from the surface are called **asperities**. The taller and more numerous the asperities, the rougher the surface and the greater the friction.

Roughness of a surface is expressed as the **mean surface roughness**, or **Ra** value, which is the average height of the asperities. Comparative Ra values for surfaces in orthopaedics are shown in *Table 25.1*. The coefficients of friction of various articulations are shown in *Table 25.2*.

Table 25.1 Mean surface roughness (Ra) of various orthopaedic surfaces

Material	Ra/μm
Articular cartilage	1–6
Charnley stem	1
Matt Exeter stem	0.7–1.3
Polyethylene cup	0.25–2.5
Metal femoral head	0.025
Ceramic femoral head	0.02
Polished Exeter stem	0.01–0.03

Table 25.2 The coefficients of friction of various articulations

Articulation	Coefficient of friction (μf)
Normal knee	0.005–0.02
Normal hip	0.01–0.04
Metal-on-polyethylene	0.02
Metal-on-metal (dry)	0.8
Aluminium-on-aluminium	2.0

Synovial fluid physiology

Synovial fluid is a dialysate of blood plasma, without clotting factors, erythrocytes or haemoglobin. Synovial fluid is clear, and sometimes yellowish and viscous, and contains **hyaluronate** (relative molecular mass [RMM] 1–2000 kDa) and **plasma proteins** (20% concentration of plasma; similar to serum). In the synovium, as in all tissues, essential nutrients are delivered and metabolic by-products are cleared by the bloodstream perfusing the local vasculature. Synovial micro-vessels contain fenestrations that facilitate diffusion-based exchange between plasma and the surrounding interstitium, which equilibrates with synovial fluid and the interstitial fluid of cartilage. Plasma proteins also enter by diffusion, but distribution favours smaller molecules due to a mechanism that limits transfer of these molecules from the plasma. The micro-vascular endothelium provides the major barrier limiting the escape of plasma proteins into the surrounding synovial interstitium, with larger molecules passing more slowly than smaller molecules. The protein path across the endothelium involves fenestrae, intercellular junctions and cytoplasmic vesicles, but the precise mechanism is yet to be determined.

In contrast, proteins leave synovial fluid through lymphatic vessels, a process that is not size-selective. Protein clearance may vary with joint disease; for example, there is more rapid removal of proteins from joints affected by rheumatoid arthritis (due to increased micro-vascular permeability) than from those affected by osteoarthritis.

Thus, in all joints there is a continuous passive transport of plasma proteins involving synovial delivery in the micro-vasculature, diffusion across the endothelium, synthesis and breakdown by the synovium and ultimate lymphatic return to plasma. The intrasynovial concentration of any protein represents the net contributions of these factors.

Synovial fluid mechanics

Viscosity is the **measure of the internal friction of a fluid**. This friction becomes apparent when a layer of fluid is made to move in relation to another layer. The greater the friction, the greater the amount of force required for this movement, known as **shear**. Shearing occurs whenever the fluid is physically moved or distributed, as in pouring, spreading, spraying and mixing. Highly viscous fluids therefore require more force to move than less viscous materials.

Isaac Newton defined **viscosity** mathematically by the formula:

viscosity = shear stress/shear rate

where **shear stress** is the force per unit area required to produce shearing action (measured in dynes/cm^2), **shear rate** is a measure of the change in speed at which the intermediate layers of fluid move with respect to each other (measured in reciprocal seconds – s^{-1}) and **viscosity** is measured in **poise**, such that a material requiring a shear stress of 1 dyne/cm^2 to produce a shear rate of s^{-1} has a viscosity of 1 poise. Newton's law of viscosity states that this ratio is a constant and so fluids that adhere to this law are called Newtonian. Non-Newtonian fluids do not follow this law, and therefore their viscosity is not constant and changes as the shear rate changes.

Viscosity of synovial fluid from normal knee joints decreases from 500 Pa.s to 0.5 Pa.s as the shear rate increases from 0.001/s to 1000/s. This **shear thinning** derives from the alignment of the hyaluronic acid molecules as shear rate increases. **Enzymatic degradation of synovial fluid in rheumatoid arthritis leads to loss of non-Newtonian properties**, making the fluid a less effective lubricant. In contrast, **hyaluronates of synovial fluids from osteoarthritic joints are not degraded and maintain their non-Newtonian properties**. These properties allow synovial fluid to act as an efficient lubricant as well as allowing nutrition of articular cartilage.

Key facts about synovial fluid

1. Non-Newtonian (shear stress is not proportional to shear rate).
2. Pseudoplastic (undergoes shear thinning).
3. Thixotropic (undergoes shear thinning with time when sheared at a constant rate).

Important definitions:

Rheology: the science of deformation and flow of matter.

Shear: the rate of deformation of a fluid when subjected to a mechanical shearing stress.

Shear stress: an applied force per unit area needed to produce deformation in a fluid.

Viscosity: a measure of the resistance of a liquid to flow (internal friction).

Newtonian fluid: a fluid or dispersion whose rheological behaviour is described by Newton's law of viscosity. Here shear stress is proportional to shear rate, with the proportionality constant being the viscosity, e.g. water, thin motor oils, synovial fluid in rheumatoid arthritis (enzymatic degradation makes it a less effective lubricant).

Non-Newtonian fluid: when the shear rate is varied, the shear stress does not vary in the same proportion (or even necessarily in the same direction). The viscosity of such fluids will therefore change as the shear rate is varied (envisioned by thinking of any fluid with a mixture of molecules with different shapes and sizes). The most common types of non-Newtonian fluids one may encounter include pseudoplastic and dilatant fluids.

Pseudoplastic: a non-Newtonian fluid whose viscosity decreases as the applied shear rate increases, a process that is also termed **shear thinning** e.g. paints, emulsions, synovial fluid.

Dilatant: a non-Newtonian fluid whose viscosity increases as the shear rate increases. The process is termed shear thickening and although rarer than shear thinning, is found in fluids containing high levels of deflocculated solids, e.g. sand/water mixtures, clay slurries.

Plastic: a fluid that behaves as a solid under static conditions, but once flow is induced with a force known as the 'yield value', the fluid may behave as either Newtonian or non-Newtonian, e.g. tomato ketchup.

Thixotropic: pseudoplastic flow that is time-dependent. When sheared at a constant rate, viscosity gradually decreases (common and seen in materials such as synovial fluid, grease, heavy printing inks and paints).

Rheopexy: this is essentially the opposite of thixotropic behaviour, in that the fluid's viscosity increases with time as it is sheared at a constant rate (rarer).

Joint lubrication

Several hypotheses have been proposed to elucidate the mechanisms of lubrication that may explain the minimal friction and wear characteristics of cartilage and artifical joints. They fall into two groups:

- **Fluid-film lubrication**: surfaces are separated by a fluid film that fully supports the applied load, preventing contact between the surfaces. The minimum thickness of the fluid film must exceed the surface roughness of the bearing surfaces in order to prevent asperity contact.
- **Boundary lubrication**: bearing surfaces are in contact but separated by a boundary lubricant of molecular thickness, which prevents excessive bearing friction and wear. In boundary lubrication, the load is carried by the surface asperities rather than by the lubricant.

The biotribological performance of a joint depends on the lambda (λ) ratio. This is the ratio of fluid-film thickness to surface roughness: a ratio of 3 represents fluid-film lubrication, while a ratio of less than 1 represents boundary lubrication.

Studies have shown that fluid-film lubrication dominates in synovial joints. In practical terms, all types of fluid-film lubrication and boundary lubrication occur in synovial joints, depending on the specific joint in question and the particular type of loading applied.

Types of fluid-film lubrication in synovial joints

Various theories of lubrication have been proposed to explain lubrication in synovial joints. These are shown in **Figure 25.1**.

Hydrodynamic lubrication

In hydrodynamic (HD) lubrication, there is no contact between surfaces and hence no wear. The surfaces are separated by a thin fluid film, which supports the applied load. The speed of sliding and the viscosity of the lubricating fluid have to be sufficient to create a thin wedge-shaped fluid film between the surfaces, and hence HD lubrication can occur only under **high speeds** and **low loads**, otherwise the surfaces come into contact. HD lubrication is a poor model for synovial joints; however, it may occur during the high-speed non-accelerating rotatory motion of the femur during the swing phase of gait.

Elastohydrodynamic lubrication

HD lubrication assumes that the cartilage is rigid and non-porous when in fact it is elastic and deformable. In elastohydrodynamic (EHD) lubrication, elastic deformation of the bearing surface **enlarges the area of the bearing surface** and **traps pressurized fluid**. An increased surface area decreases the shear rate, thereby increasing the viscosity of the synovial fluid. These factors increase the capacity of the fluid film to carry load and decrease stress within the cartilage. Using this model, the thickness of the fluid film has been calculated to be up to 1μm, which is less than the roughness of articular cartilage (Ra = 1–6 μm).

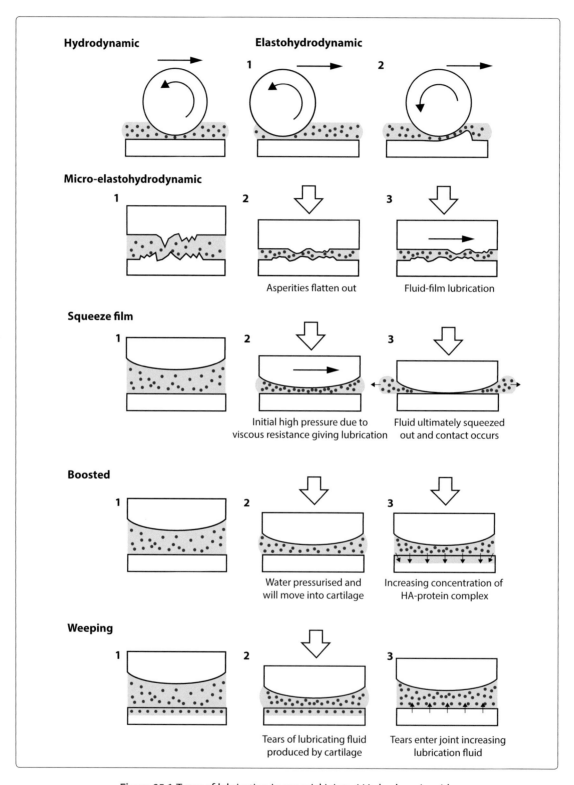

Figure 25.1 Types of lubrication in synovial joints. HA: hyaluronic acid.

Micro-elastohydrodynamic lubrication

The micro-elastohydrodynamic (MEHD) lubrication model assumes that the **asperities** of articular cartilage are **deformed under high loads**. This smoothes out the bearing surface and creates a film thickness of 0.5–1 μm, which is sufficient for fluid-film lubrication.

Squeeze-film lubrication

This occurs when **parallel bearing surfaces approach each other without relative sliding motion**, trapping the joint fluid between the approaching bearing surfaces. Because a viscous lubricant cannot instantaneously be squeezed out from the gap between approaching surfaces, pressure is built up as a consequence of the viscous resistance offered by the lubricant as it is being squeezed from the gap. This pressure is temporarily capable of supporting large loads before the fluid is squeezed out and surface contact occurs. The pressure may also deform the articular cartilage surface. Squeeze-film lubrication may occur during **heel-strike**.

Mechanisms have also been proposed concerning a localized increase or change in the composition of synovial fluid between the bearing surfaces.

Boosted lubrication

Boosted lubrication assumes that, under squeeze-film conditions, the water in the synovial fluid is pressurized into the cartilage, leaving behind a more concentrated pool of **hyaluronic acid–protein complex** to lubricate the surfaces.

Weeping lubrication

In weeping lubrication, synovial fluid is squeezed out of the areas of cartilage that are under load and fluid is reabsorbed by the areas of cartilage that are unloaded. This is an unlikely mechanism in diarthrodial joints.

Boundary lubrication in synovial joints

Prolonged standing decreases the fluid in between the joint surfaces as the lubricating fluid is 'squeezed out'. The surfaces remain coated by a gel-like surface film (thickness 5–20 nm) covering the cartilage. This hydrophobic monolayer functions like the pile of a carpet to provide a cushioning layer, decreasing the frictional force and protecting the articular surface from abrasion. This monolayer is composed mainly of the glycoprotein **lubricin** (RMM 250 kDa), but it also contains **dipalmitoyl-phosphatidyl choline**, a phospholipid. Enzymatic treatment of cartilage to remove the monolayer leads to increased coefficients of friction. Lubrication mechanisms are important during gait, and different mechanisms are thought to act at different stages of the gait cycle (*Table 25.3*).

Table 25.3 Presumed lubrication in the hip joint during the gait cycle

Phase of gait cycle	Predominant type of lubrication
Heel-strike	Squeeze-film
Stance	(M)EHD
Toe-off	Boundary, (M)EHD, weeping
Swing	Hydrodynamic
Prolonged stance	Boundary, boosted

(M)EHD: (micro-) elastohydrodynamic.

Lubrication mechanisms in prosthetic joints

Metal-on-polyethylene articulations

The fluid film is too thin in metal on ultra-high-molecular weight polyethylene (UHMWPE) articulations, therefore boundary lubrication predominates. Contact stresses can be up to 20 MPa in total hip replacements (THR) and 30 MPa in some non-conforming total knee replacements (TKR), with the velocity of sliding varying from 0 to 50 mm/s.

Lubrication occurs with a pseudo-synovial fluid, which has both a complex and variable biological composition but without the rheological properties of healthy synovial fluid.

Hard-on-hard bearing couples

For hard-on-hard bearings, the lubrication regimen is described as mixed; part of the time there is **boundary lubrication** and part of the time **HD lubrication** occurs. The factors determining the lubrication state are complex but depend upon surface roughness, sphericity and radial clearance.

- **Surface roughness**: to achieve HD lubrication, the hard-on-hard bearing surfaces must be very smooth and the Ra value very small. This situation is only appropriate in metal-on-metal and ceramic-on-ceramic bearings.
- **Sphericity**: any variation in sphericity creates points of elevation, which decrease the thickness of the fluid film at that point and promote wear.
- **Radial clearance**: defined as the difference in the radius of the head and cup. If the radius of the head is smaller than the cup, then the head will contact the inner surface of the cup at the apex of the head or polar region. Although fluid can lubricate the surfaces, **point loading at the apex** occurs. Conversely, if the diameter of the head is larger than the cup then contact occurs at the **equatorial** region of the cup; in this situation fluid cannot ingress and **jamming of the head** can occur. The ideal situation lies in between these two extremes giving mid-polar contact. In **mid-polar contact**, there is an optimum distribution of the contact loads and also good lubrication of the joint.

As well as the above factors, it also should be noted that in order for HD lubrication to occur, there has to be **angular velocity**, i.e. the joint should be in motion. Larger head sizes give rise to greater angular velocity and therefore are more likely to promote HD lubrication. At rest or during slow movement, the angular velocity is not high enough to promote HD lubrication and therefore only boundary lubrication can occur.

Ceramic-on-ceramic bearings

The surfaces of ceramic bearings can be exceptionally smooth. In general, ceramic can be described as being wettable. **Wettability describes the relative affinity of a lubricant for another material (Figure 25.2)**. It can be measured by the **angle of contact at the edge of a drop of lubricant applied to the surface of the material**. Ceramic surfaces show a greater degree of wettability than metals; as ceramics are more hydrophilic, they have improved lubrication and lower friction.

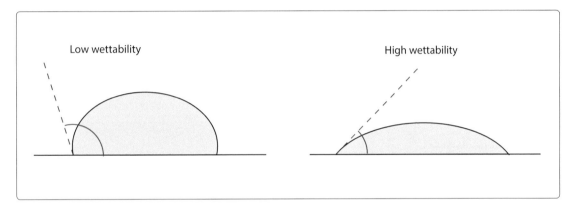

Figure 25.2 Contact angle for a fluid droplet on a solid surface

Metal-on-metal bearings

In metal-on-metal articulations, **true fluid-film lubrication** may occur with **large diameter articulations**. In metal-on-metal articulations, the effective radius is the important determinant of fluid-film thickness. A large effective radius increases contact surface area and decreases interface stress. Radial clearance between the femoral head and acetabular cup allows a large effective radius and therefore, fluid-film thickness.

Factors determining lubrication
1. Magnitude and direction of loading.
2. Geometry of the bearing surfaces/surface roughness.
3. Material properties of the surfaces, e.g. wettability.
4. Velocity at which the bearing operates.
5. Viscosity of the lubricant.

Wear

Wear of bearings is a **progressive loss of bearing substance from the material secondary to mechanical or chemical action**. The mechanical conditions under which the prosthesis is functioning when wear occurs have been classified as the four modes of wear:

- **Mode 1**: the generation of wear debris that occurs with motion between the two primary bearing surfaces, as intended by the designers.
- **Mode 2**: a primary bearing surface rubbing against a secondary surface, not intended as an articulating surface, e.g. a femoral head articulating with an acetabular shell following wear-through of the polyethylene.
- **Mode 3**: two primary bearing surfaces with interposed third-body particles, e.g. bone, cement or metal.
- **Mode 4**: two non-bearing surfaces rubbing together, e.g. back-sided wear of an acetabular liner, fretting of the Morse taper, stem-cement fretting or neck of femoral component impinging on rim of cup.

Several modes of wear often occur simultaneously, but **mode 1** accounts for the majority of wear in well-functioning hip and knee replacements.

The fundamental mechanisms of wear include **abrasion, adhesion and fatigue**.

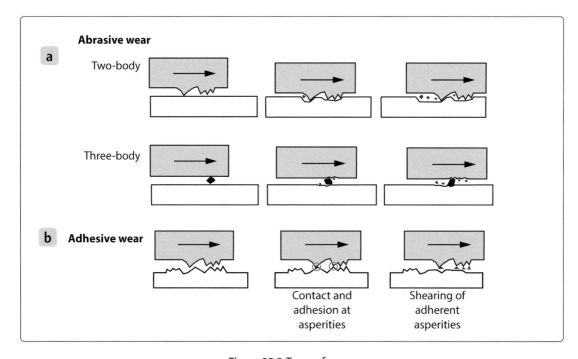

Figure 25.3 Types of wear.

Abrasive wear (Figure 25.3)

Two-body abrasive wear occurs when a **soft material** (e.g. UHMWPE) comes into contact with a **significantly harder material** (e.g. metal). Under these circumstances, the microscopic counter-face asperities of the harder material surface may plough into the softer surface, producing grooves. Some of the softer material may be detached to form wear debris. A femoral head has micro-asperities of height 0.1 μm with an Ra value of 0.025 μm.

Third-body abrasive wear (e.g. a stone in one's shoes) occurs when **extraneous material** such as metallic, ceramic (bearing or coating), bone or cement particles, or even products of corrosion, **enter the interfacial region**. Such hard material may become embedded in the polymer and abrade the femoral head. Raised regions on the originally smooth femoral head then abrade the polymer at a much greater rate than the unblemished surface. A single transverse scratch may increase the wear factor by up to ten times. This is worse with a metal head than with a ceramic head, as the latter does not form heaped-up ridges (i.e. ceramic has a better scratch profile).

Abrasive wear can be minimized by manufacturing a hard and smooth femoral head and avoiding extraneous material in the interface.

Adhesive wear (Figure 25.3)

Adhesive wear occurs when a **junction is formed between the two opposing surfaces** as they come into contact. The junction is held by intermolecular bonds between solids, and this force is responsible for friction. If this junction is stronger than the cohesive strength of the individual bearing material surface, then fragments of the weaker material may be torn off and adhere to the stronger material. UHMWPE adheres to metal, especially if dry, leading to shearing of UHMWPE.

Fatigue wear (delamination)

This is a form of failure that occurs in structures subjected to dynamic and fluctuating stresses. In these circumstances, it is possible for failure to occur at a stress considerably lower than the yield strength for a load. An important parameter that characterizes a material's fatigue behaviour is the **fatigue life**. This is the number of cycles needed to cause failure at a specified stress level, as taken from the S–n plot (**Figure 25.4**). The **endurance limit** is defined as the **stress level below which a specimen will withstand cyclic stress indefinitely** without exhibiting fatigue failure. In practice, this limit is usually **arbitrarily set at 10 million cycles**.

Volumetric and linear wear

- **Volumetric** wear is the **volume of material detached from the softer material** as a result of wear and is expressed in mm^3/year.
- **Linear wear** is the **loss of height of the bearing surface** and is expressed in mm/year.

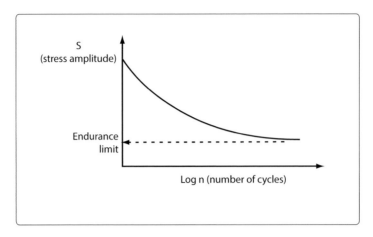

Figure 25.4 S-n curve.

Laws of wear

Volume of material (V) removed by wear increases with load (L) and sliding distance (X) but decreases as the hardness of the softer material (H) increases:

$V \propto LX/H$

$V = k'LX/3H$

$V = kLX$

Where k' is a dimensionless wear coefficient and k is the wear factor for a given combination of materials that incorporates the hardness of the softer material.

Thus, the **wear volume is greater in larger femoral heads because of the increased sliding distance**. Wear volume is also dependent on the type of articulation used.

Measurement in vitro

Volumetric wear can be measured *in vitro* using simple reciprocating pin-on-plate, rotating pin-on-disc apparatus or more complex joint simulators. Joint simulators aim to mimic the loading conditions *in vivo* by applying load cycles at 4 Hz, but often with no rest periods. The lubricant and temperature can be adjusted, and wear is measured by loss of weight of softer implant or volume of released particles. However, simulators tend to underestimate wear when compared with wear rates *in vivo*. It takes 60 days to apply 10 million cycles, with each 1 million cycles being equivalent to approximately 1 year of clinical use.

Measurement in vivo

Cup penetration is commonly measured *in vivo* by comparison between initial and follow-up radiographs, corrected for magnification, e.g. medial migration of polyethylene hip sockets in millimetres per year. A shadowgraph technique or coordinate machine can be utilized to measure this. Radiographs using the uni-radiographic method or the duo-radiographic method can also measure wear.

Volumetric wear can also be measured by direct examination of explanted cups. Gravimetric methods have been used, whereby the explants are weighed; however, UHMWPE may absorb water, making it heavier, and therefore controls are required.

Consequences of wear and wear particles

Consequences of wear particles:

- Synovitis.
- Aseptic osteolysis and loosening.
- Systemic distribution.
- Immune reaction.
- Increased friction of the joint.
- Misalignment of the joint and catastrophic failure.

Osteolysis and aseptic loosening are the most frequently recognized long-term complications of total joint arthroplasty. Both are the direct result of wear debris. Assuming the volume of wear debris is constant, then the **number of wear particles is inversely proportional to their size**. These particles exert their biological activity after phagocytosis by **macrophages** (as the particles are similar in size to bacteria), by stimulating the release of soluble pro-inflammatory mediators. Particles in the size range 0.1–10 µm are biologically active, with those in the size range 0.1–0.5 µm being the most potent. Mediators released near to bone stimulate bone resorption by osteoclasts leading to osteolysis, aseptic loosening and ultimate failure of the prosthesis. Macrophages are also thought to contribute directly to this process by the release of oxide radicals and hydrogen peroxide (**Figure 25.5**).

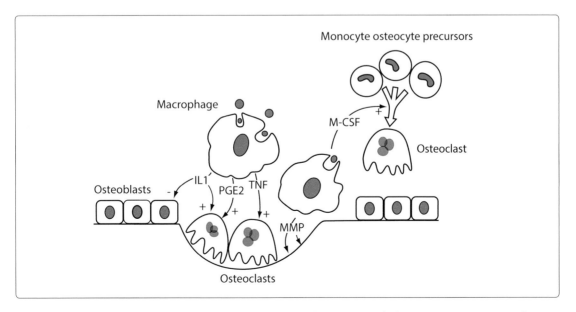

Figure 25.5 Cascade of cells and mediators involved in osteolysis. IL1: interleukin 1; M-CSF: monocyte colony-stimulating factors; MMP: matrix metalloprotinase; PGE2: prostaglandin E2; TNF: tumour necrosis factor-alpha.

Important mediators in this process may **stimulate osteoclasts** (interleukin 1 [IL-1], interleukin 6 [IL-6], tumour necrosis factor-alpha [TNF-α], prostaglandin E2 [PGE2], transforming growth factor-beta [TGF-β]) or **osteoclast precursors** (monocyte colony-stimulating factors [M-CSF] and granulocyte colony-stimulating factors [G-CSF]), **inhibit osteoblast function** (IL-1) or **directly expose bone** (metalloproteinases such as collagenase).

Several studies have suggested a critical wear volume related to osteolysis; for example, volumetric wear rates above 140 mm³/year are associated with significant osteolysis around acetabular cups. However, the severity of the osteolytic reaction may also depend on the size of the particles, their shapes and their surface areas.

The major factors that affect the extent of macrophage activation by the wear particles and thus the extent of osteolysis are:

- Volume of wear debris.
- Total number of wear particles.
- Size of particles.
- Morphology of particles (irregular shapes are more active than spheres).
- Immune response to the particles.

Wear particles are constantly produced in enormous numbers from prosthetic bearings, with a rough estimate for a 22.225 mm head being an average number of 38,000 submicron particles per step.

Locally, at the bone surface, osteolysis is self sustaining, setting up a vicious cycle: as bone resorption and prosthetic loosening progress, abrasion and fretting at the interface may produce an increased amount of particulate debris.

Systemically, wear particles, both metallic and UHMWPE, are commonly transported to the liver, spleen or abdominal lymph nodes in patients with joint replacements. Wear particles are more prevalent in the liver and spleen in patients with revision implants, implying that these organs are involved only when large amounts of wear debris are generated from mechanical failure. Usually no toxic effects are apparent from these wear particles, although rarely granulomas form in remote organs in response to heavy particulate load.

Biotribological considerations of different bearing surfaces

Metal-on-UHMWPE

The bearing surface of Charnley's original low friction arthroplasty (LFA) introduced in 1958 was stainless steel on Teflon™. Although this bearing had a very low coefficient of friction, Teflon™ had desperately poor wear characteristics and its use was abandoned in 1961. The following year, UHMWPE was introduced. UHMWPE has a slightly higher coefficient of friction than Teflon™ but much better resistance to wear. Thus, this highly successful bearing combination has become the gold standard against which other bearing combinations are compared.

The fundamental limitation of UHMWPE is **wear resistance**. A large number of factors affect the wear rate of polyethylene. These factors can be thought of as a result of manufacturing techniques, sterilization methods and shelf-life factors.

Manufacturing techniques

UHMWPE can be produced by: 1) ram bar extrusion with secondary machining; 2) compression moulding into bars with secondary machining; 3) hot isostatic pressing (HIPing) into bars with secondary machining; or 4) direct compression moulding into the shape of the desired product. Of these techniques, direct compression moulding produces UHMWPE with the best wear profile.

Sterilization methods

Sterilization methods can be divided into **non-energetic** (no radiation) and **energetic** (using radiation) methods. **Non-energetic methods** use **ethylene oxide or gas plasma** to sterilize the polyethylene (PE). Conversely, **energetic techniques** utilize **gamma irradiation** at either low or high doses. Non-energetic methods have no effect upon the cross-linking of PE. Conversely, irradiation of UHMWPE causes PE chain scission and then cross-linking of the chains. Cross-linking the UHMWPE has advantageous effects in improving the adhesive and abrasive wear resistance. The disadvantages of cross-linking are decreased tensile strength, fatigue strength, fracture toughness and increased brittleness. These factors might be particularly relevant if the polyethylene is edge loaded, e.g. in an open acetabular cup.

Irradiation should be carried out in an oxygen-free environment, such as in a vacuum or in an environment with an inert gas (such as argon); irradiation in the presence of oxygen generates free radicals that promote oxidation of the PE. This in turn leads to accelerated wear rates and PE failure.

Polyethylene may undergo secondary processing with heat annealing. In this process, the irradiated PE is heated close to its melting point. The process helps to remove the free radicals.

Shelf-life factors

Ideally storage of PE is conducted in an oxygen-free environment. If oxygen is present in the surrounding atmosphere then it can diffuse into the PE. The oxygen in turn promotes oxidation of the PE. The degree of on-shelf oxidation that occurs is dependent upon the prior level of irradiation during sterilization or manufacture, with greater radiation exposure leading to increased levels of free radicals within the PE, whether the irradiation was conducted in an oxygen-free environment, the use of secondary processing and whether the PE has been stored in an oxygen-free or -rich environment. Maximum oxidation occurs 1–2 mm below the surface, the so-called **subsurface white band**, the thickness of which increases with time.

Interestingly, cross-linked PE releases a relatively high number of **submicrometre**- and **nanometre**-sized PE particles and relatively fewer particles that are several micrometres in dimension; these submicron particles appear to have more functional biological activity in *in vitro* studies.

Therefore, the type of preparation that leads to the least amount of osteolysis is yet to be determined. The response is also dependent on the shape of the particles and on the total volumetric wear. There are many variables and all of these need to be borne out in clinical studies. Although short-term studies for cross-linked UHMWPE seem encouraging, longer follow-up is required.

Factors affecting metal/UHMWPE wear in total hip replacement

Penetration of a femoral head into an acetabular cup is a combination of **creep** and **wear**. Creep is a viscoelastic property and is defined as time-dependent irreversible plastic deformation in response to a constant load. The amount of creep depends on the applied load and is unaffected by sliding movements between surfaces. Creep usually dominates the initial penetration rate, which hip simulator studies have shown to be of the order of 0.1 mm for the first 1 million loading cycles. This equates to about 1 year of clinical use.

The **direction of creep is superomedial**, as this is the direction of the compressive joint contact force in the hip, whereas the **direction of wear is superolateral**, as this is perpendicular to the instantaneous axis of rotation.

Wear of the original polished surface of the joint replacement may lead to an increased Ra and increased friction between the joint surfaces. High wear and penetration rates of UHMWPE in acetabular components lead to impingement, which leads to wear from the site of impingement, loosening, loss of movement and dislocation.

Factors that determine wear:

- **Patient factors**:
  - weight (applied load);
  - age and activity level (applied rate of load and number of cycles over time).
- **Implant factors**:
  - *choice of material:*
    - coefficient of friction of materials;
    - roughness (surface finish);
    - toughness (abrasive wear);
    - hardness (scratch resistance, adhesive wear).
  - *type of metal:*
    - cobalt-chrome has excellent properties, particularly if cold worked, because it is hard, resistant to corrosion and resistant to fatigue;
    - stainless steel is cheaper but easily scratched;
    - titanium alloys have poor wear characteristics and a high coefficient of friction compared with cobalt-chrome. They are also sensitive to surface flaws and scratching. Although their use as a bearing surface has been abandoned, they are commonly used for femoral components, particularly uncemented, and almost always for tibial trays of fixed-bearing TKRs.
  - *UHMWPE:*
    - production: ram extrusion produces linear wear of about 0.11 mm/year and compression moulding of about 0.05 mm/year;

- gamma sterilization in air: oxidation of UHMWPE leads to increased crystallinity and reduction in fatigue strength;
- thickness: should be at least 8 mm, as contact stress, wear and amount of creep increase dramatically when thickness of PE falls below this level. Adequate UHMWPE thickness can be obtained with a 40 mm cup only by downsizing the femoral head to 22 mm.

Head size:
- the larger the head size, the greater the sliding distance and volumetric wear;
- from the tunnelling expression, volume of wear debris = $\pi r2P$, where P is the penetration and r is the radius of the femoral head. $P \propto 1/r2$, and therefore the larger the femoral head diameter, the lower the penetration.

Modularity:
- modularity is attractive because it allows screw fixation, liner exchange and the use of extended lip liners ('dial-a-prayer');
- there is increased wear in both cemented and uncemented metal-backed cups due to reduced UHMWPE thickness and increased peak stresses, particularly in the presence of incongruency and gaps between liner and metal backing;
- backside wear occurs from relative movement between liner and shell, and is worse if there is a poor locking mechanism or screw holes with sharp unpolished margins. Settling of the cup may lead to increased prominence of screws. UHMWPE may creep through holes, which provide a conduit for wear particles.

- Decreased offset of prosthesis:
  - due to increased joint reaction forces.
- *Miscellaneous factors:*
  - surface roughness:
    - damaged femoral heads have higher volumetric wear rates, higher total penetration and higher total number of particles produced over the prosthesis lifetime;
    - damaged heads generate increased numbers of small, more biologically active particles ($< 10\ \mu m$).
  - third-body wear.

Additional factors affecting metal/UHMWPE wear in TKR

Design considerations in TKR

Compared with THR, the tibiofemoral articulation of total condylar knee replacements is non-conforming. The design of fixed-bearing TKR is a compromise between reproduction of the normal knee kinematics and the reduction of contact stresses. **Unconstrained posterior cruciate ligament (PCL)-retaining round-on-flat tibial inserts** produce high contact stresses but allow rotation and femoral rollback without excessive PCL tension. This non-conformity creates areas of high contact stress within the UHMWPE that is design-specific. **Conforming PCL-sacrificing round-on-round designs** with concavity in both sagittal and coronal planes ('double-dishing') reduces contact stress but with the penalty of reduced rotation. This in turn increases the shear stress at the bone–implant interface.

The relative lack of conformity in all TKR with the associated increased stress on the PE means that fatigue wear, rather than abrasive or adhesive wear, is a major problem in TKR.

The repeated loading of the PE in the TKR causes subsurface fatigue failure of the UHMWPE at a depth of a few millimetres, at the area of maximum principal stress. Subsequently, cracks appear in the PE when the endurance limit is exceeded.

After the PE has started to crack, a surface layer of UHMWPE breaks off, producing large particles. UHMWPE has macro-asperities two orders of magnitude greater (height 1–10 μm) than the micro-asperities of metal surfaces. These macro-asperities are plastically deformed by loading and upon contact with the PE underneath, produce local contact stress concentrations above the yield stress of the UHMWPE. Subsequently the PE undergoes failure by plastic deformation and rupture. This process is known as **micro-delamination**.

Contact stresses have been shown to increase markedly if the thickness of the UHMWPE falls below 8 mm. Maximum stresses on the tibial tray is four times body weight at 15° flexion, which exceeds the uni-axial yield strength of UHMWPE of many knee replacements.

Hence a number of factors can exacerbate the fatigue wear:

- A subsurface layer of oxidation.
- Subsurface faults.
- Misaligned or unbalanced implants.
- Thin UHMWPE.

A **mobile bearing** solves the kinematic conflict by allowing a highly conforming articular surface to exist with free rotation. By eliminating the need for rotation at the femorotibial articulation and allowing rotation of the tibial PE–tibial tray interface, the contact area of the articular surface can be greatly increased, thereby reducing contact stress and wear.

Metal-backed modular tibial components were developed to provide more secure fixation, improve load transmission and decrease UHMWPE creep, but at the expense of possible undersurface wear. One method of reducing undersurface wear is by use of a more conforming implant, particularly with a highly polished cobalt-chrome base plate. However, there are insurmountable difficulties in the manufacture of polished cobalt-chrome base plates with a suitable locking mechanism for modular fixed-bearing implants. Hence, they are machined from titanium alloy, with inferior wear properties. Despite these theoretical advantages, no study has shown that mobile-bearing TKRs provide improved functional performance, greater activity in younger patients, lower revision rates for mechanical failure or lower wear rates.

Alternative bearing surfaces for THR

Ceramic-on-UHMWPE

Alumina ceramic has superior wear characteristics over metal. It is one of the hardest materials known (after diamond and carborundum), which therefore makes it resistant to scratching. It can be machined to a **smoother** surface than metal and it is **wettable**, which could explain its excellent friction characteristics under load. These characteristics can be used to explain the reduction in linear wear seen in the combination of a 22.225mm alumina ceramic head and cross-linked UHMWPE. After bedding in, the linear wear has been reported for the ceramic-on-UHMWPE as 0.022 mm/year, compared with 0.07 mm/year with standard metal-on -UHMWPE.

However, despite these tribological advantages, the ceramic-on-UHMWPE bearing still produces UHMWPE debris and has not consistently shown lower rates of osteolysis. In addition, the use of ceramic is limited by **expense** and the risk of **head fracture** (0.004% incidence with modern alumina ceramics). Head fractures are associated with small head diameters, large grain size of the alumina and suboptimal fitting of the Morse taper, although modern manufacturing has largely overcome these problems.

Ceramic-on-ceramic

First-generation ceramic-on-ceramic bearings experienced high loosening and fracture rates due to poor-quality ceramic, design faults and cemented all-ceramic acetabular components. Since the 1980s however, ceramics have gained higher purity, finer grain structure and improved mechanical properties. Ceramics are very **strong, stiff, biocompatible and bioinert and do not corrode**. They can be manufactured to a very smooth surface finish and are very **hard** (**scratch resistant**). They also have high **wettability** compared with metals and PE. Wettability describes the relative affinity of a lubricant for another material. It can be measured by the angle of contact at the edge of a drop of lubricant applied to the surface of the material (**Figure 25.5**). Ceramic surfaces show a greater degree of wettability than metals; as ceramics are more hydrophilic, they have improved lubrication and lower friction. Ceramics therefore exhibit very **low friction** and **wear**, with linear wear rates being a fraction of standard metal-on-PE (linear wear rates 0.025 μm/year). Particulate debris from well-functioning articulations is difficult to quantify, but *in vitro* studies quantify it to the order of 10 nm. Damaged bearings on the other hand release particles that are in the submicron to micron range, similar to UHMWPE, which can stimulate the inflammatory cascade. However, osteolysis is rare with ceramic-on-ceramic bearings. Ironically, although linear wear rates are very low and the size of the particulate debris is very small, the absolute number of particles shed greater than for hard-on-soft bearings.

Excellent long-term results have been demonstrated in clinical practice. However, ceramics are susceptible to **abrasive wear** and **edge-loading**, particularly if the acetabular cup is placed too open. They are also subject to **brittle fracture**, leading to catastrophic failure, although this is a very rare occurrence with modern alumina ceramics.

Three types of ceramic are utilized in joint arthroplasty: zirconia, alumina, and Oxinium™.

Zirconia is no longer used for the manufacture of femoral heads. Although it has high fracture toughness, it can undergo phase transformation at high temperatures and in wet environments, which substantially weakens the material and roughens the surface, degrading its wear properties. Zirconia is also very costly and is not licensed for use as a bearing surface with zirconia or alumina and therefore must be used with PE. In 2001, zirconia femoral heads were recalled from circulation by the Medical Devices Agency (the regulatory agency in the UK for medicines and healthcare products) because of an observed high rate of fracture.

In contrast with zirconia, **alumina ceramic** is increasing in popularity. Its quality has improved tremendously with reduction of grain size and diminished number and size of inclusions. This has been achieved with the aid of the 'HIPping' process, which has led to a denser, finer grain size in the alumina. In addition, the tapers for both the femoral head and the socket are much better designed in order to accept ceramic bearings. The advantages of a durable ceramic-on-ceramic bearing now outweigh the disadvantage of minimal fracture risk. However, care should be taken when handling this material. Trial reductions with the ceramic liner *in situ* should be avoided, and there should be no debris or protruding screw heads in the bearing/Morse taper interface. The ceramic bearings should not be struck with a hammer, and careful templating and cup positioning are required due to the reduced liner lip and neck length options.

Oxidized zirconium (OxZr, Oxinium™) was introduced in 2003 as a bearing surface for total hip arthroplasty. This is a metallic alloy with a ceramic surface. Zirconium alloy is heated in air and oxygen diffuses into the alloy and transforms the surface into ceramic, i.e. the surface is not coated. The oxidized surface reaches a depth of 5 μm, with an oxygen enriched transition layer below. Oxidized zirconium provides superior resistance to abrasion without the risk of brittle fracture, thereby combining the benefits of metals and ceramics. Cross-sectional profiles indicate a uniformly hard ceramic layer on the surface, with a gradual decrease in hardness with increasing distance from the ceramic oxide layer. This minimizes abrasive scratching. Oxidized zirconium can be used in patients with metal sensitivity, as it has undetectable levels of nickel. Knee simulator tests have shown that use of oxidized zirconium can reduce UHMWPE wear substantially.

When revising fractured ceramic femoral heads, total synovectomy, cup exchange and insertion of a cobalt-chrome or new ceramic femoral head minimizes the chance of early loosening of the implants and the need for one or more repeat revisions. The fragments of ceramic are difficult to remove from the tissues and are a major source of third-body wear to subsequent articulations. Total synovectomy is required in order to remove as much debris as possible. Damage to the Morse taper leads to increased fracture risk of an exchanged ceramic head and may be an indication for revision of a well-fixed femoral component.

Metal -on-metal

Early cemented THRs, such as the McKee–Farrar and Ring devices, featured cobalt-chrome alloy bearings. The first generation of implants had a high failure rate because high frictional torque was transmitted to the cement-bone interface, leading to loosening. In addition, there was high wear because of the thin acetabular shells and a small clearance between the socket and the ball. These early bearings were often **equatorial bearing** and could even squeak or jam (**clutch coning**). Engineering advances have allowed the manufacture of consistently **mid-polar bearing** articulations with reduction of the frictional torque. Mathematical models have shown that the ideal radial clearance between the head and the cup to reduce friction and wear should be 90–200 μm. In addition, it is hypothesized that fluid-film lubrication can exist in current surface replacements.

Metals have **good fracture toughness** and so **resist abrasive wear** well, but in order to overcome the adhesive wear the hardness must be increased. This can be achieved by using alloys such as **cobalt–chrome–molybdenum** (CoCrMo) with **high carbide** content. Carbide particles can occupy up to 5% of the surface and have been shown to increase the surface hardness by 10–20%. This reduces the wear rates to approximately 5 μm/year after the first 6 months, when the rate is approximately 10 μm/year. The metal-on-metal articulation also exhibits the ability to **self-heal**, i.e. to polish out isolated surface scratches caused by third-body particles.

However, they seem to exhibit 10–20 times greater wear-in during the initial 1–2 years, but this subsequently reaches a plateau.

The **metal wear particles** are small (50–500 nm) in comparison with those that activate macrophages (0.5–1 µm) and so do not excite such an inflammatory response. Although they are small, more particles (8×10^{12} particles/year) are produced than with UHMWPE (0.4×10^{12} particles/year). Despite this, osteolysis is rarely seen in metal-on-metal articulations. It may be that these particles are transported away from the joint capsule, and therefore this raises concerns about the observed systemic levels of **metal ions** in the body; it has been postulated that these ions may be **toxic or carcinogenic**. It is generally agreed that the levels of cobalt and chromium ions are higher in the blood and urine from patients with metal-on-metal implants than from patients without implants. Carcinomas associated with cobalt and chromium implants have been reported in some animal implantation models but, to date, epidemiological studies of patients with joint replacements have not shown a higher incidence of cancer with metal-on-metal prostheses. However, long-term data are awaited, and caution must be exercised in young and/or pregnant individuals.

Metal sensitivity is another issue, and its association with prosthetic failure is still debated. Current dermatological preoperative screening is not recommended for fear of sensitization of the individual.

Metal-on-metal articulations can be used with conventional THR or as a resurfacing implant. The Metasul™ (Zimmer, Warsaw, IN, USA) bearing system, in which the metal acetabular bearing is embedded in a PE liner, has shown good results. Wear studies have shown that there is a bedding-in period for the first 2 years when the linear wear is 10–20 µm, largely due to third-body abrasion from particles generated as scratches from the original polishing are eradicated and/or from dislodged surface carbides. The main contact zones are eventually worn smoother than the original surfaces, indicating a self-healing or self-polishing effect. This produces a reduction in wear rate, which falls to about 5 µm per year after the third year. This compares with linear wear rates of around 200 µm for metal-on-UHMWPE and 20–100 µm for ceramic-on-UHMWPE.

However, more recently, grave concerns have been raised regarding the use of metal-on-metal articulations in multiple publications. The major concerns are regarding the release of metal ions and with the discovery of aseptic lymphocyte vasculitis-associated lesions (ALVAL) in some patients with metal on metal articulation. ALVAL has been particularly associated with some hip resurfacing devices, which led to the recall of the ASR™ XL Acetabular System and DePuy ASR™ Hip Resurfacing System after data from the UK National Joint Registry indicated a high revision rate. Various associated factors have been implicated including prosthesis design, implant positioning, patient body mass index (BMI) and gender, and metallurgy. These concerns have led many surgeons to abandon metal-on-metal articulations in hip arthroplasty.

A comparison of wear rates for alternative bearing articulations is shown in *Table 25.4* and their advantages and disadvantages are summarized in *Table 25.5*. The ultimate goal is to eradicate wear from arthroplasties, for which several strategies can be employed (*Table 25.6*).

Table 25.4 Wear rates in different articulations with a 28 mm head

	Metal-on-UHMWPE	Ceramic-on-UHMWPE	Metal-on-metal	Ceramic-on-ceramic
Linear wear μm/year	150–200	75–100	5–10	Negligible
Volumetric wear mm³/year	40–80	15–20	0.1–1.0	0.004
Particle numbers	7×10^{11}	–	$4 \times 10^{12} – 2.5 \times 10^{14}$	No reports
Particle size μm	0.5–100	0.5–100	0.05–0.5	0.025

UHMWPE: ultra-high-molecular weight polyethylene.

Table 25.5 Advantages and disadvantages of alternative bearing surfaces

Bearing surface	Advantages	Disadvantages
Ceramic-on-ceramic	Low wear Biocompatible	Risk of head fracture Abrasive wear Edge loading
Metal-on-metal	Good long-term clinical results Ability to self-polish	Undetermined effect of elevated ions Undetermined cancer risk Potential metal hypersensitivity
Cross-linked UHMWPE	Reduced wear	Particles more biologically active Excess cross-linking can lead to reduced mechanical properties Short-term clinical results

UHMWPE: ultra-high-molecular weight polyethylene.

Table 25.6 Strategies to reduce wear

1) Improve the bearing surface	
a) Improved UHMWPEs	
b) Metal-on-metal	
c) Ceramic-on-UHMWPE	
d) Ceramic-on-ceramic	
2) Improved fixation	
a) Prevention of wear particle migration along the interface	
b) Seal the interface	
3) Prevent osteolysis	
a) Bisphosphonates	
b) Tissue inhibitors of matrix metalloproteinases (TIMPs)	

Corrosion

Corrosion is defined as the **unwanted dissolution of a metal in a solution**, resulting in its continued degradation. Electrochemical deterioration of a metal happens when an oxidation reaction occurs at an **anode** with a loss of electrons to produce a positively charged metal ion. These ejected electrons must be transferred to another chemical species (**cathode**) and form the reduction reaction.

In situ degradation of metal alloy implants is undesirable for two reasons:

- The degradation process may decrease the structural integrity of the implant.
- The release of degradation products may elicit an adverse biological reaction in the host.

Degradation may result from either **electrochemical dissolution** phenomena or **wear**, or a **synergistic combination** of the two. Electrochemical processes may include generalized corrosion, uniformly affecting the entire surface of the implant, and localized corrosion, affecting either seemingly random sites on the surface (**pitting corrosion**) or regions of the device that are shielded from the tissue fluids (**crevice corrosion**). Electrochemical and mechanical processes (e.g. **stress corrosion cracking, corrosion fatigue, fretting corrosion**) may interact, causing premature structural failure and accelerated release of metal particles and ions.

The most commonly used metals for implants are titanium, cobalt-chrome and stainless steel alloys. These are normally considered to be highly corrosion-resistant due to the formation of a thin passive oxide film that spontaneously forms on their surface and serves as a protective barrier to further corrosion (**passivation**). If damaged, the protective film normally reforms very rapidly. However, a change in the character of the environment may cause a passivated material to revert to an active state with a substantial increase in corrosion rates.

Generalized corrosion

Galvanic corrosion

This form of corrosion occurs when two **dissimilar metals** are **electrically coupled** together. Metals are considered to be dissimilar in this instance if their surface potential is different. The difference in potential causes electron flow between the two metals. The greater the difference in potential, the more driving force exists for this to occur. The electrochemical series can be used to predict galvanic relationships and determine unsuitable combinations. The more active alloy will become anodic and, thus, the more noble metal will be cathodic. If corrosion occurs in this situation, it will be accelerated on the more active metal, causing greater damage.

Localized corrosion

Pitting corrosion

Pitting is a form of **localized corrosion** attack in which small pits or holes form. The pits ordinarily penetrate from the top of a horizontal surface downwards in a near-vertical direction. This is an extremely insidious type of corrosion, often going undetected and with very little material loss until failure occurs. Pitting results in damage to the implant with a substantial amount of metal ion release. Pits can form at various points that are exposed to a solution containing aggressive species, and these can result from breaks in the protective film, defects in the metal/protective film or voids in the alloy or metal. Pitting can occur particularly if the solution has a low pH and contains chloride ions. Human body fluids contain approximately 0.9% sodium chloride, and so pitting can occur on metal implants. The early stage of pit formation is sudden and is accompanied by a very high current. Once initiated, the pits are self-sustaining and thus may continue to grow. Dissolution occurs within the pit, and oxygen reduction takes place on the adjacent surfaces.

Electrons flowing between the two sites can be seen. The anode of the cell is the small area of active metal, and the cathode is the large passive surface of the remaining metal. There is a large potential difference in this cell, which causes a high flow of current and rapid corrosion.

Crevice corrosion

This is caused by the formation of a **cavity or crevice** where **exchange in material** with the surrounding bulk solution is limited. This results in a change in the chemical composition of the solution within the crevice, which demonstrates a decrease in the species required for oxygen reduction, a build-up of aggressive species and an associated decrease in pH. Tighter crevices reduce the amount of electrolyte that must be deoxygenated and acidified and will thus cause more rapid attack. High concentrations of H^+ and Cl^- ions have been found in crevices, which can be particularly damaging to the passive films on metal implants.

After oxygen becomes depleted within the crevice, the metal is oxidized and the electrons migrate to areas outside the crevice, where they are consumed in the reduction reaction. As the corrosion in the crevices increases, the rest of the surface becomes cathodically protected, and corrosion is localized.

Fretting corrosion

This is a **synergistic combination** of **wear** and **crevice corrosion** of two materials in contact. It results from micro-motion between the two, which disrupts the protective film of a metal. The movement required for disruption of the passive layer can be as little as 3–4 nm and is dependent on the contact load and frequency of movement. This can cause permanent damage to the oxide layer, and particles of metal and oxide can be released into the body from fretting. For example, if the passive oxide film on CoCrMo is fractured, exposing the base alloy to an aqueous solution, then the following reactions of chromium (Cr) may occur with similar reactions involving cobalt (Co) and molybdenum (Mo):

$Cr \rightarrow Cr^{3+} + 3e^-$ (dissolution)

$2Cr + 3/2O_2 \rightarrow Cr_2O_3$ (repassivation)

$2Cr + 3H_2O \rightarrow Cr_2O_3 + 6e^-$ (repassivation)

The Cr in the alloy oxidizes into ionic form (**dissolution**) or reacts with oxygen to reform the oxide film (**repassivation**).

Stress corrosion (fatigue)

Metals that are repeatedly deformed and stressed in a corrosive environment show **accelerated corrosion** and **fatigue damage**. A metal implant would be subject to repeated mechanical loads of up to 3×10^6/year, and implants at the lower extremities must support three or four times the body weight. Furthermore, the chemically aggressive environment of the human body makes testing simulating the physiological environment very important.

Intergranular corrosion

Metals have a granular structure, with **grain** being the term for areas of continuous structure and the **grain boundary** being the disordered areas between grains. The grain is anodic and susceptible, whereas the grain boundary is cathodic and immune. Alloys are infinitely more susceptible to intergranular corrosion than are pure metals.

Intragranular (leaching) corrosion

This occurs due to electrochemical differences within grains.

Inclusion corrosion

This occurs due to the inclusion of **impurities**, **cold welding** or **metal transfer**, e.g. metal fragments from a screwdriver.

Practical examples of corrosion in orthopaedics

- Stainless-steel wire in contact with cobalt-chrome or titanium alloy stem.
- Stainless-steel head in contact with titanium alloy stem.
- Titanium alloy screw in contact with stainless-steel plate.

In the absence of relative motion, galvanic coupling of cobalt-chrome with titanium alloy is stable. However, combination of stainless steel with either cobalt-chrome or titanium alloy is unstable, with the steel being susceptible to attack. Couples of similar metals are also stable. In the presence of motion, accelerated corrosion may occur, even when similar metals are used, with its extent depending on the type of fretting motion, the chemistry of the local solution and the micro-structure of the metals.

Conclusion

This chapter provides the basic concepts and principles of friction, lubrication, wear and corrosion in orthopaedic surgery. The understanding of the basic science of natural and artificial joints is crucial to improving survivorship of implants used in the orthopaedic industry.

Viva questions

1. What do you know about synovial fluid?

2. What are the mechanisms of component wear? How can wear be prevented?

3. What is corrosion? What are the different types?

4. What are the methods of lubrication in synovial and artificial joints?

5. What is the pathological basis for osteolysis ?

Further reading

Archibeck MJ, Jacobs JJ, Black J. Alternate bearing surfaces in total joint arthroplasty: biologic considerations. *Clin Orthop* 2000;**379**:12–21.

Campbell P, Shen FW, McKellop H. Biologic and tribologic considerations of alternative bearing surfaces. *Clin Orthop* 2004;**418**:98–111.

Hall RM, Bankes MJ, Blunn G. Biotribology for joint replacement. *Curr Orthopaed* 2001;**15**:281–90.

Heisel C, Silva M, Schmalzried TP. Bearing surface options for total hip replacement in young patients. *J Bone Joint Surg Am* 2004;**85**:1366–79.

Jacobs JJ, Gilbert JL, Urban RM. Corrosion of metal orthopaedic implants. *J Bone Joint Surg Am* 1998;**80**:268–82.

26 Gait

Pramod Achan, Mark Paterson and Fergal Monsell

Introduction

Human gait is the pattern of movement of the body when involved in bipedal locomotion. This pattern can vary in a normal or physiological manner, depending on conditions such as age or speed. It may also vary as a consequence of pathological conditions such as stroke or osteoarthritis.

In order to appreciate the abnormal gait associated with disease or trauma, it is essential to have a basic understanding of normal human gait. This chapter describes the features of normal gait and the means by which it is evaluated, before discussing some of the abnormal patterns which characterize certain disorders.

Normal gait

The development of bipedal gait may have allowed humans to use their upper limbs, but it creates problems of stability. The centre of mass in the upright adult lies in front of the S2 vertebra, and must remain over the support base if a person is to stay upright. Normal gait is the result of a complex series of muscle actions that produce efficient forward movement of the body without sacrificing stability.

Gait is defined in terms of the **gait cycle**. A single gait cycle encompasses **all the events between the first contact with the ground of one foot (initial contact) and the next time the same foot contacts the ground**. **Figure 26.1** shows the key events and their approximate relative duration.

Certain concepts need to be understood before the events of the gait cycle can be fully appreciated:

- Muscle contraction may be **concentric, eccentric or isometric**. When a muscle contracts concentrically, the muscle–tendon unit shortens and kinetic energy is released. When contracting eccentrically the overall unit lengthens and energy is stored.
- The **moment** about a joint is a measure of the turning effect produced by a force about the joint. The magnitude of the moment is the product of the force and the perpendicular distance from the centre of rotation of the joint axis to the line of action of the force.

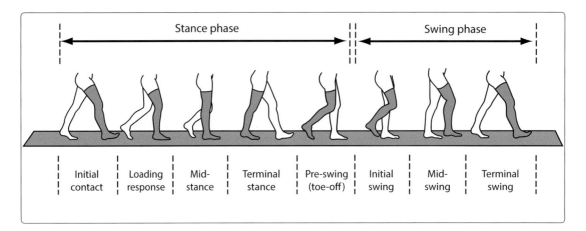

Figure 26.1 The gait cycle.

- The **ground reaction force** (GRF) is defined as the reaction to the force that the body exerts on the ground. It combines gravity's effect on the body and the effects of the body's movement and acceleration (**Figure 26.2a**). The position of the GRF in relation to each lower limb joint at any point in the gait cycle determines whether the overall moment at that joint is a flexion or extension moment, and this in turn will dictate which muscles will need to act, and in what manner, to maintain stability. The GRF is key to determining the forces required to make forward progress whilst at the same time maintaining stability.

With these basic concepts in mind, we can now look at the sequence of normal gait in more detail.

The gait cycle comprises a **stance phase** and a **swing phase**. The **stance phase starts on initial contact and ends when the last part of the foot leaves the ground. This marks the start of the swing phase, which continues until the next initial contact.** In normal walking, **stance** comprises **60%** and **swing 40%** of the cycle. From this, it can be seen that there must be periods when both feet are in contact with the ground; these **double-support** periods occur either side of the swing period and each comprise about **10%** of the cycle. Stance and swing are further divided into subphases, described below.

Stance

- **Initial contact** (IC): this is the point at which the leading foot strikes the ground; in normal gait, this contact is made with the heel. Since the other foot is still on the ground at this time, IC marks the start of the period of double-support. Heel contact means that the GRF will be behind the ankle and knee joints, creating plantarflexion and knee flexion moments, respectively. These are resisted by **controlled eccentric activity of tibialis anterior, toe extensors and the vasti.** Immediately after heel-strike, the dorsiflexors 'pay out' eccentrically to lower the rest of the foot to the ground (**Figure 26.2b, First**).

- **Loading response** (LR): this period starts when the whole foot comes into contact with the ground, and finishes at the end of double-support when the contralateral foot leaves the ground. In this period there is slight flexion of the knee, which is a weight acceptance or shock-absorption mechanism. Perry described IC and LR as the periods of the **first rocker** (**Figure 26.2a**), when the fulcrum and hence the GRF is at the heel; subsequent limb movement brings the GRF progressively further forward in the foot, as described below.
- **Mid-stance** (MS) – **second rocker**: as the body moves forward over the static foot, the lower leg or shank also moves forward so that the ankle is in passive dorsiflexion. The amount of forward movement is restrained by **eccentric contraction of the calf complex or triceps surae, and in particular the soleus component (Figure 26.2b, Second)**. In this, the second rocker, the GRF moves forward in the foot and in front of the knee. There is thus an overall extension moment at the knee, maintaining the joint in extension with minimal muscle activity being required. As the body moves further forward a stabilizing extension moment at the hip also occurs, further reducing the amount of muscle activity required at this energy-conserving stage of gait.

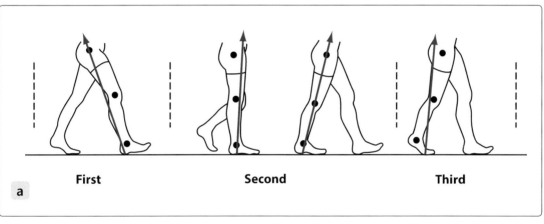

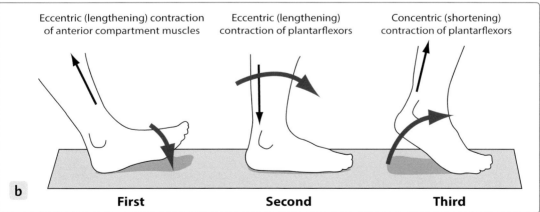

Figure 26.2 a: Gait rockers and the ground reaction force; b: the three ankle rockers.

- **Late or terminal stance** (TS) – **third rocker**: the heel begins to lift under the powerful **concentric contraction of the triceps surae (particularly gastrocnemius)** (**Figure 26.2b**, Third). This is the stage of the third rocker, with the pivot point now moving still further forward to the metatarsal heads. With the hip now extended, the ankle plantarflexes and the knee starts to flex as the GRF passes behind the knee joint (**Figure 26.2a**). The end of terminal stance is signalled by **pre-swing** or toe-off as the limb is thrust forwards into swing phase, the calf contraction coming to an end and being replaced by a short burst of concentric contraction of the hip flexors. This has the effect not only of flexing the hip but also increasing knee flexion by induced acceleration. Thus, the knee flexes rapidly as a combined result of gastrosoleus and hip flexor activity, reaching the 60° of flexion necessary to achieve clearance of the foot in the swing phase. In late pre-swing, the ankle dorsiflexors are activated to prevent the foot dropping into plantarflexion in the swing phase.

Swing

This is conventionally divided into **initial, mid-swing** and **terminal swing** (ISW, MSW and TSW). Throughout much of the swing phase, the limb moves as a pendulum under its own momentum, the hip flexors and ankle dorsiflexors having switched off by the end of initial swing. By terminal swing, the brakes are applied to the pendulum by the isometric activity of the hamstrings, and just prior to IC, the ankle dorsiflexors switch on again to control the foot on its 'landing flare'.

Coronal and transverse plane movement

The above descriptions all apply to sagittal plane movement. It is also necessary to consider how the body moves when viewed from in front or behind, and from above. A key feature of coronal movement in normal gait is the action of the hip abductors on the stance limb to correct the adduction caused by the pelvis falling on the unsupported swing side. In the transverse plane, the pelvis is seen to rotate forwards on the side of the swinging limb while the ipsilateral hip externally rotates to maintain normal foot progression. This strategy not only serves to lengthen the step but also limits the vertical excursion of the pelvis, thereby reducing energy expenditure (see below).

Prerequisites of normal gait

Perry (1985) described **five prerequisites of normal gait**, a concept subsequently popularized by Gage:

1. **Stability in stance: this requires a stable foot position and good control of body segments above the lower limbs whilst still achieving clearance and forward propulsion.**
2. **Adequate foot clearance in swing: this requires appropriate positioning of hip, knee and ankle in the stance limb with adequate flexion at the hip and knee and adequate ankle dorsiflexion in the swing limb.**
3. **Adequate step length: this follows from good balance and stability on the stance side with appropriate flexion on the swing side.**
4. **Appropriate pre-positioning of the foot in terminal swing: this follows from all the above.**

5. **Energy conservation: this is achieved by minimizing vertical excursion of the body during gait and by ensuring that joint stability is achieved wherever possible by the position of the GRF rather than by muscle activity.**

Abnormal gait is characterized by failure to meet one or more of these requirements.

Gait analysis

The assessment of gait and the identification of any deviation from normal is known as gait analysis. In its simplest form, it is a **clinical or observational analysis**, in which a subject's gait is observed in sagittal and coronal planes in a clinic setting. Video recordings make it possible to study the gait pattern more effectively and without tiring the subject.

A more objective method of assessing gait involves **instrumented gait analysis**, which in addition to video recordings in two planes, involves the following evaluations:

- Linear gait parameters.
- Kinematics.
- Kinetics.
- Electromyography (EMG).
- Energy expenditure.
- Pedobarography.

Linear gait parameters:

- **Step length**: distance between point of contact of one foot to the next point of contact of the other foot (metres).
- **Stride length**: distance between point of contact of one foot and the next point of contact of the same foot (i.e. one complete gait cycle) (metres).
- **Cadence**: number of steps per minute.
- **Velocity**: equals step length × cadence (metres/min).
- **Foot progression angle**: angle made between the direction of progression and the long axis of the foot (degrees).

Kinematics: kinematics is the measurement of the movement of the body segments involved in walking. In instrumented analysis, it is usually achieved using infra-red reflective markers with multiple cameras enabling accurate three-dimensional localization of key anatomical landmarks. Data obtained are usually presented in graphical form for sagittal, coronal and transverse motion (**Figure 26.3**).

Kinetics: the measurement of forces, moments, energy and power associated with body movements during gait. In order to determine these, data from a force plate are required in addition to kinematic data.

EMG: in gait analysis, EMG is most useful in determining the timing of individual muscle activity during the gait cycle. Either surface or fine-wire electrodes may be used.

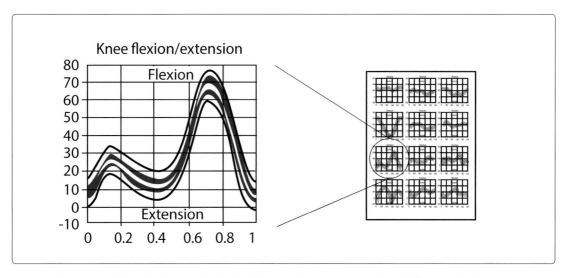

Figure 26.3 Example of normal gait data for knee flexion/extension for children aged 6–9 years.

Energy expenditure: the efficiency of a particular gait pattern in terms of metabolic energy expenditure can be estimated by measuring oxygen consumption at rest and following walking exercise. The physiological cost index is an approximate surrogate estimation of energy expenditure, based on the direct relationship between heart rate (HR) on exercise and oxygen consumption and is expressed by the formula:

$$\text{Physiological cost index} = \frac{\text{HR}_{\text{exercise}} - \text{HR}_{\text{rest}}}{\text{Walking speed.}}$$

Pedobarography: in-shoe or pressure mat systems can measure pressure and foot contact area of the foot in the stance phase.

Development of gait

When a toddler first starts to walk, there is little resemblance to the patterns and pre-requisites described above. The knees move quite stiffly and there is a wide base of support. Sutherland showed that the growing child does not develop the adult type of heel-toe gait until the age of 3.5 years.

Abnormal gait patterns

Trendelenburg gait

During stance phase, abductor muscles that are either weak or effectively de-functioned by hip pain, deformity or displacement allow the pelvis to drop on the contralateral side, seen clearly in the coronal plane. In an attempt to bring the centre of gravity back over the weight-bearing hip, the trunk leans towards the affected side.

Short leg gait

Several possible compensations are available in leg length discrepancy to enable clearance of the longer limb in swing phase. These include:

- **Circumduction** of the longer limb: the hip abducts and the limb swings around outside the normal line of progression, effectively shortening the limb.
- **Hip hitching**: abdominal and paraspinal muscles are activated to hitch the pelvis up on the longer side to gain the same advantage.
- **High stepping**: exaggerated hip and knee flexion increases the clearance of the longer limb in swing.
- **Vaulting**: plantarflexion of the ankle in the shorter limb during stance increases clearance of the longer limb whilst maintaining a level pelvis.

Antalgic gait

This is a gait pattern adopted in an attempt to minimize pain that may be coming from anywhere in that limb. The resulting limp is characterized by a shortened single support period in stance on the affected side, with a shortened swing phase on the contralateral limb, and increased double support times. In the clinic, this asymmetry of gait is frequently identified most easily by listening to the rhythm of the footsteps.

Gait deviations seen in neurological conditions such as cerebral palsy, polio and myelodysplasia are complex and varied, and detailed consideration of these is beyond the scope of this chapter. Key to understanding these abnormalities is the acknowledgement that normal gait requires normal rotational and angular alignment of the lower limb segments or 'levers'. Torsional deformity of the femur or tibia or hip displacement will interfere with the normal hip, knee and ankle kinematics, and planovalgus foot deformity will prevent normal operation of the three rockers. This kind of problem is referred to by gait specialists as '**lever-arm dysfunction**'.

Viva questions

1. What are the pre-requisites of normal gait?
2. During gait, how may a person compensate for a leg length discrepancy?
3. Give examples of eccentric and concentric activity of the gastrocnemius muscle during the gait cycle.
4. What are the three rockers of gait?
5. What are the causes of a positive Trendelenburg gait?

Further reading

Baker R. *Measuring Walking. A Handbook of Clinical Gait Analysis.* MacKeith Press, London, 2013.

Chambers HG, Sutherland DH. A practical guide to gait analysis. *J Am Acad Ortho Surg* 2002;**10**:222–31.

Gage JR, Schwartz MH, Koop SE, Novacheck TF. *The Identification and Treatment of Gait Problems in Cerebral Palsy. Clinics in Developmental Medicine* 180–181. MacKeith Press, London, 2009.

Saunders JBM, Inman VT, Eberhart HD. The major determinants in normal and pathological gait. *J Bone Joint Surg Am* 1953;**35**:558.

Sutherland DH, Olsen R, Cooper L, Woo L. The development of mature gait. *J Bone Joint Surg Am* 1980; **62**:336–53.

27 Prosthetics

Manoj Ramachandran, Imad Sedki, Jo Dartnell and Linda Marks

Introduction

A basic knowledge of the definition, terminology, components of prostheses and complications of amputations is essential for the orthopaedic surgeon. This chapter concerns exoprostheses, e.g. artificial arms and legs, but not endoprostheses, e.g. joint replacements.

A prosthesis is a **device or artificial substitute** designed to **replace**, as much as possible, the **function or appearance** of a missing limb or body part. Prosthetics is defined as the specialty relating to prostheses and their use.

The aim of **prosthetic rehabilitation** is to enable the patient to achieve maximum functional independence with the prosthesis, taking into account the patient's pre-morbid abilities, lifestyle and expectations. Note that this aim is not the same as for amputee rehabilitation, which includes wheelchair mobility for patients who are unable to walk. Many might reconsider using prostheses at a later stage as their needs change. For example, a lady born with a congenital deficiency at the level of proximal radius managed all her life without a prosthesis until she became blind at age 70 years. At this stage, she approached the prosthetic centre asking for a prosthesis that is attached to a cane as a terminal device, to free her remaining hand to carry her shopping.

Successful outcome with prosthetic use is dependent on the following:

- **Patient**:
  - pre-morbid level of activity;
  - level of amputation;
  - ability to learn new skills;
  - pathology in contralateral limb;
  - static and dynamic balance;
  - sufficient trunk control (and upper-limb strength);
  - other comorbidities.

- **Prosthesis**:
  - comfortable to wear;
  - well suspended with minimal pistoning movement;
  - easy to don (put on) and doff (take off);
  - appropriate components;
  - lightweight, durable and reliable;
  - cosmetically pleasing.
- **Teamwork**:
  - appropriate communication between the surgical and rehabilitation team is essential. Typically the team should include a surgeon, a rehabilitation physician, prosthetist, specialist physiotherapist, occupational therapist and psychologist. A pre-amputation assessment with the rehabilitation team is very beneficial when the patient's medical condition allows it, enabling the patient to make a fully informed decision regarding surgery. Post-operatively, prompt therapy is critical for maximizing function and independence and this can start as soon as the patient is medically fit, possibly within the first week. The patient's motivation and participation in the programme are pivotal. Patients are followed up long-term by these centres as adjustments and new prostheses are needed. Patient's rejection of their prosthesis can be as high as 50% for upper limbs and can be minimized by meticulous preparation and support. In congenital deficiencies, rehabilitation starts at the pre-natal stage by providing counselling to the parents;
  - the surgeon should operate with the prosthesis in mind in order to fashion an organ of locomotion and thus create an optimal stump for limb fitting (see below).

Amputations

Upper-extremity amputations are generally more common in the young male population secondary to trauma, while **lower-extremity amputations** are more common in an older population secondary to medical disease (peripheral vascular disease, diabetes, thromboembolism). *Table 27.1* lists the most common indications for amputation. Manually skilled workers are at the highest risk of upper limb amputation, 50% of them occurring whilst

Table 27.1. Upper limb referrals to prosthetic centres

Cause	Number of referrals	Percentage
Trauma	113	37
Congenital absence	92	30
Peripheral vascular disease	23	7
Neoplasia	22	7
Infection	12	4
Other	45	15
All	307	100

(Source: The National Amputee Statistical Database for the United Kingdom 2006/2007).

at work. Early fitting of a prosthesis, within the first 60 days, not only improves function but also improves the likelihood and speed of return to work. Female, older amputees and those not using prostheses are less likely to return.

Obtaining a pain-free limb prior to amputation has been shown to significantly reduce the rate of phantom limb pain, anxiety and improve the rehabilitation potential of the patient. Epidural anaesthesia for at least 24 (ideally 72) hours pre-operatively is shown to reduce phantom pain and anxiety at 6 months but is often not practically feasible.

For **trans-osseous amputations**, the following should be borne in mind in order to create an ideal stump for limb fitting:

- The **scar** should be **well healed and mobile**, away from subcutaneous bony edges and underlying neuromata.
- The **skin** should be as **sensate** as possible and split thickness skin grafts should be avoided.
- The **stump** should have a **cylindrical or conical shape** at closure.
- **Excessive soft tissue** distal to the bone section should be **avoided**.
- **Traumatized tissue** must **not** be retained in the **stump**.
- **Nerves** should be **sectioned cleanly** under gentle tension and allowed to retract into proximal soft tissue to prevent neuroma formation in an inappropriate location.
- All **bone ends** should be **bevelled or contoured**.
- **Myoplastic techniques** (suturing muscles to periosteum) should be attempted with secure multiple sutures, although **myodesis** techniques (direct suture of muscle to bone) may be of use in trans-femoral and trans-humeral amputations. These should be performed with the proximal joint in full extension to avoid creating muscle contractures. A detached myoplasty is a common reason for surgical refashioning of the residium.
- **Non-absorbable sutures** must be avoided.

The **optimum level** for amputation to allow limb fitting must be achieved, a common error being that the stump is left too long. For the four main sites of trans-osseous amputation, the levels are as follows:

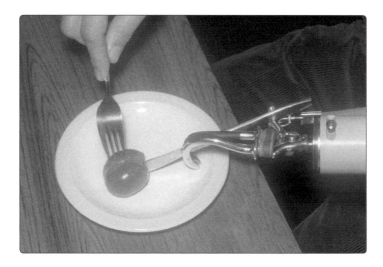

Figure 27.1 Wrist rotary prosthesis.

- **Trans-radial (forearm)**:
  - optimum: junction of proximal two-thirds and distal third of forearm;
  - shortest: 3 cm below insertion of biceps brachii;
  - longest: 5 cm above wrist joint, to allow space for wrist rotary prosthesis (**Figure 27.1**).
- **Trans-humeral (upper arm)**:
  - optimum: middle third of arm;
  - shortest: 4 cm below anterior axillary fold;
  - longest: 10 cm above olecranon, to allow space for elbow mechanism (**Figure 27.2**).
- **Trans-femoral (thigh)**:
  - optimum: middle third of thigh;
  - shortest: 8 cm below pubic ramus;
  - longest: 15 cm above medial knee joint line, irrespective of the patient's height, to allow space for knee mechanism (**Figure 27.3**).
- **Trans-tibial (leg)**:
  - optimum: 8 cm for every 1 m of height;
  - shortest: 7.5 cm measured from the medial knee joint line;
  - longest: level at which a myoplasty can be performed (junction between the Achilles tendon and muscle belly).

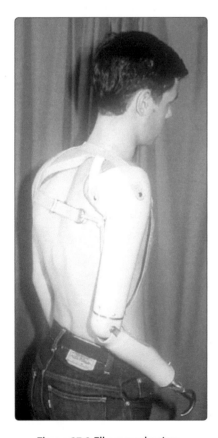

Figure 27.2 Elbow mechanism.

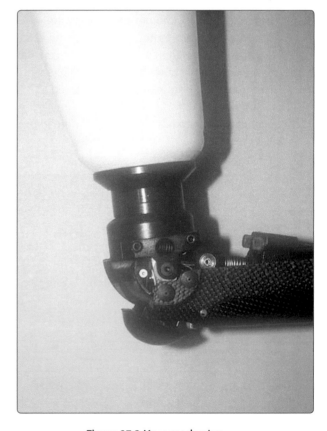

Figure 27.3 Knee mechanism.

For **disarticulation amputations**, the advantages and disadvantages should be considered when fitting prostheses.

Advantages include the following:

- The residual limb retains a distal weight-bearing surface.
- The bulbous shape assists suspension of the prosthesis.
- The proceedure is quicker with less bleeding due to the lack of bone sections, particularly important in medically compromised patients.
- All the muscles controlling the residual limb are retained and balanced.
- Overcomes the problem of bone overgrowth in paediatric patients.

Disadvantages include the following:

- The amputation can compromise the choice and/or fitting of prosthetic components.
- The prosthesis can appear bulky. An exception to this rule is in the case of Symes amputation for congenital absence of the fibula with associated leg shortening. The shortening of the leg allows the bulb of the stump to be masked within the shaping of the external calf prosthesis.

Prostheses

Lower limb prostheses

Lower extremity amputations are more common in an older popluation secondary to medical disease (peripheral vascular disease, diabetes, thromboembolism), representing over 70% of referrals. It is reported that up to 56% of those patients will require a contralateral limb amputation within 3 years with a survival rate of 40% at 5 years. Other reasons include trauma, infection and congenital deficiency, where patients have far greater potentials to achieve higher activity levels. The trans-tibial level is the most common level of amputation and the most proximal level providing near normal function.

Upper limb prostheses

The most common reasons for referrals to prosthetic centres in the UK are traumatic loss or congenital deficiency (*Table 27.1*). Unlike lower limb prostheses where the prosthesis is essential for ambulation, an upper limb prosthesis falls short of replacing the various gross and fine motor functions of the missing limb. Therefore, the prosthesis is usually considered a targeted function prosthesis, or a tool to facilitate a range of functions. Congenital upper limb deficiency patients often abandon prostheses as they are able to perform most activities of daily living one handed.

Classification of prostheses

Prostheses can be classified according to the following:

- **Level of amputation**: e.g. trans-femoral, trans-radial.
- **Structure**: e.g. exoskeletal (where the strength of the prosthesis is in the rigid external structure and all parts are fitted on to or within this structure) or endoskeletal, also known as modular (where the individual components are linked by internal struts and the whole assembly is covered with a soft external cosmesis (**Figure 27.4**).
- **Function**: e.g. cosmetic, functional.

Often a combination of these descriptors is used, e.g. 'cosmetic trans-radial prosthesis', 'exoskeletal trans-tibial prosthesis'.

Common elements of prostheses

All prostheses have some common elements (**Figure 27.5**):

- **Socket/interface:** the connection between the residual limb (known as the residium) and the prosthesis. This protects the residium and transmits the forces necessary for function. The socket can either be manufactured using a plaster mould of the residium as a template or it can be manufactured directly from mapping of the residium using computer-assisted technology. The socket may need to be serially adjusted as the volume of the residium changes.
- **Suspension mechanism:** attaches the prosthesis to the residium. There has been significant developments in methods of suspension over recent years. The ideal method of suspension has the following qualities:
  - easy to don and doff;
  - results in a minimal degree of pistoning: there is always a small degree of movement between the residium and the socket – this movement is called pistoning. This happens on moving, loading or unloading the prosthesis. Excessive pistoning results in the prosthesis feeling heavier, reduces comfort and causes pressure sores.

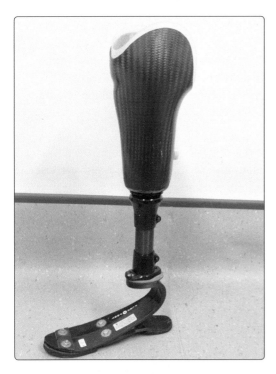

Figure 27.4 Endoskeletal prosthesis.

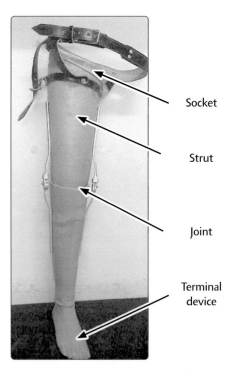

Figure 27.5 Components of a prosthesis.

Suspension mechanisms can be classified as:

- **anatomic or self suspension**: uses the bulbous shape of the residium, or the joint proximal to it, e.g. knee disarticulation sockets use the femoral condyles, and trans-radial and trans-tibial sockets extend to grip above the condyles of the elbow or the knee (supracondylar suspension). This is relatively quick and easy to manage, but restricts joint movements and does not work well in obese patients;
- **belts, straps or sleeves**: one of the simplest methods of suspension, and allows the patient to wear the socket with cotton socks. The number of socks can be varied if the volume of the residium changes, which makes this the favoured system for the first prosthesis following amputation, as oedema is expected to subside. It is simple to use, but might allow pistoning as the fit gets looser;
- **roll-on locking liners**: devised in the 1980s by the Icelandic company (Ossur) and called the ICEROSS system. The patient wears a liner on the residium made usually from silicon. Silicon attaches firmly on the skin and does not slide, so must be rolled on and off. A threaded pin attaches to the end of the liner and engages in a lock at the bottom of the socket when the patient dons the prosthesis. A button is pressed to unlock and doff the prosthesis. Advantages are that it is secure, and the socket brim can be lowered allowing maximum joint movement. Disadvantages are pistoning due to the elongation of the soft tissues of the residium due to the weight of the prosthesis, skin problems associated with wearing silicon liners and lack of evaporation of sweat, and distal discomfort due to the pin in bony residiums;
- **suction suspension**: a valve allows air to be expelled when the socket is donned. The brim of the socket is sealed using an external sleeve or just the soft tissues (skin suction), creating negative pressure between the residium and the socket. To doff the prosthesis, the valve is opened or sleeve removed. An advantage is minimal pistoning so is favoured by highly active amputees. The disadvantages include restriction of proximal joint flexion and the need for sleeves/liners, which prevent sweat evaporation causing skin irritation or infections.
- **The link**: connects the socket with the terminal device and may just be a metal or carbon fibre pilon, e.g. trans-tibial prosthesis, or might include articulating joints, e.g. trans-humeral prosthesis that includes an elbow and a wrist. It might also include dynamic devices to allow shock absorption or torque to facilitate playing golf, for example.
- **Terminal device**: most distal part of the prosthesis. See below for individual descriptions.

Prosthetic fitting

In the immediate post-operative period, the key issues are adequate wound healing, pain management and early therapy for mobility, strength and activities of daily living training. To prepare the residium for the prosthesis, a skin-desensitization programme may be beneficial, consisting of **massage** (to reduce excessive scar formation), **oedema control** (with elastic compression) and **gentle tapping** (on the distal aspect of the residium to mature the site). Pre-prosthetic training may include the use of an early training device, e.g. a pneumatic post-amputation mobility aid (PPAMaid) or an upper-limb gauntlet with a rudimentary terminal device.

The timing of prosthetic fitting is highly dependent on the condition of the wound and the shape of the residium, as it is not possible to fit an oedematous bulbous residium. However, new evidence shows improved wound healing and reduced oedema with the use of early walking aids, probably as a result of improved circulation. It is therefore not essential for the wound to be fully healed to start walking training, as long as infection is ruled out. Once the patient achieves good balance and restores sufficient cardiovascular abilities to manage walking, casting for a prosthesis should be considered.

Common prostheses

Trans-tibial prostheses

Socket

The socket of choice used to be the **patella tendon-bearing** (PTB) prosthesis (**Figure 27.6**). A plaster cast is taken of the residium (negative cast), then a positive cast is made to match the exact shape of the residium. The positive cast is then rectified by the prosthetist to take account of pressure-sensitive areas (using reliefs – concavities within the prosthesis) and pressure-tolerant areas (using build-ups – convexities within the prosthesis). More commonly, sockets are now **total-contact** and, increasingly, **total surface-bearing**, where there is less PTB and weight is distributed more evenly over the entire surface of the residium.

Suspension

Any of the above suspension mechanisms.

Terminal device

In the trans-tibial prosthesis, this is the foot/ankle component or a specialized device. Types of prosthetic feet/ankles include:

- **Non-energy-storing**, e.g.
  - solid ankle cushioned heel (SACH): A small degree of plantarflexion is simulated by compression of the heel that also acts as a shock absorber. This is mainly prescribed to low-activity users as it is light in weight, cost effective and requires little maintenance;
  - multi-axial foot and ankle, which adds inversion, eversion and rotation during stance phase. This is useful over uneven ground.
- **Energy-storing**: these feet are generally made of carbon fibre and contain deforming components in the keel (and sometimes heel), which, when compressed at rollover, want to return to their normal configuration and provide some energy return at toe-off (or heel-strike). These feet also mimic ankle movement during stance and allow inversion/eversion movement when fitted with a split keel. These are the most prescribed type of ankle/foot components with a very wide range of commercially available products (**Figure 27.7**).
- **Energy-storing with hydraulic ankle**: a new category of prosthetic ankle/foot components that allows slow ankle movement as it returns to neutral during swing, thus simulating ankle dorsiflexion to clear the ground. They also provide enhanced ankle flexibility to adapt to uneven surfaces (**Figure 27.8**).
- **Motor-powered ankles**: the motor is powered by a rechargeable battery and controlled by a micro-processor with feedback from sensors that detect load, walking surfaces and

speed (**Figure 27.9**). These improve walking ability and distance by reducing the energy requirements of walking. Battery life, weight and high cost remain significant limiting factors.

- **Specialized**: these devices are highly specialized for specific functions and may not look like feet at all. They often contain carbon-fibre composites and are most commonly used for running and sprinting. Others include waterproof feet, diving ankles (allowing 90° planterflexion to attach a fin) and cycling attachments.

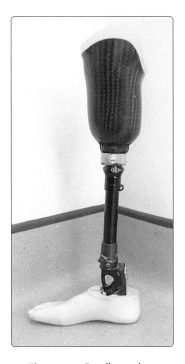

Figure 27.6 Patella tendon-bearing prosthesis.

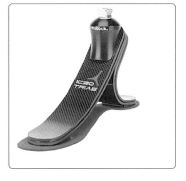

Figure 27.7 Energy-storing Trias foot with the foot shell. (Courtesy of Otto Bock Healthcare Plc.)

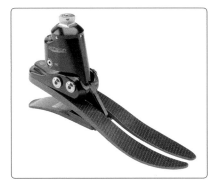

Figure 27.8 Energy-storing foot with hydraulic ankle. Echelon Foot. (Courtesy of Chas A Blatchford and Sons Ltd.)

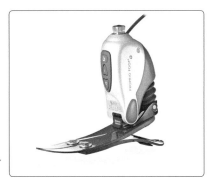

Figure 27.9 Proprio powered foot and ankle. (Courtesy of Össur.)

Trans-femoral prostheses

Socket

The socket brim shape is important here, as it conveys how body weight is transferred to the socket through the ischial tuberosity. As the cut end of the femur is weight intolerant, the socket needs to transfer the forces directly to the pelvis bypassing the femur. Old designs such as the H and quadrilateral socket were generally uncomfortable but relatively easier to make. The soft tissues of the residium are now believed to behave like fluid under pressure, and new designs aim to load those soft tissues more uniformly through total contact, which reduces pistoning and improves control and proprioceptive feedback. Computer-assisted manufacture (CAD/CAM) sockets replace casting by measuring or 3D scanning the surface of the residium. Special software and a carver create a final positive cast, which is then used to produce the socket using conventional techniques.

In general, trans-femoral sockets restrict hip rotation and abduction and prevent excessive hip flexion. They are therefore less comfortable in the seated position, making it harder to sit in a low chair and interfering with car transfers.

Suspension

There are several options:

- **Rigid pelvic band**: limits hip to flexion and extension.
- **Total elastic suspension** (TES) belt: allows all planes of hip movement.
- **Suction socket**.
- **Roll-on locking liner**: attached with a distal lock or, if less available space in the case of a long residium, a lanyard, which replaces the pin with a cord.

Terminal device

The terminal devices are ankles and feet, as per trans-tibial prostheses.

Articulating joint

This is a knee joint. Prosthetic knee joints can be either locked or free. Locked knees are prescribed to patients with balance problems or muscle weakness, and the lock can be released to allow knee flexion in the seated position. Free knee joints can be classified as:

- **Weight activated**: the knee is free during swing but locks once weight is applied, i.e. during stance (hence it is called a stance control knee). This provides improved stability and safety.
- **Multi-axial joints**: instead of a single axis for flexion–extension, the knee has variable axes that depends on the flexion angle, in a similar way to the human knee. Advantages are that the knee resistance to flexion is angle dependent, so being stable in extension (in stance) and more free in flexion (mainly during swing), and upward translation of the shin during flexion allows ground clearance during swing by making the prosthesis shorter as the knee flexes (**Figure 27.10**).
- **Hydraulic or pneumatic knees**: single or multi-axial (**Figure 27.11**). A piston controls the resistance of the knee to movement and is speed dependent. This gives enhanced stumble control as the knees becomes rigid if the patient lands on the prosthesis in high

velocity. Some allow gradual smooth slow flexion during stance (yielding knees), which is particularly useful in walking downstairs or down a slope. These knees are prescribed to patients with higher activity levels to facilitate outdoors walking.

- **Micro-processor controlled knees**: all current designs are single-axis hydraulic knees (**Figure 27.12**). The knee includes electronic sensors and a battery powered micro-processor that constantly modifies the resistance of the hydraulic piston, depending on walking speed and surfaces. Advantages are improved energy requirements and also safety, by reducing the risk of falls. Disadvantages are high cost, weight and battery life.
- **Powered prosthetic knees**: new development that includes a micro-processor controlled knee plus a motor to assist in knee extension (**Figure 27.13**). These have the potential to improve walking abilities and significantly reduce the energy requirements for walking, in addition to protecting the contralateral limb from excessive wear and tear. Battery life, weight and cost are still significant limiting factors.

Knee and ankle disarticulations

For these disarticulations, two different types of socket with anatomic suspension are available:

- **Differential socket**: the socket is made up of an outer hard cylindrical socket and an inner liner. The liner is made from a plaster cast of the stump and rectified to increase the pressure (grip) over the isthmus of the residium (this is also known as a differential liner). A vertical split allows ingress and egress of the bulb of the stump. The outer aspect of the liner is built up to slide smoothly into the outer cylindrical socket.
- **Windowed socket**: a removable window is cut out of the narrowest area of the socket in order to allow the bulb of the residium to pass through and the socket to be closed, thus maintaining suspension.

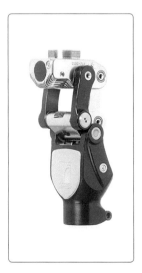

Figure 27.10 Multi-axial Total knee. (Courtesy of Össur.)

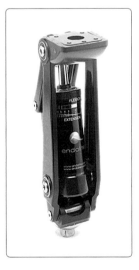

Figure 27.11 KX06 hydraulic multi-axial knee. (Courtesy of Chas A Blatchford and Sons Ltd.)

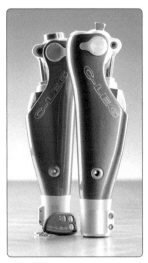

Figure 27.12 Micro-processor controlled knee. C Leg. (Courtesy of Otto Bock Healthcare Plc.)

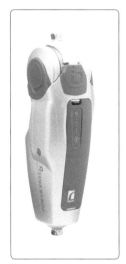

Figure 27.13 Power Knee. (Courtesy of Össur.)

Hip disarticulations and trans-pelvic amputations

Prostheses for this level of amputation are bulky (**Figure 27.14**). Gait can be grossly abnormal, as the lumbar spine has to be used to swing the prosthesis through for heel-strike. The energy requirements are high (*Table 27.2*) and can be twice as much compared to mobilizing with crutches. Therefore, many amputees abandon the prosthesis at a young age and then request to use one years later, due to shoulder or back problems.

The general components of such prostheses are as follows.

Socket and suspension

- **Hip disarticulations**: the ipsilateral ischial tuberosity is available for weight bearing and the ipsilateral iliac crest for suspension (although the socket is usually suspended over both iliac crests). Note that short trans-femoral residual limbs with the femur shorter than 5 cm are fitted with a hip disarticulation socket.
- **Trans-pelvic amputations**: the extent of the amputation is quite variable and is dictated by the underlying pathology (most commonly malignancy). The patient weight bears mainly through the contralateral ischial tuberosity and partially through the soft tissues on the ipsilateral side. The weight is transmitted through the pelvis to the spine through the contralateral sacroiliac joint, often resulting in low back pain.

Terminal device

The terminal devices are ankle/foot components, as per trans-tibial prostheses.

Articulating joint

These are knee joints, as per trans-femoral prostheses, but hip joints can be:

- **Conventional**: joint lies directly under the socket but causes extra bulk under the socket and asymmetry in sitting.

Table 27.2 Energy consumption above normal, following amputation

Long trans-tibial	10%
Average trans-tibial	25%
Bilateral average trans-tibial	20–40%
Short trans-tibial	40%
Average trans-femoral	65%
Hip disarticulation	>300%
Bilateral trans-femoral	>300%

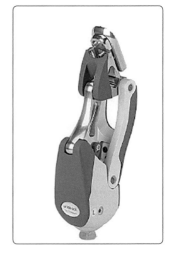

Figure 27.14 Helix Hip. (Courtesy of Otto Bock Healthcare Plc.)

- **Four-bar**: sited anteriorly on the socket and folds away anteriorly for sitting, thus avoiding asymmetry. The connecting tube at the hip and knee joints slants posteriorly to ensure that the prosthetic trochanter–knee–ankle (TKA) line passes behind the hip joint axes and in front of the knee joint axes for stance stability.

Upper limb prostheses

These are generally passive or active.

- **Passive** – cosmetic with no actively moving parts but have some important functions:
  - some bimanual tasks, e.g. used to steady a piece of paper for writing or hold a light weight object;
  - simple functions when the other hand is occupied, e.g. turn on the light switch;
  - restore some symmetry to the trunk muscle – reduce future neck and back problems;
  - improve gait symmetry, especially in more proximal amputations;
  - protect the residual limb, e.g. with a hypersensitive scar in digits;
  - improve the patient's body image.
- **Active** – functional prostheses usually include an active terminal device that is either body- or electric-powered (see below).

Socket and suspension

Body-powered: a harness with cables attaching to the patient, which produces movement in the terminal device on movement of a neighbouring non-injured bodypart. The harness is usually attached in a figure of 8 configuration to the contralateral axilla. The terminal device control cable is tensioned either by biscapular abduction (increasing the distance between the two scapula), which allows the terminal device to be relatively static, or by ipsilateral glenohumeral joint flexion, which also moves the terminal device forward with the limb as it opens or closes, depending on the type.

- **Advantages** – ability to graduate power, better proprioceptive feedback, cheap, low weight and high reliability.
- **Disadvantages** – poor cosmesis, the control harness restricts the proximal joint (usually shoulder) and is less efficient if the shoulder is too flexed or abducted. This makes it harder to perform functions with the terminal device above the head.

Articulating joint

These are an elbow and/or a wrist. Prosthetic elbows are usually hinged joints that could be locked or unlocked by either the other hand or a cable connected to the harness. The most commonly prescribed prosthetic wrists are rotational friction units. Sufficient friction is applied to prevent the terminal device rotation under load, yet not so much that the amputee cannot manually rotate it with the remaining hand.

Terminal device

Note that there are five different types of grip recognized for hand function, making it difficult for prostheses to replicate such complex movements. Therefore, the ability of the terminal device reflects the greatest need of the individual patient.

A split hook provides improved fine motor control, while a body powered hand provides improved cosmesis. Two main types of body powered terminal devices exist:

- **Voluntary opening device**: the device remains closed by rubber bands or springs, and the amputee tensions the cable to open the device. An object is held with a pinch force proportional to the number of rubber bands or springs by releasing the cable. The number of rubber bands can be varied by the amputee depending on the muscle strength and the performed function; however, the pinch force cannot exceed the strength of the bands (**Figure 27.15**).
- **Voluntary closing device**: a weak spring keeps the device open, and the amputee can close the device by tensioning the cable. The pinch force could be varied widely as it is not limited by the number of bands or springs. However, the amputee must apply continuous force to maintain the grasp.

Myoelectric prostheses

Myoelectric prostheses have been available for decades and were hoped to revolutionize prosthetics for patients with missing hands. Range of movement and cosmetic appearance are improved from conventional prostheses. They are best and most cost-effectively used by unilateral trans-radial amputees, improving their functional ability and reducing their time off work. Each patient is unique but it may take months to learn how to operate the device effectively.

Electrodes within the socket are placed specifically to detect individual voluntary muscle electromyography (EMG) signals within the residual limb. These are amplified, passed through a micro-processor and used to operate the terminal device. The patient learns to contract the muscle(s) at different speeds or a certain number of times to control different features of the terminal device, e.g. finger flexion – sustained grasp or brief movement. The power of muscle contraction affects the force or speed of movement of the device.

The newer generations of myoelectric prostheses are called multi-articulating hands. They provide a wider range of functions, such as individual digital movements and thumb rotation for gesturing and different grips. Reliability and cost effectiveness are still not proven. Examples are Bebionic (RSL Steeper), iLimb (Touch Bionics) and Michaelangelo (Otto Bock) (**Figure 27.16**).

Disadvantages include the signals are affected by skin condition, sweating within the socket and the lack of proprioceptive sensory feedback. The prosthesis is relatively heavy as it incorporates a motor and a battery, in addition to higher cost and need for regular maintenance. They are complex, expensive and heavy devices, and successful rehabilitation relies on appropriate patient selection.

They rely heavily on:

- An experienced multi-disciplinary team.
- Appropriate timing and fitting of the prosthesis.
- On-going training and support to improve function.
- Technical support.

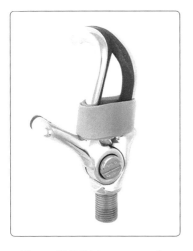

Figure 27.15 Voluntary opening hook. (Courtesy of Otto Bock Healthcare Plc.)

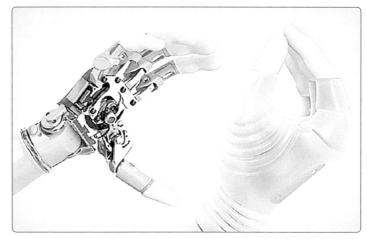

Figure 27.16 Michelangelo hand. (Courtesy of Otto Bock Healthcare Plc.)

A patient must meet all of the following criteria to be considered for a myoelectric device:

- Sufficient neurological, myocutaneous and cognitive function to allow effective operation of the device.
- No confounding medical comorbidites, e.g. neuromuscular disease.
- The residual limb has kept a sufficient microvolt threshold to allow function of the device.
- Be comfortable wearing a socket with a passive function prosthesis before progressing to a myoelectric.
- The patient's environment will not damage or impair the device's function e.g. wet.

Prosthetic cosmesis

Patients either aim for a natural looking prosthesis or prefer a more 'bionic' look. Body image issues are common and counselling is often required. Achieving good function where the patient moves and uses the prosthesis in an intuitive natural manner greatly enhances cosmesis, even without any special covers. Nevertheless, an upper limb user holding the prosthesis in an awkward manner might draw more negative attention in spite of using a well-matching high-definition silicon cover.

High-definition silicon cosmesis

Exceptionally life-like cover of prostheses using silicon is now available, providing better cosmesis and excellent psychological benefits to the patient (**Figure 27.17**).

- Advantages:
  - allows the patient's natural skin colour, tone, markings and even hair to be matched;
  - strong;
  - long-lasting;
  - resilient;
  - allows nails to be painted and the polish removed without detrimental effect to the silicon.

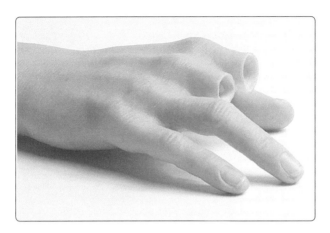

Figure 27.17 Livingskin. (Courtesy of Touch Bionics.)

- Disadvantages:
  - heavy – making it optimal for digit or partial hand/foot amputations, but potentially cumbersome for whole limbs.
  - difficult to use over articulating prosthetic joints and may affect their functionality;
  - colour matching is a one off event and obviously will not match seasonal or even daily changes related to skin temperature, blood circulation or sun tanning;
  - silicon can wear and stain and is difficult to repair when damaged. It is more expensive than off the shelf options.

Latest developments

Osseo-integrated implants have been developed allowing the prosthesis to be directly connected to the bone, but are not yet widely available. These are ideal for patients unable to use conventional sockets and provide improved proprioceptive feedback and joint range of movement. A new technique using intraosseous transcutaneous amputation prosthesis (ITAP) utilizes an implant with hydroxyapatite coating that integrates with both bone and skin, reducing the risk of infection. This technique is currently being researched, but complication rates, specifically infection, appear to be lower.

Complications of amputations

Complications can be either **psychosocial** (related to the initial operative procedure, i.e. amputation, and the use of a prosthesis and the perceived associated stigma) or **physical**. The more common physical complications seen are:

- **Dermatological problems**: including callosities, blisters or skin ulcers, contact dermatitis, scar problems, excessive sweating, recurrent folliculitis and infected epidermoid cysts. Severe dermatological problems mean that a small proportion of patients are unable to use a socket-based prosthesis.
- **Phantom sensation**: sensation that part or whole of the amputated limb is still present. The patient might be able to move the phantom limb which might feel shorter over time (telescoping) or fade away. Phantom sensation does not usually cause distress or require treatment.

- **Phantom pain**: sensation of pain originating in the amputated part of the limb. The pain can be either continuous or periodic, and is mainly described as shooting, stinging, burning, cramping or sometimes felt as troublesome pins and needles. The pain is usually worse at night affecting ability to sleep and improves with distraction, and rarely wakes patients up once they are asleep. It is important to acknowledge that this is 'real' and not imaginary pain and to offer reassurance and appropriate treatment. The phenomena is not well understood but evidence shows a relation to neural plasticity following amputation. Treatment includes non-pharmacological methods such as mirror therapy, meditation and motor imagery. Pharmacological treatment is mainly with anticonvulsants, antidepressants, or simple analgesics (or combinations of these). For the majority of amputees, phantom pain is temporary, is not affected by prosthetic use and does not interfere with function.

- **Painful neuromas**: every cut nerve will eventually form a neuroma. If amputation is performed correctly, these neuromas will be initially covered by muscle. Over time, the muscle bulk in the residium will decrease as a result of the loss of the distal joint, and the neuroma might become compressible on bone or by the socket. An adherent scar around the neuroma also fixes the neuroma in one position, making it more vulnerable to pressures. Treatment is by early scar management, socket modifications to avoid local pressures, anti-inflammatories and simple analgesics. In a few cases, surgery is required to cut the nerve at a higher point to allow a new neuroma to form at a less vulnerable location.

- **Choke syndrome**: venous outflow obstruction of the residium occurring as a result of narrow proximal part of the socket, in combination with an empty space more distally in the socket. This is one of the reasons why total-contact/total surface-bearing sockets are preferred. Acutely, choke syndrome presents with red indurated skin with prominent skin pores ('orange-peel' appearance). Chronically, haemosiderin deposition and venous stasis ulcers may occur.

- **Increase in energy requirements of walking**: may limit ambulation and is not related specifically to use of the prosthesis itself. The level of amputation, the aetiology leading to the amputation and the aerobic capacity and cardiopulmonary efficiency of the patient affect energy expenditure. In general, the increased levels of energy consumption (percentage above normal) by amputation level are as given in *Table 27.2*. The rehabilitation team and patients prefer to have a high trans-tibial amputation with a short stump rather than trans-femoral, due to the great increase in energy consumption for the higher level. Therefore every attempt possible should be made to preserve the knee joint.

- **Weight gain and increased long-term cardiovascular risk**: Although energy requirements of walking increase, amputees in general spend less energy due to reduced activity levels. Most lower limb amputees gain weight following amputation and it is essential to encourage active cardiovascular exercise in the long term.

Viva questions

1. What is a prosthesis?
2. What are the indications for fitting a prosthesis?
3. Tell me about this prosthesis.
4. As a surgeon, what do you have to consider when fitting a prosthesis?
5. What are the complications of prosthetic use?

Further reading

Colwell MO, Spires MC. Lower extremity prostheses and rehabilitation. In: M Grabois (ed). *Physical Medicine and Rehabilitation: The Complete Approach*. London: Blackwell, 2000, pp. 583–607.

Highsmith MJ, Kahle JT, Bongiorni DR, *et al*. Safety, energy efficiency, and cost efficacy of the C-Leg for transfemoral amputees: a review of the literature. *Prosth Orthotics Int* 2010;**34**(4):362–77.

Karanikolas M, Aretha D, Tsolakis I, et al. Optimized perioperative analgesia reduces chronic phantom limb pain intensity, prevalence, and frequency: a prospective, randomized, clinical trial. *Anesthesiology* 2011;**114**(5):1144–54.

Leonard JA, Jr, Meier RH, III. Upper and lower extremity prosthetics. In: JA DeLisa (ed). *Rehabilitation Medicine: Principles and Practice*. Philadelphia, PA: Lippincott, Williams & Wilkins, 1998, pp. 669–96.

Luff R. Amputations. In: J Goodwill, M Chamberlain, C Evans (eds). *Rehabilitation of the Physically Disabled Adult*, 2nd end. Cheltenham: Nelson Thornes, 1997, pp. 172–99.

Martin C. Upper limb prostheses. A review of the literature with a focus on myoelectric hands. 2011 Work Safe BC evidence-based practice group: www.worksafebc.com/evidence

Smith DG, Michael, JW, Bowker, JH. *Atlas of Amputations and Limb Deficiencies: Surgical, Prosthetic and Rehabilitation Principles*, 3rd edn. Rosemount, IL: American Academy of Orthopaedic Surgeons, 2004.

28 | Orthotics

Manoj Ramachandran, Kyle James and Lisa Mitchell

Introduction

This chapter reviews the definition, nomenclature and ideal characteristics of orthoses. Furthermore, their functional and biomechanical effects, the materials used in their manufacture and the complications associated with their use are defined.

An **orthosis** is "a **device** that is **externally applied** or **attached** to a body segment and that **facilitates or improves function by supporting, correcting or compensating for skeletal deformity or weakness**" (Department of Health and Social Security [1980]).

Orthotics is defined as the specialty relating to orthoses and their use. The word 'orthosis' seems to be derived from a combination of the words 'orthopaedic' and 'prosthesis'. It has now replaced the older terms 'splint', 'brace' and 'calliper'.

Nomenclature

Traditionally, orthoses have been named after a part of the body, a person, a place or an institution, but rarely after function. In the 1960s, the American Academy of Orthopaedic Surgeons (AAOS) set up a task force to suggest standard reproducible terminology for orthoses. According to the AAOS nomenclature (*Table 28.1*), an orthosis is described first by the joint or region of the body that it encompasses and second by a biomechanical analysis of its function. Built into the nomenclature is the ability to indicate functional hinge requirements at each joint. In the USA, prescription charts are in use on which are recorded in diagrammatic form

Table 28.1 Regions of the body in American Academy of Orthopedic Surgeons (AAOS) nomenclature

Upper limb	Lower limb	Spine
S – Shoulder	H – Hip	C – Cervical
E – Elbow	K – Knee	T – Thoracic
W – Wrist	A – Ankle	L – Lumbar
H – Hand	F – Foot	S – Sacroiliac

the patient's functional impairment, treatment objectives and orthotic recommendations. In the UK, the use of a combination of AAOS and eponymous nomenclature has persisted.

Thus, FO = foot orthosis, KO = knee orthosis and KAFO = knee–ankle–foot orthosis (note the term is KAFO, not K.A.F.O).

Control of designated function

- F: free motion allowed.
- A: assist, i.e. application of an external force to increase range or velocity of a desired motion.
- R: resist movement by external force.
- S: stop, i.e. static unit to deter motion in one plane.
- H: hold, i.e. elimination of all motion in prescribed plane.
- L: lock, i.e. optional lock.

Orthoses

Orthoses inevitably have to strike a balance between the often-conflicting requirements of function, cosmesis and acceptability. The practical ideal orthosis should aim to have the following characteristics:

- Biomechanically effective.
- Lightweight.
- Durable.
- Cosmetically pleasing.
- Easy to put on (don) and take off (doff).
- Rapid provision and replacement.
- Inexpensive.
- Washable.
- Adjustable.
- Comfortable.
- Free of pressure areas.

Functional characteristics of orthoses

The main groups of functions for which orthoses are used are:

- **Provision of support**: to prevent weak muscles or ligaments being stretched, or to support joints by substituting for weakened muscles or ligaments, e.g. thoracolumbar orthosis (TLO) to support a collapsing osteoporotic spine, or KAFO to relieve weight from the lower-leg skeletal mass.
- **Limitation of motion**: e.g. KO to prevent hyperextension.
- **Correction of deformity**: to force the affected joint(s) into near-alignment and redirect growth if possible, e.g. thoracolumbar sacral orthosis (TLSO) to correct an idiopathic scoliosis, or ankle–foot orthosis (AFO) in cerebral palsy. Serial splinting describes the regular readjustment of orthoses to gradually improve the position or range of movement of a joint contracture.

- **Assistance of motion**: e.g. hip–knee–ankle–foot orthosis (HKAFO) to aid walking in myelomeningocele.
- **Miscellaneous**: e.g. warmth, placebo effect.
- **Combination**: many orthoses combine several functions, e.g. KAFO for a leg afflicted by polio gives support, limits movement at the knee (and perhaps the ankle), may help to correct a varus ankle and may have a spring to assist ankle dorsiflexion.

An alternative functional classification of orthoses comprises two main groups:

- **Static (passive)**: has no moving parts and is used to immobilize a part of the body in a particular position.
- **Dynamic (active)**: has moving parts, but movement is controlled by an energy store, e.g. an elastic band. An example is a post-operative outrigger for mobilizing tendon repairs of the hand. Maintaining mobility in joints has advantages in prevention of joint stiffness and muscle wasting, and hastening repair of bone, tendon and ligaments.

For all orthoses, at least **three points of pressure** are needed for proper control of a joint. For **supportive orthoses** of the resting splint type, the joint must be maintained in optimum anatomical position during rest periods. For **corrective orthoses**, the purpose of the orthosis is to impose or control a set of forces on the body part. Each force has both magnitude and direction, and the resultant must be worked out. The three-point principle (as proposed by Sir John Charnley for fracture immobilization) has long been accepted. Dynamic requirements of an orthosis are less well defined.

Basic biomechanical concepts

A basic understanding of biomechanics is essential when prescribing orthoses. Newton's third law of reaction, which states that for every **reaction** there is an **equal and opposite reaction**, is vital for comprehension of the principle of **ground reaction force** (GRF) (see Chapter 16). If an orthosis is to be used to modify gait, the prescriber must also be aware of the normal gait cycle in order to diagnose abnormal gait patterns (see Chapter 26). Complex gait problems may require the use of a gait laboratory to determine specific muscle-group inadequacies.

It is important to understand the effects of GRF during the gait cycle (**Figure 28.1**). The GRF is the force exerted by the ground on the body. It is equal in magnitude, but opposite in direction, to the force exerted on the ground by the body. If the GRF does not pass through the centre of a joint, then it produces a moment (turning force) on that joint. In mid-stance, the GRF is posterior to the hip, resulting in a hip extension moment that is counterbalanced by the gradual tightening of the anterior hip capsule. The GRF falls anterior to the knee, causing a knee extension moment that is resisted by the tight posterior knee capsule (**Figure 28.1A**). The GRF falls anterior to the ankle, resulting in an ankle dorsiflexion moment that is resisted by contraction of the gastrocnemius–soleus muscle complex. Thus, in balanced mid-stance, very little muscle activity is needed in order to maintain upright posture. During pre-swing, the force passes behind the knee and acts as a flexor, thus reducing the work requirements for knee flexion (**Figure 28.1B**).

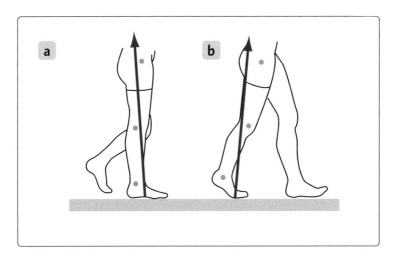

Figure 28.1 Ground reaction force and its line of action during (a) mid-stance and (b) pre-swing.

Forces and moments generated about a particular joint may be calculated using the concept of free-body diagrams (see Chapter 16). Knowledge of such forces and moments is essential when designing an orthosis.

Biomechanics of orthoses

Orthoses function by application of mechanical forces to the musculoskeletal system. Their success depends on a thorough understanding of biomechanical principles and their correct application.

Regardless of whether the body is stationary or moving, it is always subject to a system of external forces and moments. Normally, the effects of the external moments acting on the body are restricted or controlled by forces generated internally, either in passive tissues such as capsules, ligaments and articular cartilage, or in active tissues such as muscles. Injury or disease of one of these (e.g. ligament rupture, muscle atrophy, spasticity, contractures) can lead to an inability to produce the appropriate force to resist the system of external forces. Modifying the system of external forces and moments acting about one or more joints of the body by using an orthosis may restore a more normal function.

There are four ways by which an orthosis may modify the system of external forces and moments across a joint. The first three are direct (the orthosis surrounds the joint being influenced) and the last is indirect (modification of an external force occurs beyond the physical boundary of the orthosis):

- **Control of moments about a joint**: this is the most common reason for prescribing an orthosis. By modifying the moments about a joint, an orthosis may partially or totally restrict the rotational movement at the joint (**Figure 28.2**). The end result is either a decrease in the range of movement about a particular axis or a limitation of the number of axes about which motion may occur. For an orthosis to be effective in controlling rotation, it must consist of a rigid framework incorporating straps and pads, which apply three forces to the limb. This **three-point fixation** involves one force acting over the joint centre,

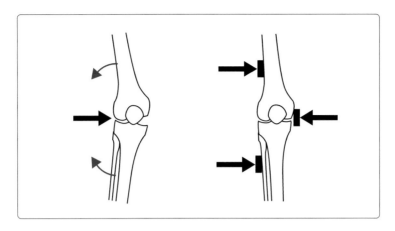

Figure 28.2 Control of moments about a joint.

and the other two forces acting in the opposite direction to the first, placed proximally and distally to the joint. An example is a KO used for medial collateral ligament rupture of the knee, which is designed to eliminate motion in either the coronal or the transverse plane, while allowing motion in the sagittal plane.

- **Control of translation forces across a joint**: translational instability arises only when there are significant shear forces acting across the joint (**Figure 28.3**). **Four-point fixation** is required to prevent translation. The orthosis can be hinged to allow rotation. An example is a KO used to prevent translation in the transverse plane in posterior cruciate ligament (PCL) rupture of the knee.
- **Control of axial forces across a joint**: this is achieved by load sharing between the anatomical structures and the orthotic exoskeleton and is particularly useful for reducing pain in arthritic joints (**Figure 28.4**).

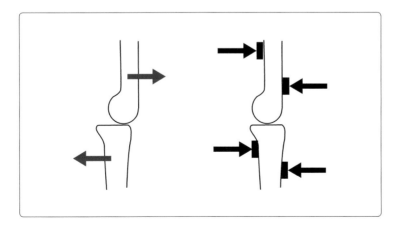

Figure 28.3 Control of translational forces about a joint.

- **Control of line of action of GRF**: this involves modification of the point of application and line of action of the GRF during either static or dynamic weight bearing and is relevant only to the lower limb (**Figure 28.5**). It is particularly useful in modifying abnormally high moments about a joint, but it can also be used to change the alignment of a joint. An example is the use of a lateral heel wedge, which can transfer the GRF from the medial aspect of a varus degenerate knee to the intercondylar eminence or lateral joint line.

Materials used in orthotics

Traditionally, orthoses were made from **leather, rubber, metal or plaster of Paris**. These orthoses tended to be bulky, unsightly and unacceptable to the patient. Leather, such as cattle hide, continues to be used for shoe construction, as it conducts heat and absorbs water well. Rubber has tough resiliency and shock-absorbing qualities and is still used for padding in body jackets and limb orthoses. Metals, such as stainless steel and aluminium alloys, are adjustable and can be used for joint components, metal uprights and bearings. Plaster of Paris continues to be used as the initial mould taken from the patient for the preparation of orthoses.

Gordon Yates in 1968 first described the use of lightweight and more cosmetically pleasing plastic materials in the manufacture of orthoses. The three major materials now in use are:

- **Thermosetting plastics**: e.g. polyester resins, which can be moulded into permanent shape after heating and do not return to their original consistency, even after being reheated. They are formed by pouring liquid plastic resin into a mould, which is then mixed with

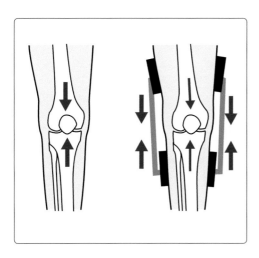

Figure 28.4 Control of axial forces across a joint.

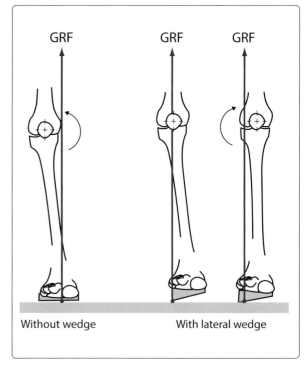

Figure 28.5 Control of the line of action of the ground reaction force.

catalyst that polymerizes the resin to set into a rigid form. They are more commonly used in prosthetics than orthotics, where greater rigidity is required.

- **Thermoforming plastics** (thermoplastics): these soften when heated (allowing reshaping by application of pressure) and harden when cooled. They can be reshaped many times and are subdivided according to their moulding temperatures:
  - **high-temperature thermoplastics:** require moulding temperatures 120–190°C. Great skill is required in their manufacture. They are ideal for high-stress activities. These orthoses are made by heating a sheet of polyethylene (e.g. Vitrathene™, Subortholen™, Ortholen™) or polypropylene (e.g. Vitralene™) in a hot oven. The final product is then either vacuum-formed or moulded over a positive plaster of Paris cast. Plastics differ in molecular weight, tensile strength, fatigue resistance and mouldability. They are commonly used for making more rigid orthoses such as AFOs and TLSOs;
  - **moderate-temperature thermoplastics:** require moulding temperatures of 100–120°C. An example is Plastozote™ foam made from polyethylene of closed-cell construction. It is very lightweight and, after heating in a hot-air oven, it can be moulded directly on the patient, as it has low heat conductivity and its surfaces cool rapidly. It is commonly used for making custom-made cervical collars and pressure-distribution pads;
  - **low-temperature thermoplastics:** require moulding temperatures below 80°C and so can be moulded in a water bath or hot-air oven. Ideal for use in acute splinting by occupational therapists. They can be moulded directly on to the patient, with minor modifications made using a heat gun or hair dryer. As a group, these thermoplastics are less rigid and less durable than other plastics; however, they are cheaper, because less time, skill and equipment are required for fabrication. Note that they may also soften in direct sunlight or near a fire. The common types of polymers in use are trans-polyisoprene (Orthoplast™) and polycaprolactone (Polyform™, Aquaplast™), to which synthetic rubber may be added (many types of Sansplint™). The plastics differ in setting times, rigidity, impact strength and transparency.
- **Self-generating polyurethane foam**: used in Neofract™ corsets and braces, this freshly prepared foam is poured into a cotton pattern and distributed evenly with a roller. The filled pattern is allowed to harden directly over the patient. The custom-made cast is prepared in minutes and is donned and doffed by using a zip fastener. Polyurethane foam is also used to make moulded cushions for wheelchairs and can be used as filler in KAFOs and shoes.

Common orthoses

Foot orthoses

Insoles are commonly prescribed for a variety of foot pathologies. Insoles can be classified into three groups:

- **Simple insoles**: either off-the-shelf or fabricated without casting. Provide poor surface area contact and little if any biomechanical control.
- **Total contact insoles**: made initially by taking an imprint of the patient's foot and then casting this imprint with plaster of Paris. A thermoplastic is then moulded from the positive plaster of Paris cast. These are the most commonly used foot orthoses.

- **Functional/biomechanical orthoses**: corrective insoles introduced by Mervon Root, a podiatrist, in the 1960s. The foot is held in its corrected position when the cast is taken. The insole obtained therefore acts to correct the underlying foot deformity when the deformity is flexible. For fixed deformities, an accommodative insole is used.

When the limits for the use of insoles are reached, **custom-made shoes** are considered. Again, these can be corrective or accommodative, with respect to the deformity. A custom-made shoe often requires many fittings before it is satisfactory. Shoes can be modified either externally or internally in order to reduce pressure on sensitive areas by redistributing weight towards pain-free areas. For **external** shoe modifications, **heels** can be of the following types:

- **Cushioned**: wedge of compressible rubber used to absorb impact at heel-strike or, with a rigid ankle, to allow more rapid ankle plantarflexion by reducing the knee flexion moment.
- **Flared**: medial to resist eversion and lateral to resist inversion.
- **Wedged**: medial to promote inversion and lateral to promote eversion.
- **Extended**: e.g. a Thomas heel projects anteriorly on the medial side to provide support to the medial longitudinal arch.
- **Elevated**: shoe lift to compensate for fixed equinus deformity or leg-length discrepancy of more than about 0.65 cm.

For **external** shoe modifications, **soles** can have the following:

- **Rocker bars**: convex structure placed posterior to metatarsal head, shifting rollover point from head to shaft. Used for ulcers over metatarsal heads in diabetes mellitus.
- **Metatarsal bars**: bar with flat surface placed posterior to metatarsal head to relieve pressure on heads.
- **Wedges**: medial to promote supination and lateral to promote pronation.
- **Flares**: medial to resist eversion and lateral to resist inversion.

For **internal** shoe modifications, the **heels** can have the following:

- **Cushion relief**: soft pad with excavation placed under painful point of heel.
- **Cups**: rigid plastic insert covering the plantar surface of heel and extending posteriorly, medially and laterally to prevent lateral calcaneal shift in the flexible flat foot.
- **University of California at Berkeley Laboratory** (UCBL) insert: rigid plastic insert fabricated over a cast of the foot held in maximum manual correction and encompassing the heel and midfoot, with rigid posterior, medial and lateral walls. Used to control hindfoot valgus and midfoot pronation.

For **internal** shoe modifications, the **soles** can have the following:

- **Metatarsal pads**: domed pads designed to reduce stress from metatarsal heads by transferring load to metatarsal shafts in metatarsalgia.
- **Inner sole excavations**: soft pad filled with compressible material placed under metatarsal heads.
- **Arch supports**: e.g. medial arch support extending from half inch posterior to first metatarsal head to anterior tubercle of the os calcis.

Ankle–foot orthoses

AFOs are used to prevent or correct deformities and reduce weight bearing. The position of the ankle indirectly affects the stability of the knee, with ankle plantarflexion providing a knee extension force and ankle dorsiflexion providing a knee flexion force. AFOs have been shown to **reduce the energy cost of ambulation** in a wide variety of conditions, such as the spastic diplegic form of cerebral palsy, the lower motor neuron weakness of poliomyelitis and the spastic hemiplegia of stroke.

Plastic AFOs consist of a shoe insert, a calf shell, a heel-retaining strap and a calf strap attached more proximally. Examples include the following:

- **Posterior leaf spring**: narrow calf shell and narrow ankle trim line behind the malleoli to allow some flexibility. Used for compensating for weak ankle dorsiflexors – dorsiflexion assist – by preventing excessive equinus at heel-strike or drop-foot in swing. Allows the tibia to progress forwards during the second rocker of stance phase. Has no mediolateral control.
- **Solid AFO**: wider calf shell with trim line anterior to the malleoli. Prevents ankle dorsiflexion and plantarflexion, as well as varus and valgus deviation and controls foot position.
- **Hinged AFO**: adjustable ankle hinges can be set to the desired range of ankle dorsiflexion or plantarflexion. Commonly, a hinged AFO prevents plantarflexion but allows relatively full dorsiflexion during the stance phase of gait. This orthosis is contraindicated in severe foot deformity as it allows movement in the subtalar joint, worsening the foot deformity.
- **Ground reaction AFO** (GRAFO): made with a solid ankle at neutral. The upper portion wraps around the anterior part of the tibia proximally to provide strong ground reaction support for patients with weak triceps surae. Prevents knee hyperextension by creating a flexion moment at the knee (**Figure 28.6**). The requirements for use of a GRAFO are full knee extension, ankle dorsiflexion to neutral with an extended knee and no significant rotational deformity in the tibia or foot.
- **Dynamic AFO** (DAFO) or **tone-reducing AFO** (TRAFO): broad footplate used to provide support around most of the foot, extending distally under the toes and up over the medial

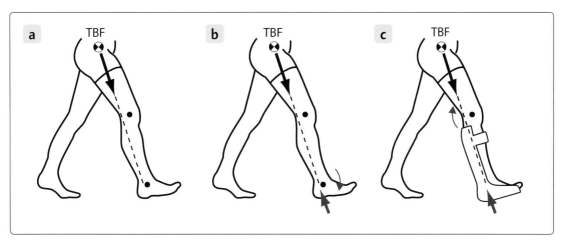

Figure 28.6 Ground reaction force (GRF) control in the sagittal plane. a: Before heel contact, no GRF acts on the lower extremity; b: at heel contact with no orthosis, the GRF control acts to plantarflex the ankle; c: at heel contact with an ankle–foot orthosis, the GRF control acts to flex the knee. TBF: total body force.

and lateral aspect of the foot in order to maintain the subtalar joint in normal alignment. There is some evidence that in cerebral palsy, these are capable of reducing tone in muscle groups above the area braced and, therefore, by reducing tone, improving function; this is the principle of inhibitive casting.

- **Metal and metal–plastic AFOs**: consist of a shoe or foot attachment, ankle joint and two metal uprights (medial and lateral), with a calf band connected proximally. The mechanical ankle joints can control or assist ankle dorsiflexion or plantarflexion by means of stops (pins) or assists (springs). The mechanical ankle joint also controls mediolateral stability.

Knee–ankle–foot orthoses

KAFOs consist of an AFO with metal uprights, a mechanical knee joint and two thigh bands. They can be used in **quadriceps paralysis** or weakness to maintain knee stability and control flexible genu valgum or varum. They can be manufactured from metal, e.g. double upright metal KAFO (most common) and Scott–Craig metal KAFO (used for spinal cord injury patients with paraplegia), or from plastic, e.g. ischial weight-bearing KAFO.

Trunk–hip–knee–ankle–foot orthoses

A trunk–hip–knee–ankle–foot orthosis (THKAFO) consists of a spinal orthosis in addition to an HKAFO (a hip joint and pelvic band in addition to a KAFO) for control of trunk motion and spinal alignment. A THKAFO is indicated in patients with paraplegia and is very difficult to don and doff. An example is the reciprocating gait orthosis (RGO).

Patients who require KAFOs or higher orthoses for ambulation require much more energy expenditure and have slower walking speeds than unimpaired individuals.

Miscellaneous examples

Weight-bearing orthoses

These orthoses are designed to eliminate weight bearing through the lower extremities, e.g. PTBO for use in the treatment of diabetic ulcers, neuropathic joints and insensate feet.

Charcot restraint orthotic walker (CROW)

Used in the end-stage foot disease of diabetes, syphilis and leprosy.

Fracture orthoses

Stabilizes the fracture site and promotes callus formation, while allowing weight bearing and joint movement. Motion at the fracture site is prevented through circumferential compression of the soft tissues (**Sarmiento's hydrostatic compression principle**).

Angular and deformity orthoses

An example is the Denis Brown orthosis used during the bracing portion of the Ponseti treatment for congenital talipes equinovarus.

Hip orthoses for paediatric disorders

Used to maintain the hip in a flexed and abducted position in order to hold the femoral head within the acetabulum, e.g. Pavlik harness, von Rosen splint. Other types are used to maintain the hip in abduction and keep the femoral head in the acetabulum, e.g. the Scottish Rite, Toronto and non-skeletal-bearing trilateral orthoses.

Complications of orthoses

Complications can be **psychosocial** (related to the use of an orthosis, particularly any perceived associated stigma) or **physical**. The following are the more common physical complications seen:

- **Compression phenomena**: tight orthoses can encircle limbs, resulting in compression of nerves, arteries and veins, and resulting in pain, paraesthesia, impaired distal circulation and oedema.
- **Heat and water retention**: leading to maceration of skin, impaired wound healing and skin infection, particularly in close-fitting orthoses such as spinal braces.
- **Patient–orthosis interfacial effects**: this interface is defined as the junction between the body tissues and the orthosis and/or the support surface through which forces are transmitted. Forces may arise at this interface, either because of equal and opposite forces imposed on the body by the support surface (Newton's third law), or because an orthosis has been designed specifically to hold one or more joints in a particular position. These forces may lead to tissue necrosis and skin breakdown, especially if the compressive and shear forces generated are distributed in a non-uniform manner, e.g. over bony prominences with thin overlying subcutaneous tissues (**extrinsic factors**), or if there are contributory patient factors, e.g. decreased skin sensation, decreased level of consciousness, paralysis, dehydration, peripheral vascular disease, malnutrition or systemic disease (**intrinsic factors**). To decrease the pressure effects of an orthosis, the following can be attempted:
  - proper contouring increases contact area and decreases the tendency of the orthosis to move;
  - good mechanical design, e.g. increased lever arm to reduce the amount of force exerted on the skin (**Figure 28.7**);
  - forces applied perpendicular to limb segment to reduce shearing;
  - adequate padding and large contact areas over which the forces can act. Note that a maximal conforming support area will provide a uniform distribution of pressure. This can be applied in two ways. First, the support surface, made of a relatively high modulus material, can be matched in shape to the area of the body it interfaces with, e.g. a spinal brace. Second, the support surface can be flat but made of relatively soft material, which can deform under load, e.g. in seating applications.

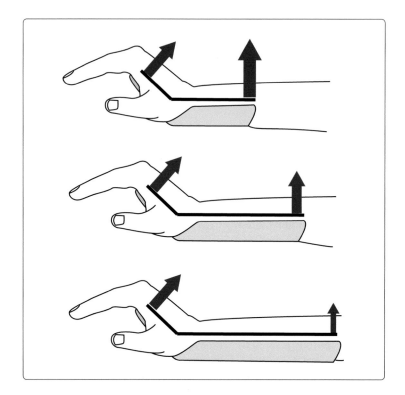

Figure 28.7 Increased lever arm of orthosis decreases pressure at the orthosis–patient interface.

Viva questions

1. What is an orthosis?
2. How do orthoses work?
3. Describe this orthosis to me. How does it work?
4. From what materials are orthoses manufactured?
5. Explain how a GRAFO works.

Further reading

Department of Health and Social Security. *Classification of Orthoses*. London: HMSO, 1980.

Engen TJ, Lehmkuhl LD. Lower extremity orthotics. *Curr Orthop* 1989;**3**:194–200.

Jain AS. Upper limb orthotics. *Curr Orthop* 1990;**4**:259–62.

Ewing Fess E, Gettle KS, Philips CA, Janson JR (eds). *Mechanical Principles*. In: *Hand and Upper Extremity Splinting,* 3rd edn. Saint Louis: Mosby, 2005, pp. 161–83.

Morrish G, Whittle MW. Spinal orthoses. *Curr Orthop* 1989;**3**:122–7.

Waters RL, Mulroy S. The energy expenditure of normal and pathologic gait. *Gait Posture* 1999;**9**(3):207–31.

Yates G. A method for the provision of lightweight aesthetic orthopaedic appliances. *Orthopaedics* 1968; **1**:153–62.

29 Inside the Operating Theatre

Manoj Ramachandran, Steve Key and Alan White

Introduction

Joseph Lister wrote in 1867: "When it had been shown by researchers of Pasteur that the septic property of the atmosphere depended on minute organisms suspended in it, it occurred to me that decomposition in the injured part might be avoided by applying some material capable of destroying the life of the floating particles".

Lister went on to develop his practice of antisepsis, including carbolic acid (phenol) spraying of the air around the operation site, instrument sterilization and washing of the surgeon's hands. Since Lister's time, much effort has been spent in trying to provide an environment in which orthopaedic surgery, especially joint arthroplasty, can be performed with minimum risk of subsequent infection. This chapter summarizes these efforts and provides a framework for the orthopaedic surgeon when considering the operating theatre environment. There is also a discussion of the general operating theatre equipment and protocols common to many orthopaedic procedures that allow surgery to proceed safely.

Operating theatre basics

The operating theatre should be located **close** to other **related facilities**, e.g. the Intensive Therapy Unit (ITU), the Accident and Emergency (A&E) department, the radiology department, the pathology department and the wards. Areas of **public circulation** and **non-essential departments** should be **avoided**. Independent orthopaedic theatres are desirable for maintenance of an aseptic environment, efficacy and speed of surgical procedures and organization of theatre lists.

Theatre design

Operating theatres should be of sufficient size to accommodate theatre personnel, the patient and the necessary theatre equipment. Most operating theatres are designed in theatre suites linked by a double or single corridor. It is conventional to think of theatres in four zones:

- The **outer zone** includes the rest of the hospital and theatre reception.
- The **clean zone** comprises the area from the theatre reception up to the theatre doors.
- The **aseptic zone** (**Figure 29.1**).
- The **disposal zone**.

Theatre design is based around the operating table. Areas that require access to and from the operating table include the anaesthetic room, scrub area, disposal zone and recovery area. To provide optimal conditions for patients and staff, **temperature, humidity, light and ventilation** must all be controlled carefully.

Temperature and humidity

Patients are at risk of **hypothermia** from **paralysis, cool intravenous fluids** and **large exposed wounds**. To prevent hypothermia, theatre temperatures of 24–26°C are recommended. However, ideal working temperatures for surgeons are between 19 and 20°C. Therefore, a compromise is achieved by creating a **warm microclimate** for the patient using **warming blankets** or **airflow mattresses**. There is, however, a potential effect on airflow systems in theatre with such devices. Temperature control is particularly important during cementation

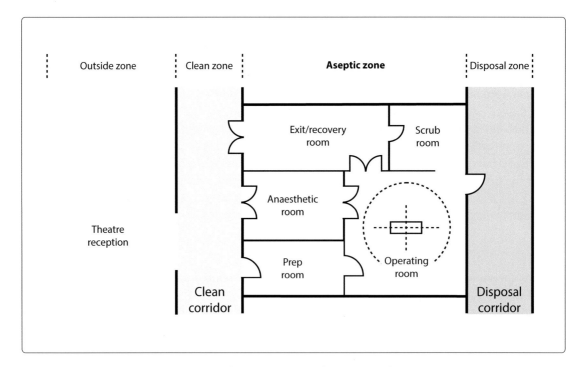

Figure 29.1. The aseptic zone in the operating theatre.

of arthroplasties, as the temperature affects the polymerization of polymethyl-methacrylate (PMMA) cement: **higher ambient temperatures can significantly reduce bone cement working times** and the surgeon should be familiar with the product literature regarding the working times for the cement they are using. A working time of only 2–3 minutes is common at temperatures of 25°C, and may be prohibitively quick at temperatures higher than this. Maintaining a constant temperature is also important when operating on young children.

Relative humidity in the theatre should be capable of adjustment in the range 40–60%. Higher humidity will also reduce PMMA working time and the surgeon should be cognisant of this. Both humidity and temperature are controlled most readily by alterations made in the ventilation of the theatre.

Illumination

High-quality artificial illumination **without shadows** is required in the operating room. The light source should be capable of producing a minimum of 40,000 lux at the incision site. Its direction and focus should be **easily adjustable** by the surgical team. Satellite lights are usually employed; however, these create heat and subsequent convection currents and may, therefore, alter local airflow patterns.

Ventilation

A surgical wound can become contaminated from a variety of sources in the operating theatre (**Figure 29.2**). In general, there are four main sources of infection in the operating room:

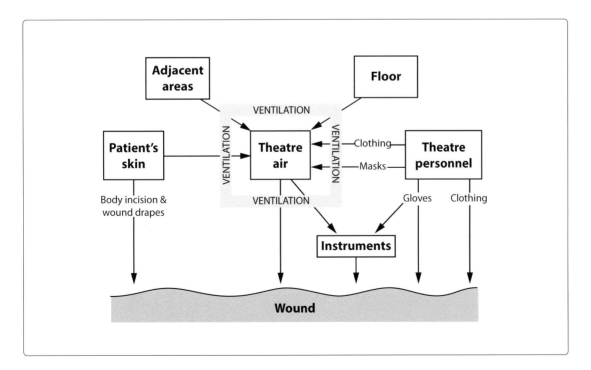

Figure 29.2 Routes and sources of infection in the operating theatre.

- Direct contact from the surgical team.
- Instruments.
- Airborne contamination.
- The patient.

Airborne contamination originates almost exclusively from personnel within the theatre. Ninety-five per cent of wound contamination can be accounted for by the airborne route. An individual may shed 3000–50,000 micro-organisms per minute, depending on activity and clothing. Bacteria from the upper respiratory tract (e.g. *Streptococcus, Staphylococcus* spp.) are dispersed by, for example, talking and coughing. The skin is regularly contaminated with *Staphylococcus*, which is shed into clothing and the surrounding environment. The axillae and groins are colonized particularly heavily. Ninety per cent of all bacteria emissions come from below the neck level.

It is the role of the ventilatory system in theatres to reduce airborne bacteria to a minimum. The result is judged by the **air cleanliness**, expressed as **bacteria-carrying particles per cubic metre** (BCP/m³) or **colony-forming units per cubic metre** (CFU/m³). This is measured most accurately with a **microbiological volumetric slit sampler**, e.g. Casella slit sampler (Casella London Ltd, London, UK), or with settle plates. Slit samplers draw in a set volume of air per minute (30–70 L/min) past culture plates; the plates are incubated for 48 h at 37°C and the colonies formed are counted. According to British Standards, air sampling is recommended in plenum-ventilated operating theatres at commissioning or after refurbishing. In ultra-clean operating theatres, air sampling is recommended on a regular basis several times a year (the standard is every 3 months) and should be done inside and outside the enclosed area.

In terms of definitions of cleanliness, in a standard plenum ventilated operating theatre lying empty, there should be less than 35 CFU of bacteria/m³ of air and less than 1 CFU/m³ of *Clostridium perfringens* and *Staphylococcus aureus*. During operative procedures, there should be less than 180 CFU of bacteria/m³. In ultra-clean laminar flow theatres, there should be less than 20 CFU/m³ at the periphery of the enclosure and less than 10 CFU/m³ at the centre.

Ventilatory systems

To reduce airborne contamination, ventilatory systems must ideally provide a bacteria-free source of air and produce positive pressure to displace contaminated air away from the operational site and to prevent entry of bacteria from contaminated areas. Air is usually taken in at the **roof level** of the theatre suite. It is drawn by a series of **fans** through filters capable of removing bacteria-carrying particles. It is also humidified and warmed or cooled. **High-efficiency particulate air** (HEPA) filters are commonly employed. These are capable of filtering particles of 0.5 μm in size with 99.97% efficiency. Ventilatory systems are of two types, plenum and laminar flow.

Plenum

In this system, pressure inside the theatre is greater than that outside. Clean air is fed via wall or ceiling diffusers and let out of vents placed just above floor level. Air also passes out around doors and other openings. In theory, air from contaminated areas should not enter the aseptic zone. However, the opening of doors and the movement of personnel within theatres makes the system less efficient. For example, opening a standard theatre door transfers 2 m³ of air across the opening, and turbulence is created by such activity. Doors to the operating room should be kept closed, except as needed for the passage of equipment, personnel and the patient. Essential equipment should be stored in the operating room to decrease theatre traffic; the frequency of theatre door-opening is a positive predictor of raised bacterial counts. Standard positive-pressure ventilated operating theatres deliver around **15–25 air changes per hour**.

Laminar flow

A laminar airflow room is a room in which laminar airflow characteristics predominate throughout the entire air space with a minimum of eddies. **Laminar airflow characteristics involve the entire body of air within a designated space moving with uniform velocity in a single direction along parallel flow lines**. True laminar airflow is not achieved unless there is close to 100% HEPA filter coverage in the ceiling grid system. There are three main types of theatre airflow:

- Horizontal laminar flow.
- Vertical laminar flow.
- Ex-flow or exponential flow (Howorth enclosures).

However, theatres are usually designed with a vertical downward airflow concept. Only specific processes require horizontal airflow.

It is common for laminar flow to be restricted to an area in the centre of the operating theatre – the **room-within-a-room principle**. The flow of air is around 0.3 m/s and is not perceptible to the individual in the airflow path. The flow is broken around obstructions such as operating lights but quickly reforms. Laminar flow theatres deliver around **300–500 air changes per hour**.

Horizontal laminar flow

Here, HEPA filters form a wall or part of a wall. The positioning of the scrub team is important, and the use of equipment such as image intensifiers may be restricted (**Figure 29.3**). Horizontal laminar flow is easier to install than vertical laminar flow in a pre-existing theatre. Of interest, Salvati *et al.* (1982) found that although horizontal laminar flow reduced the incidence of deep joint sepsis following total hip arthroplasty, sepsis rates following total knee arthroplasty increased, probably due to difficulties with intra-operative personnel placement.

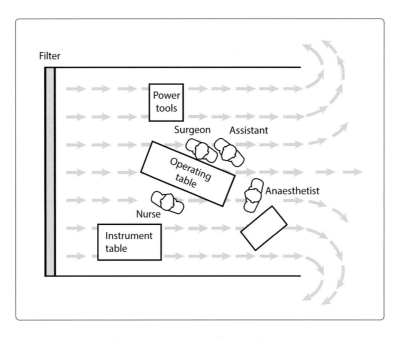

Figure 29.3 Horizontal laminar flow.

Vertical laminar flow

An enclosure is formed with panels extending from the ceiling to within 2 m (although this is variable) of the floor. Air is passed through HEPA filters in the ceiling and directed towards the operative field in a vertical direction. Entrainment of the flow, however, can occur from personnel moving within the periphery of the laminar flow area (**Figure 29.4**). Such entrainment can deflect contamination inwards towards the wound. Full enclosures, however, are free of this problem.

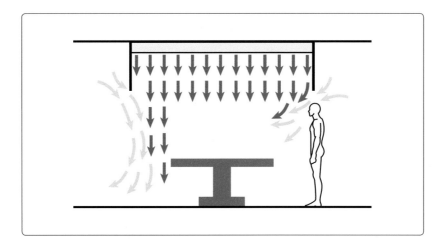

Figure 29.4 The effect of entrainment on vertical laminar flow.

Ex-flow system (Howorth enclosure)

Howorth (1980) described a flow of clean air from the operating theatre in the shape of an inverted trumpet (**exponential flow or ex-flow**) (**Figure 29.5**). The air moves downwards and outwards. Peripheral entrainment therefore cannot occur as with vertical laminar flow systems. This system is theoretically more efficient than laminar flow and, as such, requires fewer changes of air per hour.

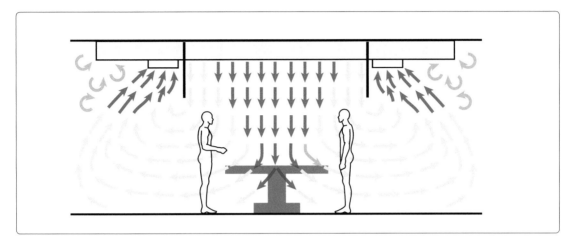

Figure 29.5 Exponential air flow (ex-flow) in a Howorth enclosure.

Clinical effects of laminar flow

Following the introduction of vertical laminar flow, Charnley (1972) reported a reduction in the incidence of deep infection from 7% to 0.5% in the period 1960–70, during which time 5800 total hip arthroplasties were performed. Charnley attributed the decreased incidence to air factors in combination with better surgical wound closure and surgical apparel. A Medical Research Council (MRC) prospective randomized trial reported by Lidwell *et al.* (1982) confirmed a significant reduction in wound contamination and deep joint sepsis in ultra-clean air theatres and found that vertical laminar flow was more effective than horizontal laminar flow. Certain prophylactic measures (*Table 29.1*) were also effective in reducing deep joint sepsis.

Table 29.1 Prophylactic measures identified by the Medical Research Council (MRC) trial

Prophylactic measure	Factor
Antibiotic loaded cement	11
Systemic antibiotics	4.8
Ultra-clean air	2.6
Plastic isolators	2.2
Body exhaust suit	2.2

Clothing and drapes

The ideal surgical clothing would prevent airborne bacteria dispersion, act as an effective barrier even when wet, and allow air and water vapour circulation. To date, this ideal clothing has not been found. Dispersion of bacteria from clothing may occur at apertures, e.g. at the neck and arm openings; this is significant particularly when combined with local convection currents set up by the radiation of body heat. Direct migration of bacteria may occur through clothing, especially when wet; this is known as moist bacterial strike-through.

Clothing types

Standard (balloon) cotton clothing

This is **comfortable**, as it is made of an **open weave**, which allows for easy air circulation. However, the pore size is 80 μm and it is therefore inefficient at preventing migration of bacteria-carrying particles. **Moist bacterial strike-through** is a particular problem.

Ventile™

This is a cotton product with a **close weave**, giving a pore size of 20 μm. It is effective in reducing bacterial dispersion but is **uncomfortable** to wear as it inhibits air circulation. It has also been employed as a front pad to prevent moist bacterial strike-through from the abdominal and lower thoracic areas of the surgeon.

Gore-Tex™

This is woven polyester laminated to a film of polytetrafluoroethylene (PTFE). The **open structure** allows for air exchange, but the pore size of 0.2 μm acts as an **effective barrier**. Dispersion via neck and arm apertures still occurs, and therefore Gore-Tex suits with seals at the neck and arms must be worn. However, such garments tend to be uncomfortable during prolonged procedures.

Disposable non-woven clothing

This is the most common type of surgical gown used in joint arthroplasty. These fabrics, e.g. spun laced fibres, are **unwoven** and appear microscopically as a random mat. Bacteria tend to get entrapped within the fibres. Because of its open structure, air circulation is not impeded. Unfortunately, these gowns are single-use only and therefore are expensive, although the overall cost may be beneficial when compared with reusable cotton gowns.

Body exhaust systems

These work by maintaining a **negative pressure** within the gown, which prevents the admission of bacteria-carrying particles by the wearer. In Charnley's all-enveloping gown and mask, air is drawn off at the helmet by a body exhaust unit. As the gown–helmet system is impermeable, air is drawn in around the operator's legs and passes over the body, cooling the operator. Operators communicate via a special audio system. Disadvantages include feelings of claustrophobia and inability to use microscopes. A variation in the Charnley body exhaust system is the **neck lace** and **mandarin gown**, which exclude the head of the operator. This system works on the basis that 90% of bacteria-carrying particles are admitted below neck level.

Clinical effects of clothing

The MRC trial showed a 50% reduction in deep joint sepsis in operations performed in ultra-clean-air theatres. A further 25% reduction was achieved by combining ultra-clean operating theatres with body exhaust systems. The lowest incidence of all (0.06%) was achieved using ultra-clean air, body exhaust systems and antibiotics. The effects of these variables were found to be independent and cumulative.

Skin preparation and surgical drapes

Skin antisepsis

Antiseptics are disinfectants used in living tissue. Their use results in a reduction in the number of viable organisms but not the complete destruction of all viable micro-organisms; unlike the process of sterilization, some viruses and bacterial spores may remain. Three solutions are commonly used for hand washing and skin antisepsis prior to surgery:

- **Iodophors**: iodine complexed with solubilizing agent, such as povidone, resulting in free iodine release when in solution. They are **potent, broad-spectrum and rapid-acting** bactericidal agents, also active against spores, fungi and viruses, but **inactivated by blood, faeces and pus**. They work through the destruction of microbial proteins and deoxyribonucleic acid (DNA). They may be irritant and cause hypersensitivity reactions. In aqueous form, they are safe on open wounds and mucous membranes.
- **Alcohols**: used in 70% concentration, **rapidly active** against a **broad spectrum** of gram-negative and gram-positive bacteria. They have some antiviral activity but are relatively inactive against spores and fungi. They work by evaporation and protein denaturation, but have no residual activity. Use on open wounds and mucous membranes is contraindicated.
- **Chlorhexidine**: a **bisbiguanide** compound with bactericidal and bacteriostatic activity against a **broad spectrum** of gram-positive and gram-negative bacteria, fungi, and lipophilic viruses. It acts through membrane disruption. It is deactivated by many **topical skin products, cleansers and hand sanitizers**; it is active in the presence of blood, soap and pus, but its effectiveness may be reduced. Use on mucous membranes or in body cavities is contraindicated. *Pseudomonas* may grow in stored contaminated solutions.

Both iodophors and chlorhexidine can be used in either aqueous or alcoholic solutions. Alcoholic solutions provide rapid acting, broad-spectrum, durable skin antisepsis but cannot be used on open wounds, delicate skin or mucous membranes, and have the disadvantage of being flammable; alcoholic solutions must be dry before continuing, and pooling must not be allowed to occur. The optimal contact time for skin antisepsis is not known. There is no evidence that a scrub longer than 2 minutes offers any additional benefit. Equally, the evidence for iodophors versus chlorhexidine is equivocal, but alcoholic solutions are preferred for patient skin preparation whenever possible. For hand washing, the UK National Institute for Health and Care Excellence (NICE) recommends the use of iodophor or chlorhexidine antiseptic solution prior to the first case, but alcoholic hand rubs alone are sufficient between subsequent cases, provided the hands are not visibly soiled.

The use of brushes and razors disrupts the deep skin flora and may increase infection rates. **Brushes** should only be used on the nails **when hand washing prior to the first case**. They should not be used between subsequent cases unless the nails are visibly soiled. If the patient needs to be **shaved** then this should be performed **immediately prior to surgery** and **electrical clippers** with a fresh blade should be used. Hair removal is important prior to the use of alcoholic skin antiseptics since thick hair may prevent adequate evaporation of the alcohol, rendering it less effective and posing a combustion risk.

Surgical drapes

Skin preparation with antiseptics is augmented by the use of isolation drapes, of which there are three types:

- **Body drapes**: disposable non-woven drapes are preferred in theory to traditional cotton fabrics, for the reasons given in the previous section.
- **Incisional drapes**: these have been adopted widely, chiefly in order to hold down the surgical drapes. There is no evidence that their use reduces the rate of wound infection. If incisional drapes are employed, then it is important that they remain adherent to the wound edge throughout the operation. NICE guidance on surgical site infection recommends that if incisional drapes are to be used then they should be **iodophor-impregnated**, unless the patient is allergic to iodine; it advises against the use of non-iodophor-impregnated incisional drapes as they may increase the risk of surgical site infection.
- **Wound-edge drapes**: these cover the incised wound. Bacteria persisting in the wound edge may lead to subsequent wound contamination. These drapes are not currently used in orthopaedics.

Masks and gloves

Masks

Micro-organisms liberated from the upper respiratory tract of theatre personnel may contaminate theatre air. The level of air contamination caused, however, is low compared with that produced from the skin of the same individual. Even so, **all members of the surgical team** must wear masks when operating on trauma and orthopaedic cases. The main purpose is to protect the wound from direct contamination and, in particular, the projectile effects of talking and breathing. Masks should be **changed after each operation**, as they are easily contaminated. There is no evidence to suggest that there is any need for non-scrubbed personnel to wear masks if they are not in the operating area, but the British Orthopaedic Association (BOA) guidelines recommend that all theatre personnel wear masks during orthopaedic operations.

Gloves

Gloves are worn to **protect the surgical wound** from contamination by any residual bacteria remaining after the surgical scrub. They also function to **protect the surgeon** from haematogenous spread of viral disease. **Glove perforation** during orthopaedic procedures has been recorded to be as high as 40%. **Surface colonization** of gloves during joint arthroplasty has also been noted. For these reasons, **double gloving** together with the changing of top gloves before implant handling is advocated, and is recommended by NICE for arthroplasty surgery. The use of **dark undergloves** improves the detection of glove perforation. In addition, there is a significant incidence of contamination of glove tips at the end of skin preparation. Gloves should, therefore, be changed before making the skin incision, or the incision site must be prepared separately, before draping the patient.

Surgical gloves can be made from **natural rubber latex** or **synthetic materials**. Latex gloves have the advantage that they provide an excellent barrier to infection whilst offering great comfort, natural tactile properties and high resistance to tears or punctures. Synthetic gloves do not contain latex but generally have inferior physical characteristics and are more expensive than latex. Some of the common glove materials and their properties are shown in *Table 29.2*.

The principal advantage of synthetic gloves is the absence of latex protein found in natural rubber. Latex can provoke a **type I**, immunoglobulin E (IgE)-mediated, immediate systemic **hypersensitivity** reaction that can be life threatening. In addition, chemicals used in the manufacturing process of latex or synthetic gloves can cause a **type IV**, T-cell mediated, delayed localized dermatitis. Type IV reactions are more common, reported in up to 17% of healthcare workers in some series. UK estimates of latex allergy amongst healthcare workers are around 1%. Onset of symptoms may be preceded by months or even years of symptom-free exposure. Symptoms often become increasingly severe with repeated exposure, so sensitized individuals must seek occupational health advice and avoid further contact with the allergen. Additionally, those with type I reactions may wear a Medic-alert bracelet and carry an Epi-pen.

Table 29.2 Properties of common surgical glove materials

Material	Advantages	Disadvantages
Natural rubber latex	Effective barrier against infection Excellent sensitivity, elasticity and comfort Strong and durable	Can be highly allergenic in susceptible individuals Hydrocarbon-based emollients weaken the rubber
Polychloroprene (Neoprene)	Latex free High strength	Lower level of elasticity and comfort than latex More expensive than latex
Nitrile	Excellent strength and chemical protection	Poor elasticity, comfort and softness, but can be mixed with latex to improve these properties
Polyisoprene	Latex free Excellent elasticity, sensitivity, comfort and strength, similar to latex	Very expensive
Polyurethane	Latex free Excellent strength Reasonable sensitivity, elasticity and comfort	Expensive

Patients with known latex allergy should, whenever possible, be first on an operating list. All latex containing equipment should be removed from the theatre (or covered, where removal is not possible) and all remaining equipment is washed with a mild detergent to clear any possible contamination. The theatre is subsequently rested for a minimum of 30 minutes for plenum theatres, or 15 minutes for laminar flow theatres, to allow sufficient air changes to remove all airborne protein. Notices are positioned to warn all staff in the vicinity.

Non-allergic irritant contact dermatitis may be caused by direct mechanical disruption of the skin due to **rubbing** of the gloves themselves, **chemicals** used in their manufacture, **powder** or **sweat**. Cornstarch powder added to gloves to ease donning is a direct irritant and can also **bind to latex protein**, enabling the **allergen to become airborne** and be **inhaled**, which can cause a hypersensitivity reaction in susceptible individuals even without direct contact. For these reasons many gloves are now manufactured to be easily donned without the need for powder; powdered gloves are rarely found in current practice. Hand washing after gloves are removed, and regular use of moisturizers, can help to reduce irritation. The use of gloves with moisturizers included in their manufacture can also help.

Antibiotic prophylaxis

The use of prophylactic antibiotics may be the single most important factor in the prevention of deep infection following lower limb arthroplasty (see *Table 29.1*). Antibiotics may be administered systemically, or locally in cement.

Systemic antibiotics

There is insufficient evidence of a significant difference in the efficacy of cephalosporins, teicoplanin or penicillins, though cephalosporins have been associated with *Clostridium difficile* colitis, especially in the elderly. Systemic antibiotic prophylaxis should be given **on induction of anaesthesia**, and **at least 5 minutes before the inflation of a tourniquet**. Infection rates have been shown to be lowest in patients receiving antibiotics within 2 hours of the incision, and there is **no difference between 1- and 3-day courses**. NICE recommends a single dose of antibiotic at the start of anaesthesia for all clean surgery involving placement of a prosthesis or implant, with a repeat dose when the operation is longer than the half-life of the antibiotic; local policy should be followed when choosing a specific antibiotic regimen.

Antibiotic-loaded bone cement

Antibiotic delivery in PMMA cement allows a high local concentration to be achieved without a significant rise in systemic concentration and, therefore, reduced side-effects and toxicity. Suitable antibiotics should be **heat stable**, predictably **eluted from the cement**, **active** against relevant organisms, have **low toxicity and incidence of allergy** and **not detrimental to the physical properties of the cement**. Those commonly used include gentamicin or tobramycin, clindamycin, vancomycin and cephalosporins. Antibiotic-loaded cement is commercially available, or the antibiotic can be mixed in theatre. Mechanical strength of the cement may be reduced by higher doses of antibiotic (>2.5 g antibiotic per 40 g cement), liquid (rather than powder) forms of the antibiotic, and by inhomogeneous mixing of the antibiotic with the cement by hand in theatre, which may also reduce working time. Such effects should not be relevant when using vacuum mixed commercially prepared antibiotic-loaded cement, but may occur when the antibiotic is added in theatre. Only about 10% of the antibiotic is actually eluted from the cement, and the elution rate decreases exponentially after the first day, over approximately 6–8 weeks. In cases where antibiotic concentration is more important than cement strength, as in spacer implantation for a staged revision of infected arthroplasty, then non-vacuum, hand mixing of a high dose of antibiotic in theatre is preferable as this increases antibiotic elution, albeit at the expense of cement strength. Combining different antibiotics also improves elution.

Use of antibiotic-loaded bone cement has not been universally adopted in primary arthroplasty due to concerns over its **mechanical properties, toxicity, allergic reactions, cost,** and the **development of resistant bacterial strains**. Systemic toxicity and allergic reactions have not yet been reported with the use of antibiotic-loaded bone cement. Data from the Norwegian and Swedish registries have shown the use of both antibiotic-loaded cement and systemic antibiotics together to be more effective in preventing deep hip infection than either alone. Moreover, gentamicin-loaded cement was found to be associated with the lowest revision rates after total hip arthroplasty, and consequently cost-effective.

Prevention of cross-infection

Local policies should be observed when dealing with patients who pose a known or suspected risk of cross-infection. Between all cases, the **floor** and any surface that has come into **direct contact** with the patient should be **decontaminated with detergent**. Contamination with blood or bodily fluids should be dealt with promptly with detergent for small spills, or chlorine-releasing agents for larger spills. **Personal protective equipment** should be used by staff in all cases.

Patients with known or suspected infection, including **methicillin-resistant** *Staphylococcus aureus* (MRSA) colonization, should be placed last on the list and recovered in theatre, or an area well away from other patients, wherever possible. Equipment and staff in theatre should be kept to a minimum. Normal hand washing procedures may be followed and there is no need to change non-sterile theatre clothing between cases, unless it is contaminated with bodily fluids. A terminal clean of all surfaces, fixtures and equipment is undertaken with detergent and chlorine-releasing agents after all infected cases; the theatre is ready to use again once all surfaces are dry, except following known or suspected transmissible spongiform encephalopathies (TSEs), in which case repeated wetting with detergent throughout a 1 hour exposure period is required. Specimens from patients with known or suspected blood-borne viral infection, tuberculosis (TB) or TSE must be labelled as posing an infection risk. The handling of used instruments also requires consideration. Those used in patients with a known or suspected blood-borne viral infection must be sealed and labelled as posing an infection risk before being sent to the sterile services department. In patients with a known TSE the instruments should be single use and incinerated after exposure. If TSE is suspected, then instruments should be quarantined until the diagnosis is confirmed or excluded; if the diagnosis is confirmed then the instruments should be incinerated.

General theatre equipment

The following is a discussion of the basic science, safe use and function of some of the general equipment commonly employed during orthopaedic operations.

Diathermy

Diathermy works through the passage of high frequency alternating current (AC) through body tissue at high local current density to generate temperatures of up to 1000°C. Neuromuscular tissue is not stimulated at AC frequencies above 50 kHz; diathermy uses frequencies of **400 kHz to 10 MHz**, at which currents of up to 500 mA are safely passed.

Monopolar diathermy

A high power unit (400 W) generates high frequency current that passes through the **active electrode** held by the surgeon, through the body and returns through the patient **plate electrode**. The plate must have a contact surface area of at least **70 cm²** and is placed on dry, shaved, well vascularized skin away from bony prominences, scar tissue and metallic implants to promote heat dissipation and avoid burns. In **cutting mode** the output is continuous and low voltage, causing high local temperatures to vaporize water and cause tissue destruction. In **coagulation mode** the output is pulsed; lower temperatures are generated leading to desiccation of tissue, denaturing of protein and vessel coagulation, with minimal tissue disruption.

Bipolar diathermy

A lower power unit (50 W) passes current between the **two limbs of the diathermy forceps** held by the surgeon. There is no plate electrode, and the current passes only through the tissue within the forceps. Bipolar diathermy is inherently safer due to the local nature of the current, and is used in extremities where high current densities passing to a plate electrode may cause ischaemic damage. Only **coagulation mode** is possible, however, and it is not possible to use the diathermy to 'buzz' other instruments.

Diathermy safety

Causes of diathermy burns include:

- Incorrect plate electrode placement.
- Patient touching earthed metal objects – most modern machines do not have an earthed reference electrode so this is only really a problem with older machines.
- Combustion of inflammable agents – pooling of spirit-based skin prep, or inflammable gases.

Additionally, the active electrode should be in contact with the target tissue and in view, and the lowest practicable power setting should be selected to avoid inadvertent injury to adjacent tissues. Monopolar diathermy must not be used on pedicles due to the risk of distal ischaemic injury. Diathermy may interfere with pacemaker function or cause cardiac burns; bipolar is preferred, with careful electrocardiography (ECG) monitoring, or if monopolar is essential the plate electrode should be positioned such that the current does not pass near the heart and only short bursts of less than 2 seconds should be used.

Tourniquets

Tourniquets are used to create a **bloodless field** in which to operate. This aids **visualization** and **improves cementation**. Pneumatic tourniquets are most often used and allow control of the pressure applied. Use of tourniquets can be hazardous, and the **minimum pressure** should be applied for the **minimum length of time** possible. The widest tourniquet possible should be used, and it should be at least half the diameter of the limb to reduce the risk of local pressure complications. When selecting tourniquet length there should be at least 3 inches (7.6 cm) of overlap of the tourniquet ends for sufficient hold, but ideally no more than 6 inches (15.2 cm) to avoid skin wrinkling under the tourniquet and possible local pressure complications related to this. It is applied well away from the operative field over two layers of padding; more layers of padding may reduce pressure transfer to the vessels and negate the effectiveness of the tourniquet. **Contoured tourniquets** can be useful in particularly obese or muscular patients to improve contact area. Systemic antibiotic prophylaxis must be administered at least 5 minutes before cuff inflation.

Prior to cuff inflation the limb is **exsanguinated** with the use of an exsanguinator, Esmarch bandage or by elevation. Accepted tourniquet pressures are **100 mmHg** above systolic blood pressure in the **lower limb** and **50 mmHg** above systolic blood pressure in the **upper limb**. The maximum tourniquet time should be no more than **120 minutes** in the **lower limb**, and **90 minutes** in the **upper limb**. If a longer tourniquet time is required then the tourniquet should be deflated for 10 minutes to allow reperfusion after the maximum time has elapsed. The limb can then be reexsanguinated and the cuff reinflated.

Contraindications to tourniquet use

- High risk of thromboembolic complications.
- Peripheral vascular disease.
- Diabetes.
- Sickle cell disease – the resulting ischaemia may provoke a crisis. Sickle cell trait is a relative contraindication; if a tourniquet is used then care must be taken to ensure optimal oxygenation, hydration and acid–base status throughout.
- Presence of arterio-venous fistula.
- Local anaesthesia – relative contraindication due to patient discomfort.
- Local sepsis is not a contraindication to tourniquet use, but exsanguination should be by elevation rather than the use of a mechanical exsanguinator.

Complications of tourniquet use

- Local:
  - skin injury – **pressure necrosis** often due to a poorly fitting or poorly applied cuff, or **chemical burns** caused by skin prep; skin prep must not be allowed to pool under the tourniquet;
  - neurapraxias;
  - arterial injury or thrombosis.

- Distal:
  - ischaemic injury;
  - thrombosis – deep vein thrombosis (DVT) or arterial thrombosis;
  - post-tourniquet syndrome – ischaemia and reperfusion injury leading to oedema, pallor, stiffness, weakness without paralysis and subjective numbness;
  - haemorrhage – intraoperative due to inadequate tourniquet pressure leading to venous congestion without complete arterial occlusion, or post-operative due to unrecognized vessel injury after tourniquet deflation;
  - compartment syndrome.
- Systemic:
  - haemodynamic effects – elevated blood pressure at inflation, and decreased blood pressure at deflation;
  - metabolic effects – hypoxia, hypercarbia, acidosis, hyperkalaemia, rhabdomyolysis and myoglobinuria can occur after tourniquet deflation, particularly after prolonged use;
  - hypercoagulability;
  - pulmonary embolus.

Due to the haemodynamic and metabolic effects it is important to inform the anaesthetist when the tourniquet is being inflated and deflated. Systemic complications are more common with bilateral tourniquet use, and deflation in particular should be staggered by 30–45 minutes where possible.

Autologous blood transfusion systems

The transfusion of autologous blood has gained popularity for its potential to reduce the risks associated with allogeneic blood transfusion. In addition to transfusion of pre-donated blood, systems exist for the reinfusion of blood salvaged from surgery either intra- or post-operatively. There are three general types of salvage procedure:

- **Washed cell salvage processors**.
- **Direct transfusion** – for reinfusion of blood from extracorporeal circuits.
- **Ultrafiltration of whole blood** – does not remove all potentially harmful contaminants, unlike cell processors, but does have the advantage of reinfusion of all blood elements including platelets and clotting proteins.

Washed cell processing systems use a double lumen suction tube attached to the surgical suction device or post-operative drain to **aspirate fluid and mix it with anticoagulant**. The fluid is collected in a sterile reservoir before being separated in a **centrifuge**. The separated red cells are then washed to remove residual damaged cell stroma, free haemoglobin, plasma and plasma proteins, platelets and white cells. Washed red cells are then transferred to the reinfusion bag for autotransfusion within **4 hours of washing**. Processed red cells have a good safety profile but the removal of platelets and coagulation factors can promote a coagulopathy if reinfused in large volumes.

During intraoperative cell salvage, suction of blood should be from pooled blood with the suction tip held below the air–blood interface, and suction tip obstruction should be avoided to reduce haemolysis of the red cells. Autotransfusion is **contraindicated in the case of sepsis or malignancy**. Cell salvage should not be used while topical antibiotics are present because they are typically not plasma bound and consequently not removed during the wash phase; they can be concentrated to the point of toxicity. Similarly, cell salvage should not be used with topical coagulant products or with bone cement before it has set; standard suction should be employed until the coagulant has been washed out of the wound or the cement has set, after which cell salvage can be resumed.

A recent meta-analysis found that post-operative autologous transfusion after hip and knee arthroplasty significantly reduced the need for **allogeneic transfusion, length of hospital stay and cost of hospitalization**. Furthermore, although **Jehovah's Witnesses** may refuse to accept allogeneic or pre-donated autologous transfusion, the process of autotransfusion may be accepted if explained, and the circuit can be modified to provide continuous contact of the blood with the body if required.

Mechanical thromboprophylaxis

Patients assessed as being at increased risk of venous thromboembolism should be offered thromboprophylaxis. Mechanical devices can **reduce thrombosis risk without increasing the risk of bleeding** and include:

- **Graduated compression stockings**.
- **Intermittent pneumatic compression devices** – foot, calf or thigh pumps.
- **Electrical muscle stimulation devices**.

All such devices work by reducing venous stasis and have been shown to reduce thromboembolic complications when used alone or in combination with chemical thromboprophylaxis. No difference has been demonstrated between the levels of compression and their efficacy, or between uniform versus sequential compression. They must be measured and fitted correctly, ensuring the compression/stimulation is applied to the muscles to promote venous return. Caution must be exercised in patients with known or suspected peripheral vascular disease, fragile skin, ulcers, peripheral neuropathy, unusual leg size or shape, oedema, or deformity preventing correct fit and known allergy to any of the materials.

Sutures

Sutures are classified as:

- **Natural** vs. **synthetic**.
- **Monofilament** vs. **braided**.
- **Absorbable** vs. **non-absorbable**.

The ideal suture material would possess the following properties:

- Maintain its **tensile strength** until its purpose is served, and be predictably absorbed if relevant.
- Induce **minimal tissue reaction** (synthetic better than natural, and non-absorbable better than absorbable).
- Sterile and **not encourage bacterial ingrowth** (monofilament better then braided).
- **Handle well**.
- **Knot securely** (braided better than monofilament).
- Not allergenic, carcinogenic, electrolytic or demonstrate capillary action.
- Cheap and readily available.

Examples of some of the commonly used suture materials are shown in *Table 29.3*.

Table 29.3 Suture materials commonly used in orthopaedic surgery

Material	Classification	Notes
Polyglactin	Synthetic, absorbable, braided (Vicryl™) or monofilament (Monocryl™)	Little tissue reaction Hydrolyzed between 56 and 70 days, but provides wound support for only 30 days Vicryl Rapide™ is more rapidly degraded, providing wound support for only 10 days
Polydioxanone (PDS™)	Synthetic, absorbable, monofilament	Slowly hydrolyzed over approx. 180 days, providing tissue strength for up to 56 days
Polyamide (Nylon™)	Synthetic, non-absorbable, monofilament (e.g. Ethilon™) or braided	Can be difficult to knot and handle due to memory Minimal tissue reaction and good resistance to infection in monofilament form Loses 15–20% of tensile strength per year
Polyester (Ethibond™ or TiCron™)	Synthetic, non-absorbable, braided	May be coated to reduce tissue trauma Minimal tissue reaction, high tensile strength and good handling
Polypropylene (Prolene™)	Synthetic, absorbable, monofilament	Can be difficult to knot and handle due to memory Minimal tissue reaction and good resistance to infection Slides excellently causing minimal tissue damage Inadvertent crushing will reduce tensile strength by 90%

Suture **strength** depends on the **material** and **diameter**. Suture size nomenclature developed historically from the limitations of early manufacturing techniques. As such, there is no simple arithmetic conversion to metric diameters; the relationship between designated size and actual diameter also varies between suture classes, but can be found on standard tables if required.

Sutures may additionally be **dyed** or **undyed**. Dyed sutures have the advantage of improved visibility, but can lead to tattooing so should not be used superficially in the skin.

Skin clips are usually stainless steel, with implications for metal allergies and magnetic resonance imaging (MRI). They have not been shown to offer any particular advantage over sutures in terms of healing, but are faster and more consistent to use.

Suture needles

Most suture needles are now pre-swaged, i.e. the suture is already attached to the needle with no need to thread the suture through an eye by hand. This is safer for staff and causes less tissue damage during use. Suture needles are described by the following characteristics:

- **Shape**:
    - straight;
    - curved – described as the proportion of the circumference of a circle;
    - special – e.g. 'J'-shaped, for deep sutures with difficult access, or compound curves.
- **Size**.
- **Tip**:
    - cutting – triangular cross-section, with apex on the concave surface, used in tough tissues such as skin;
    - tapered;
    - blunt.
- **Body**:
    - cutting;
    - reverse cutting – apex of triangular cross-section is on the convex side of the needle to reduce tissue cut-out;
    - round.

Image intensifier

The fluoroscopy system used in theatre is composed of a **C-arm** with an **X-ray tube** at one end and the cylindrical receiver, or **image intensifier** (II), at the other (**Figure 29.6**). The receiver consists of a photocathode that captures the X-ray energy and converts it into light, then detected by a closed-circuit video system to produce the image on screen. There are three basic parameters that can be varied by the X-ray generator:

- **X-ray tube current** (mA) controls the **quantity** of X-rays produced and therefore exposure.
- **X-ray tube voltage** (kV) controls the **energy and penetration** of the X-rays produced. Increasing the voltage reduces the dose required but also reduces contrast, and should therefore be optimized for the procedure being performed.
- **Duration of exposure** – the '**beam-on-time**'. The generator is activated for as long as the switch is depressed. Radiation exposure is directly proportional to the length of time the unit is activated.

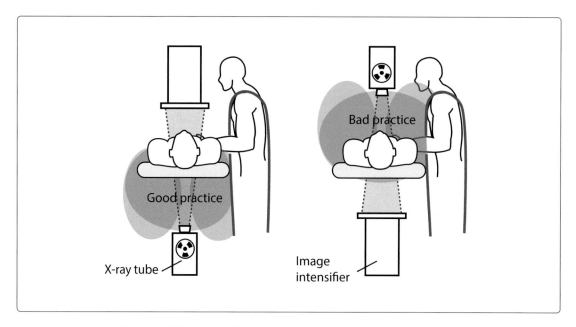

Figure 29.6 Fluoroscopy C-arm showing scatter relative to tube position.

Modern systems incorporate an **automatic brightness control** whereby the X-ray intensity at the II is constantly monitored and controls the current and/or voltage. This allows panning across different tissues and body parts, but may impair image quality when materials with large differences in radiodensity are present in the same field. **Image magnification** is achieved by electronic expansion of a small II input area over a larger II output area; the result is a reduction in image brightness and consequently an automatic compensatory increase in radiation production and exposure. **Collimation**, or **coning**, employs lead shutters to reduce the field size. This has the advantages of reducing irradiated tissue, reducing scatter and therefore image noise and degradation, and improving image quality.

The **damaging effects** of radiation depend on **dose received, rate of exposure, tissues exposed** and **age**. Highly metabolically active, rapidly dividing, undifferentiated cells are the most susceptible, such as the **haemopoietic** and **lymphoid tissues, gonads** and **intestines**. Skin and other epithelial-lined tissues, including the cornea, are also sensitive, while mature bone, muscle and neural tissue are the least sensitive. The **developing embryo is highly susceptible** so pregnancy status must be checked and radiation exposure must be avoided wherever possible. **Stochastic** effects are those occurring by chance, the probability increasing with exposure, such as **late carcinogenesis, genetic effects** and **cataracts. Non-stochastic** effects, on the other hand, occur acutely and predictably after exposure exceeding a definite threshold dose, which is usually very high and delivered over a short period of time. Such effects include **burns, hair loss, sterility, cataracts, bone marrow ablation, central nervous system (CNS) disruption** and **death**.

In order to reduce the risk of potentially harmful effects of fluoroscopy, efforts must be made to keep exposure **as low as reasonably achievable**. No part of the operator's body should be in the primary beam, therefore exposure is primarily from scatter of the beam from the patient, and less from constant leakage of radiation from the X-ray tube. Exposure can be minimized in the following ways:

- Keep **total beam-on-time to a minimum**.
- **Positioning** – **scatter is highest on the X-ray tube side of the patient** (**Figure 29.6**), and decreases with distance from the patient according to the inverse square law, to be negligible by a distance of 2 m:
  - stand as far away from the patient as possible;
  - X-ray tube positioned underneath the table, or on the opposite side of the table from the operator for lateral and oblique views;
  - the machine positioned as close to the patient as possible – reducing the air gap between the II and patient will decrease scatter, and, through the automatic brightness control, decrease dose of radiation delivered while image quality is improved. Increasing the patient–II gap will increase image size but reduce its quality, and brings the X-ray tube closer to the patient, increasing patient exposure.
- **Reduce the use of magnification**.
- **Use collimation**.
- **Shielding** – can reduce exposure by over 90%, though this will be less at higher voltages. It is most effective when placed close to the patient, though this is often impractical in the theatre situation so **personal protective equipment** is used instead:
  - lead apron – should be 0.5 mm lead equivalent and required by all staff within 2 m;
  - thyroid shields;
  - optically clear wrap-around lead glasses – threshold for cataract development is high, so only recommended if very high fluoroscopy workload;
  - leaded gloves – offer relatively little protection and compromise tactility and comfort, so not generally used. Hands should be kept out of the X-ray beam.

WHO Surgical Safety Checklist

In June 2008 the World Health Organization (WHO) launched its 'Safe Surgery Saves Lives' Global Patient Safety Challenge. The Surgical Safety Checklist is part of this initiative. It should be completed for every patient undergoing a surgical procedure, and be entered in the patient notes or electronic record by a registered member of the team. It is designed to reduce the number of errors and complications resulting from surgical procedures by improving team communication and by verifying and checking essential care interventions. The checklist is performed in three stages:

Sign in

Prior to the induction of anaesthesia:

- Patient confirms his/her **identity, site, procedure and consent**.
- Check the **surgical site** is marked.
- Confirm **anaesthetic safety check** is completed.

- Confirm presence or absence of known **allergies**.
- Check if **airway difficulties** or **aspiration risk** is anticipated.
- Check if **>500 mL blood loss (>7 mL/kg in children)** is anticipated.

Time out

Immediately prior to the start of surgery:

- Confirm all team members have **introduced** themselves by name and role.
- Check **patient identity, site and procedure**.
- Anticipated **critical events**:
  - surgical – including anticipated blood loss and specific equipment requirements;
  - anaesthetic – including American Society of Anesthesiologists (ASA) grade and monitoring or other support required.
- **Sterility** of instruments and any other **equipment issues** is confirmed.
- **Antibiotic prophylaxis** is given.
- Patient **warming** is in place.
- **Hair removal** is performed if required.
- **Glycaemic control** is in place.
- Check venous **thromboembolism prophylaxis** is in place.
- Ensure essential **imaging** is displayed.

Sign out

Before any team member leaves the theatre:

- **Procedure performed** is confirmed and recorded.
- Correct instruments, swabs, and sharps counts is **verified**.
- Ensure all **specimens are labelled** correctly.
- **Equipment problems** are identified.
- Key **anaesthetic and surgical concerns** for the recovery and further care of the patient are identified.

The checklist may be adapted through local clinical governance arrangements to support local or specialty specific practice.

Though not integral to the WHO Surgical Safety Checklist, a **team briefing** and **debriefing** are considered good practice and, together with the three stages of the checklist, complete the National Patient Safety Agency's 'five steps to safer surgery'. The team briefing is usually performed before the start of the list, and is an opportunity for all team members to introduce themselves and to discuss the list as a whole, including a discussion about each patient and any anticipated problems or challenges. The debrief is undertaken at the end of the list as an opportunity to discuss any issues that have arisen, for example equipment problems.

Viva questions

1. What is the layout of an operating theatre department?
2. What are the main sources of infection in an operating theatre environment?
3. What different types of ventilatory system are used in theatres?
4. What factors can be altered in operating theatres in order to help reduce the incidence of deep joint sepsis following joint arthroplasty?
5. What is moist bacterial strike-through? How can it be prevented?

Further reading

British Orthopaedic Association. *British Orthopaedic Association Recommendation on Sterile Procedures in Operating Theatres.* London: British Orthopaedic Association, 1995. www.boa.ac.uk.

Charnley J. Postoperative infection after total hip replacement with special reference to air contamination in the operating room. *Clin Orthop Relat Res* 1972;**87**:167–87.

Howorth FH. Air flow patterns in the operating theatre. *Eng Med* 1980;9:87–92.

Johnson R, Jameson SS, Sanders RD, *et al*. Reducing surgical site infection in arthroplasty of the lower limb. A multi-disciplinary approach. *Bone Joint Res* 2013;**2**:58–65.

Lidwell OM, Lowbury EJ, Whyte W, *et al*. Effect of ultraclean air in operating rooms on deep sepsis in the joint after total hip or knee replacement: a randomised study. *Br Med J (Clin Res Ed)* 1982;**285**:10–14.

National Institute for Health and Care Excellence. Clinical Guideline 74: Surgical Site Infection. NICE, 2008. www.nice.org.uk/nicemedia/live/11743/42378/42378.pdf.

National Patient Safety Agency. Alert: NPSA/2009/PSA002/U1 WHO Surgical Safety Checklist. Supporting Information. NPSA, 2009. www.nrls.npsa.nhs.uk.

Salvati EA, Robinson RP, Zeno SM, *et al*. Infection rates after 3175 total hip and total knee replacements performed with and without a horizontal unidirectional filtered air-flow system. *J Bone Joint Surg Am* 1982;**64**:525–35.

30 | Basic Science of Osteoarthritis

Chethan Jayadev and Andrew Price

Introduction

Osteoarthritis (OA) is the most common musculoskeletal disorder affecting over 8 million people in the UK. Its prevalence increases with age. OA is uncommon in people under the age of 40 years, but is seen in up to 80% of people over 75 years. It causes considerable pain, disability and psychological distress to individuals and places a significant socio-economic burden on healthcare providers and government resources. In this chapter, we review the pathophysiology and biological treatment of OA.

Definition

OA is a complex degenerative disorder of the entire synovial joint characterized by progressive loss of articular cartilage and subchondral bone remodelling.

OA primarily involves the knee, hip, hand, spine and foot. The wrists, shoulders and ankles are less frequently affected. The clinical features of OA include joint pain, tenderness, limited movement, crepitus, occasional effusion, deformity and variable degrees of low-grade inflammation without systemic effects.

The classic radiographic features of OA are:

- Loss of joint space.
- Osteophyte formation.
- Subchondral sclerosis.
- Subchondral cysts.

Additional features may include loose bodies, ankylosis, deformity and subluxation. **Figure 30.1** depicts the pathological features of OA.

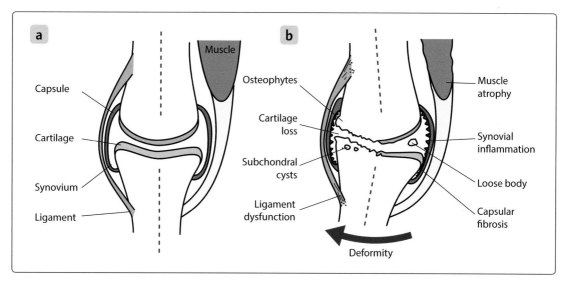

Figure 30.1 Pathological features of osteoarthritis. a: A normal synovial joint; b: an osteoarthritic joint.

Aetiology and classification

OA occurs in normal joints experiencing abnormal loads or abnormal joints experiencing normal loads. OA can be classified according to underlying cause:

- **Primary (idiopathic) OA** by definition has no identifiable cause and is the most common form. Risk factors include advancing age, genetic predisposition, female gender (menopause), obesity and abnormal joint loading.
- **Secondary OA** develops as a result of an antecedent joint condition or systemic disorder. These include trauma, infection and a number of hereditary, developmental, metabolic, endocrine and neurological conditions (*Table 30.1*).

The distinctions between primary and secondary OA have become increasingly blurred. OA represents a heterogeneous spectrum of disorders initiated by multiple factors with a final common pathway. OA is also commonly classified according to the distribution of joint involvement, being either localized (mono-articular or oligo-articular) or generalized (poly-articular).

Pathogenesis

OA is a mechanically driven but biologically-mediated process that is modulated by genetic and acquired risk factors (**Figure 30.2**).

Mechanical and biological events **disrupt the normal equilibrium** between **degradation and synthesis of articular cartilage and subchondral bone**. The loss of homeostasis results in both the biological and biomechanical failure of the entire synovial joint.

Table 30.1 Causes of secondary osteoarthritis (OA)

Trauma	Infection
Acute joint trauma	Septic arthritis
Intra-articular fracture	
Chronic occupational/recreational overuse	
Meniscectomy	

Instability	Inflammatory arthritis
Joint dislocation	Rheumatoid arthritis
Ligamentous injuries	Ankylosing spondylitis
Joint hypermobility	Psoriatic arthritis
Ehlers–Danlos' syndrome	Reactive arthritis

Bone and joint disorders	Metabolic and endocrine disorders
Slipped upper femoral epiphysis	Alkaptonuria (ochronosis)
Legg–Calve–Perthes' disease	Haemochromatosis
Blount's disease	Wilsons's disease
Leg length inequality	Gaucher's disease
Osteonecrosis (avascular necrosis)	Acromegaly
Paget's disease	Hyperparathyroidism
Osteochondritis	Hypothyroidism
Osteopetrosis	

Dysplastic and hereditary conditions	Neuropathic disorders (Charcot joint)
Developmental dysplasia of the hip	Diabetes mellitus
Multiple epiphyseal dysplasia	Tabes dorsalis
Chondrodysplasias	Leprosy
Stickler's syndrome	Syringomyelia
	Meningomyelocele

Crystal deposition disorders	Bleeding disorders
Gout	Haemophilia
Calcium pyrophosphate deposition	Von Willebrandt's disease
Basic calcium phosphate	(recurrent haemarthrosis)
Oxalate deposition (dialysis)	

Haemoglobinopathies	Miscellaneous
Sickle cell disease	Kashin–Beck disease
Thalassemia	

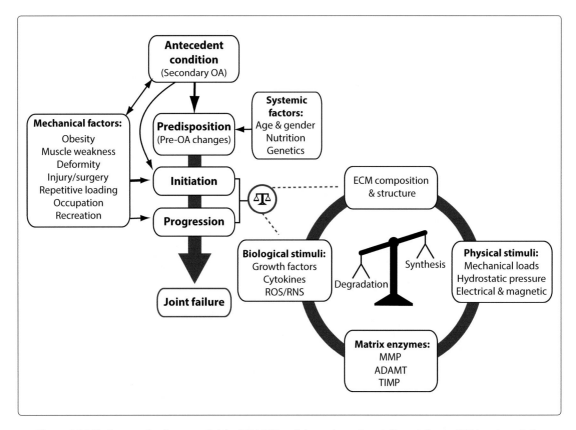

Figure 30.2 Pathogenesis of osteoarthritis. ADAMT: a disintegrin and metalloproteinase; ECM: extracellular matrix; MMP: matrix metalloproteinase; RNS: reactive nitrogen species; ROS: reactive oxygen species; TIMP: tissue inhibitor of matrix metalloproteinase.

OA is not a disease of cartilage alone. All tissues of the synovial joint act in concert to preserve joint homeostasis, integrity and function. These mechanisms eventually fail, leading to progressive joint deterioration over several years. The initiation and progression of the events that lead to joint failure remain incompletely understood. Studies into the basic science of OA have concentrated on articular cartilage and subchondral bone. We shall therefore focus the chapter on these tissues.

Changes in OA cartilage

Pathological features

The macroscopic changes of articular cartilage in OA are **softening, fibrillation, pitting, erosion (ulceration), delamination** and eventually **denudation** to subchondral bone. This sequence produces the cardinal radiographic feature of progressive joint space narrowing. Indian ink can reveal fibrillation in cartilage with a macroscopically normal appearance.

Microscopic features include (**Figure 30.3**):

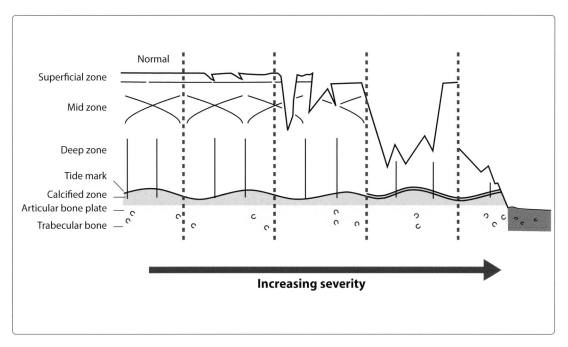

Figure 30.3 Schematic of the microscopic features of osteoarthritic cartilage.

- Reduction in metachromasia when stained for proteoglycan (i.e. toluidine blue, Alcian blue, Safranin-O). This can be observed before any surface changes.
- Vertical fissures and deep horizontal clefts.
- Chondrocyte proliferation (clustering), hypertrophy and death – seen initially in the superficial zone.
- Tidemark irregularities – discontinuities, duplication (advance) and vessel perforation.

Matrix changes

The typical biochemical changes in the extracellular matrix (ECM) are:

Loss of proteoglycans and reduced aggregation

Loss of the large aggregating proteoglycan, aggrecan, is a consistent and early biochemical finding. There is a rapid loss of proteoglycan that progresses with disease severity. This is due to a combination of leaching from the damaged collagen network and enzymatic breakdown. There is a compensatory increase in proteoglycan synthesis by chondrocytes, particularly in early OA. This leads to changes in glycosaminoglycan (GAG) composition: the ratio of chondroitin sulphate to keratan sulphate (KS) is increased, and there is relatively more choindroitin-4 sulphate than chrondroitin-6 sulphate. As OA progresses, the proteoglycan chain lengths are shorter. Aggregation is reduced due to proteolytic activity at the hyaluronic acid binding region of the core protein.

Reduced quality and integrity of the collagen network

The ultrastructure and organization of the type II collagen mesh is significantly disturbed. Fibre size and orientation become variable and disordered. Cross-linking is reduced. The content of collagen is maintained in early OA by an increase in synthesis by chondrocytes. In the later stages there is a reduction in both quality and content, but the relatively greater loss of proteoglycan means the tissue concentration of collagen is effectively increased. The relative content of minor collagens such type I, III, VI and X can increase with OA progression.

Increase in water content

An increase in water content is one of the earliest detectable changes in OA, albeit by only a few per cent over normal cartilage. OA cartilage always swells (gains water) despite the loss in proteoglycan. This is due to the increased porosity of the weakened type II collagen meshwork. The collagen network is less able to resist the swelling pressure of the existing proteoglycans.

ECM changes predominantly occur in the interterritorial matrix and start in the superficial zone, extending deeper with progression. These changes are summarized in **Figure 30.4.**

Biomechanical changes

The biochemical and structural alterations in the matrix of OA cartilage result in inferior mechanical properties compared to normal articular cartilage. In particular, resistance to compression (bulk modulus) is reduced and there is failure of load bearing function.

The inferior quality of the type II collagen network results in reduced tensile stiffness and strength of the solid matrix. Disruption of the solid matrix leads to increased water content (porosity) and a significant increase in permeability. Consequently, there is a loss of interstitial fluid pressurization that normally provides a significant component of the load support in compression. Load support shifts more to the solid matrix, predisposing to further damage and cartilage degeneration by fatigue wear. The increase in permeability also allows loss of lubricant leading to greater interfacial wear.

Cellular and molecular mechanisms

Chondrocytes

Chondrocytes respond to physical and biological changes in their microenvironment, i.e. mechanical load (static and dynamic), osmotic pressure, matrix composition and soluble mediators (cytokines, growth factors, reactive oxygen species [ROS]).

Chondrocytes in OA cartilage are more metabolically active than those in normal cartilage:

- Increased deoxyribonucleic acid (DNA) synthesis and proliferation.
- Increased proteoglycan and collagen synthesis.
- Increased production of degradative matrix enzymes (see below).
- Chondrocyte death by apoptosis.

The upregulation of both anabolic and catabolic activity is an attempt to repair and remodel the articular cartilage. The tipping of this balance to catabolism subsequently leads to degeneration.

Phenotypic shifts have also been described with production of matrix proteins seen during development, e.g. type IIA pro-collagen, hypertrophy of deep zone chondrocytes with production of type X collagen, matrix metalloproteinase (MMP)-13 and matrix calcification (cf. hypertrophic zone of growth plate).

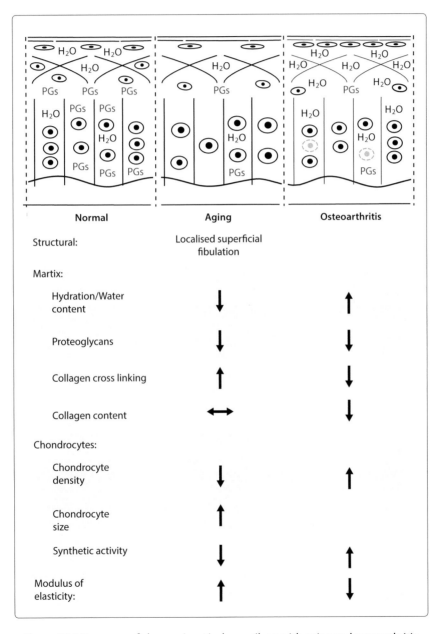

Figure 30.4 Summary of changes in articular cartilage with aging and osteoarthritis.

Matrix enzymes

The MMP and ADAMTS (a disintegrin and metalloproteinase with thrombospondin motif) families of proteolytic enzymes are responsible for matrix degradation in OA. Both are zinc and calcium dependent.

- Proteoglycan is predominantly broken down by aggrecanase (ADAMTS-4, ADAMTS-5) and MMP-3 (stromolysin-1).
- Type II collagen is broken down by MMP-13 (collagenase-3) and MMP-1 (collagenase-1). MMP-13 is the most potent type II collagenase and levels are significantly increased in OA.

Tissue inhibitors of MMPs (TIMPs) attenuate MMP activity. Tissue plasminogen activator/plasmin and cathepsins (B and D) stimulate MMPs in normal cartilage. The expression, release and activity of MMPs and aggrecanase are increased in OA, facilitated by inflammatory cytokines and ROS.

Inflammatory cytokines

Inflammatory cytokines are critical mediators in the disturbed metabolism and enhanced catabolism of OA. Interleukin (IL)-1β seems to be the main pro-catabolic cytokine involved in the pathophysiology of OA, complemented by tumour necrosis factor (TNF)-alpha and IL-6. They enhance the production and activity of MMPs and aggrecanase, and reduce chondrocyte synthesis of proteoglycan and type II collagen. IL-4 and IL-10 are thought to have a chondroprotective function.

These cytokines are produced by chondrocytes and synovial cells (synoviocytes and mononuclear cells), and act in an autocrine/paracrine fashion. They are also produced by inflammatory cells, secondary to bleeding or infection, and can contribute to rapid joint deterioration.

Reactive oxygen species

ROS play an important role in normal cartilage physiology and homeostasis. They include superoxide anions (O_2^-), hydroxyl radicals (OH), nitric oxide (NO) and their derivatives. ROS production is increased by mechanical stress and pro-inflammatory cytokines. Saturation of intrinsic antioxidant mechanisms produces a state of oxidative stress that promotes chondrocyte death, matrix degeneration and further increases pro-inflammatory cytokines.

Growth factors

Anabolic factors attempt to increase collagen and proteoglycan synthesis and attenuate catabolic mechanisms. These factors include bone morphogenetic proteins (BMPs), insulin-like growth factor (IGF)-I, transforming growth factor (TGF)-β and fibroblast growth factor (FGF). However, the chondrocyte response to such factors is eventually diminished by pro-inflammatory cytokines and ROS.

Aging

Advancing age is a strong risk factor for development of OA. Articular cartilage undergoes structural and compositional changes with aging. These features are summarized in *Table 30.2* with comparison to OA. Despite some similarities, aging and OA should not be considered the same process.

Changes in OA subchondral bone

Subchondral sclerosis, bone cysts and osteophytes are cardinal radiographic findings of established OA.

The articular cartilage and peri-articular bone form a functional unit in both health and disease. There is emerging evidence for molecular cross-talk between cartilage and bone that increases during the progression of OA. Subchondral bone changes begin very early in the disease process. They develop and evolve simultaneously with cartilage changes.

Bone remodelling

Increased bone remodelling occurs due to a combination of mechanical loading, micro-fractures and soluble mediators. This is associated with increased vascularity and cellular metabolism. Modification of the trabecular architecture, thickening of the subchondral cortical plate and mineralization lead to **subchondral sclerosis** and **eburnation**. The increase in stiffness reduces the protective shock absorbing capacity of the subchondral bone, predisposing the overlying cartilage to damage from repetitive loading. The remodelling process becomes increasingly abnormal and disordered. The weakened bone undergoes **attrition** and collapse under compression.

Osteophytes

Osteophytes develop at the joint margin adjacent to areas of increased joint loading and may contribute to maintaining joint stability. Their formation is initiated by proliferation of periosteal cells at the joint margin that differentiate into chondrocytes. Subsequent endochondral ossification produces an enlarging bony protrusion. Osteophytes grow in the path of least resistance guided by capsular traction. Mechanical factors, subchondral bone vascularization and local production of TGF-β and BMP-2 are implicated in the pathogenesis of osteophyte formation.

Subchondral cysts

Subchondral bone cysts represent micro-fractures of the subchondral trabecular bone at various stages of healing and remodelling with gelatinous replacement of the marrow. Synovial fluid may also be forced into the degenerating micro-fracture through cartilage fissures and an increasingly permeable solid matrix.

Bone marrow lesions

Bone marrow oedema-like lesions (BMLs) are non-cystic, ill-defined areas of high intensity adjacent to the subchondral bone plate on magnetic resonance imaging (MRI) (T2 or proton density-weighted) images (**Figure 30.5**). BMLs are observed in both early and established OA, and in particular knee OA. They correlate spatially with areas of increased cartilage degeneration, bone remodelling, subchondral cyst formation and subsequent bone attrition.

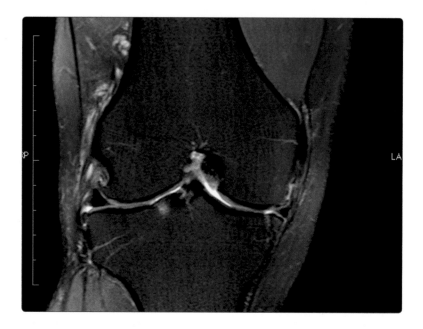

Figure 30.5 Bone marrow oedema-like lesion (BML). Proton density MRI sequence showing a BML under an area of cartilage loss at the junction of the lateral tibial articular surface and tibial spine.

The natural history of BMLs is controversial, but there is evidence that they are predictive for pain and progression in knee OA.

Changes in other tissues

The roles of synovium, muscles and ligaments in OA are probably underestimated and have not been as extensively studied. Other important factors include joint stability, balance and proprioception, which are essential for homeostasis at an organ, tissue and molecular level.

The synovium becomes hyperplastic and there is an increased mononuclear cell infiltrate. It represents a reactive component of the joint capable of generating cytokines in response to intra-articular damage and pathology. There is increasing evidence for the role of synovitis in the pathophysiology of OA and many of the clinical features reflect synovial inflammation (e.g. joint swelling, effusion, stiffness, erythema).

OA is also characterized by **joint capsule fibrosis**, **muscle atrophy** and **ligament dysfunction**.

Biological treatment of OA

The patient's symptoms and the clinical severity are often discordant with their radiographic and biological features. There is no cure for OA and current therapeutic approaches are largely palliative, being targeted at symptomatic relief. The goals of non-surgical therapy are:

- **Protection of the joint** from mechanical overload through weight loss, walking aids and lifestyle modification.

- **Prevention of muscle wasting** and improve **proprioception** through targeted exercise and physiotherapy. Maintaining loading and physiological loading is essential for cartilage nutrition.
- **Analgesia** to relieve pain and facilitate the above.

Arthroplasty is clearly established as a successful intervention for late stage OA in patients in the later stages of life. However, it is not without its risks and some individuals will require revision surgery. We will focus on biological treatments for OA.

Intra-articular glucocorticoid

Intra-articular injection of glucocorticoid for OA provides rapid but short-lived (<4 weeks) improvement in pain and function. Their mode of action is through anti-inflammatory transcriptional regulation. National Institute for Health and Care Excellence (NICE) recommends their use as an adjunct to core treatment for the relief of moderate to severe pain in people with OA.

Most basic science experimental data suggest that glucocorticoids have a detrimental effect on cartilage metabolism, i.e. inhibition of chondrocyte proliferation, decreased collagen and proteoglycan synthesis and impaired response to important to growth factors. However, there is little clinical evidence of these negative effects.

Intra-articular viscosupplementation

Hyaluronic acid (HA) is a high-molecular weight (MW) GAG. It is a critical component of synovial fluid and is required for normal joint homeostasis. In OA, both the concentration and molecular weight of the endogenous HA are decreased, which reduces the viscoelasticity of the synovial fluid.

Intra-articular injection of HA aims to restore the viscoelasticity and augment the flow of synovial fluid. Additional biological effects may include inhibition of degradation and improved synthesis of endogenous HA, effects on cytokine production and function and inhibition of nociception.

The literature supports the therapeutic efficacy and safety of intra-articular HA in knee OA with beneficial effects on pain, function and patient global assessment. The improvement in symptoms has a delayed onset, but prolonged duration (from 5 to 13 weeks post-injection), when compared to intra-articular corticosteroid. The evidence is more limited for hip OA. Studies on intra-articular HA have been subject to publication bias and there remains controversy over their use. Current NICE guidelines do not recommend their use.

Commercially available formulations vary in MW and cross-linking, e.g. Hyalgan™ (low MW), Orthovisc™ (intermediate MW, but lower than normal synovial fluid) and Synvisc™ (high MW and cross-linked). These differences are thought to influence volume and frequency of injections, half-life within the joint and biological activity. However, there are few randomized head-to-head comparisons. It is not possible to draw conclusions regarding the relative value of different products.

Glucosamine and chondroitin

Glucosamine is an amino-monosaccharide that is a component of the GAGs, KS and HA. Chondroitin sulphate is itself a GAG. Consequently, both agents are constituents of articular cartilage proteoglycans. The rationale for glucosamine (hydrochloride or sulphate) and chondroitin sulphate supplementation in OA is that improved substrate availability may increase proteoglycan synthesis. Glucosamine has a better gut absorption than chondroitin sulphate, but both need to be taken in high oral doses.

The *in vitro* and *in vivo* effects of these compounds remain highly controversial, although their safety is rarely disputed. Glucosamine has been more extensively studied. There is evidence from cell culture, explant and animal studies that glucosamine increases proteoglycan synthesis and attenuates IL-1-mediated cartilage catabolism in OA. A recent large network meta-analysis suggests that glucosamine, chondroitin or their combination do not reduce joint pain or have an impact on joint space narrowing in comparison to placebo. Current NICE guidelines do not recommend the use of glucosamine or chondroitin products in OA.

Future prospects

The development of disease-modifying OA drugs (DMOADs) is currently receiving considerable academic and commercial attention. DMOADs aim to retard or halt the progression of biological and structural changes and ideally reverse the balance between degradative and synthetic processes within the joint.

A number of DMOADs are currently in phase II and III clinical trials, but there are a vast number being tested in pre-clinical *in vitro* and animal models. Potential DMOADs include:

- Vitamin D3 (phase II and IV).
- Calcitonin (phase III).
- Inhibitors of inducible nitric oxide synthase (phase II).
- Growth factors, e.g. BMP-7 (phase II) and FGF-18 (phase II).
- Antioxidants, e.g. vitamin C.
- Cytokine inhibitors, e.g. IL-1 inhibitors.
- MMP and aggrecanase inhibitors.
- Doxycycline (inhibits activity of collagenases in animal studies).

There are numerous challenges to DMOAD development: the complex and heterogeneous biological and clinical nature of OA; the lack of suitable biomarkers and sensitivity of radiological endpoints; the poor relationship between biological and structural progression with clinical endpoints; the slow natural history of OA, and the need for long-term follow-up.

Viva questions

1. Define osteoarthritis. What is the fundamental principle in its pathogenesis?

2. Describe the biochemical changes seen in the extracellular matrix of osteoarthritic cartilage.

3. Describe and explain the biomechanical changes in osteoarthritic cartilage.

4. What is an osteophyte? Explain how they form.

5. Outline some of the biological mechanisms involved in the development of osteoarthritis.

Further reading

Abramson SB, Attur M. Developments in the scientific understanding of osteoarthritis. *Arthritis Res Ther* 2009;**11**(3):227.

Arden N, Nevitt MC. Osteoarthritis: epidemiology. *Best Pract Res Clin Rheumatol* 2006;**20**(1):3–25.

Buckwalter JA, Mankin HJ, Grodzinsky AJ. Articular cartilage and osteoarthritis. *Instr Course Lect* 2005;**54**:465–80.

Nuki G. Osteoarthritis: a problem of joint failure. *Zeitschrift Rheum* 1999;**58**(3):142–7.

Pearle AD, Warren RF, Rodeo SA. Basic science of articular cartilage and osteoarthritis. *Clin Sports Med* 2005;**24**(1):1–12.

31 Biomechanics of Fracture Fixation

Nick Aresti, Paul Culpan and Peter Bates

Introduction

Although the principles of biomechanics have been covered previously in chapters 13 and 17, this is the perfect point in this book to revisit them as they apply to fractures and fracture fixation. This chapter aims to bring together all the pertinent concepts that will allow the orthopaedic trainee to approach the common problem of fractures and their management that is seen in everyday practice from a basic scientific point of view.

Forces, moments, stress, strain

Stress

Stress is the measure of force applied to a structure per unit area. In engineering terms, there are two types of stresses: normal and shear. Normal stresses are created when a force acts perpendicular to a plane, and can either be tensile (force acts away from a plane) or compressive (force acts towards a plane). Shear or torsional stresses are generated when a force is directed parallel or oblique to the plane of reference.

Clinical example

The stress that is experienced by a **distal femoral locking plate** can be thought of as the weight a patient puts through the leg, divided by the cross-sectional area of the plate. Note that this **stress is independent of the working length**. It is a common misconception that plating constructs that have long bridging segments (many screw holes left empty over the fracture or a 'long working length') experience less stress when they are loaded, because the force is spread over a greater length of plate. In fact, for a given amount of weight bearing, the force per cross-sectional area is the same regardless how many screw holes are left empty across the fracture. What does change in a long segment bridge plate is the amount of movement (strain) that takes place each time the patient takes a step or moves the leg. The **stress on the plate** is governed purely by the amount of **weight bearing (force)** and the **thickness of the plate (cross-sectional area)**.

Moments

A moment is created when a force is applied to an object some distance away from a pivot point (or fulcrum). When pulling on a cupboard door, force goes through the handle and because the door pivots on its hinges, the door rotates open or closed. As the force applied to the door-knob creates a 'turning effect', it is known as a 'moment' of force. This can be calculated by multiplying the force applied, by its distance from the fulcrum (the lever arm). The greater the force or the distance from the pivot point, the greater the turning force or moment. The further the door handle is from its hinge, the easier the door is to open.

Clinical example

A **plate bender** with longer handles creates a greater 'turning moment' for a given force applied and therefore less force is required to create the required bend, compared with a shorter equivalent. Similarly, **T-handles** allow the surgeon to generate more torque than ordinary straight-handled screwdrivers.

Bending moments

A bending moment is created when a turning force is applied to a structure to make it bend. One side of the structure, the convexity, will be under tension and the concavity under compression.

Clinical example

When a bending force is applied to bone, the tension side typically fails first, leading to a transverse or short oblique fracture pattern. With greater energy applied, there is often a wedge or butterfly fragment associated. However, in situations where the degree of mineralization is less than it is in a normal adult, bones typically fail in compression rather than tension, e.g. the 'torus' buckle fractures of the distal radius in children. Similarly, osteoporotic fractures involving vertebrae, a tibial plateau or distal radius tend to fail in compression.

Torsional moments

A torsional moment is created when a turning force is applied to a structure. When this is applied to bone, a spiral fracture configuration tends to result.

Clinical example

The classical ankle fracture, a supination, lateral rotation injury (Weber B type), occurs when the foot becomes planted in an inverted position and is then forced to rotate externally under the leg (or the tibia above it rotates internally). This mechanism produces a very predictable spiral fracture pattern of the lateral malleolus, which starts anteriorly around the level of the syndesmosis and exits posteriorly and proximal to it.

Different materials have varying tolerance to tension, compression, torsion and shear. For example, steel and collagen fibres are strong in tension, whereas ceramics such as concrete and hydroxyapatite are stronger in compression. Bone is a **composite material**, meaning that it benefits from the combined mechanical properties of all its constituents. The collagen fibres allow it to tolerate tensile forces whilst also resisting fracture lines propagating through, i.e. it makes them less brittle and gives an improved fatigue resistance. The hydroxyapatite is strong in compression and so allows bones to be weight-bearing structures. In this way, bone is strong enough in compression to allow skeletal weight bearing, but is also tough and resilient enough to allow bending, shear and rotational forces acting through it.

Strain

When stress is applied to a structure, it will cause it to deform. The degree of deformation, or strain, is the change in length of the structure as a ratio of its original length (change in length/ original length). Strain has no given units as it is a length–length ratio, and is therefore portrayed as a percentage.

The concept of strain can be used to describe the mechanical properties of various biomaterials. However, in orthopaedics, strain most commonly refers to movement at a fracture site.

When tissue is damaged, the repair process involves proliferation of mesenchymal stem cells (MSCs). The cell lineage they go on to differentiate into will dictate the type of tissue that subsequently forms. Following a fracture, the degree of movement present between the bone ends is a major determinant in this cell differentiation. At the fracture site, movement can be described as **strain**, which is experienced by the tissues surrounding the bone ends. Perren and Cordey's (1980) original strain theory described the concept of 'strain tolerance' to predict how a fracture would respond to movement, i.e. different tissue types were able to tolerate different amounts of strain. This is actually the wrong way around; in fact the strain itself **drives** the type of tissue precursor that proliferates. In other words, the amount of movement at a fracture site decides which cell type the MSCs proliferate into, and thus which tissue forms there. *Table 31.1* demonstrates the amount of strain that stimulates the production of various tissue types.

Strain is not only governed by the degree of movement at a fracture site (change in length), but also by the surface contact area of the broken fragments (original length). A simple transverse fracture has a small contact surface area when compared to a highly comminuted one. The same amount of movement will therefore create less strain at a comminuted fracture site because it is shared along a greater surface area of fracture (**Figure 31.1**).

Table 31.1 Strain amount and the tissue produced at fracture sites

Strain	Tissue type differentiated (phenotype)
100%	Granulation tissue
17%	Fibrous connective tissue
10%	Fibrocartilage
2–10%	Woven bone
<2%	Lamellar bone

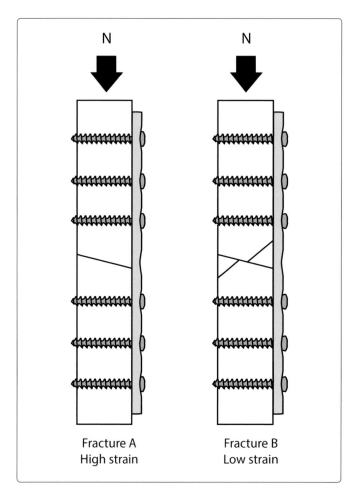

Figure 31.1 For a given loading force (N) acting on similar constructs A and B, both will deform equally, but the fracture strain will be less in B because any movement is shared along the greater surface area of fracture.

Types of fracture healing

Several factors determine the amount of movement at a fracture site and therefore the degree of stability. Traditional teaching has described fracture healing as taking place in the presence of either **absolute** or **relative stability**.

Absolute stability

In absolute stability conditions where physiological loading leads to minimal strain (<2%), the complete lack of movement means that bone callus formation is inhibited. As stated above, the callus 'cascade' (haematoma, granulation, soft callus, hard callus, etc) is ultimately delivered by MSCs and these are strain-sensitive cells that respond to ambient movement. If there is no movement, then the sequence cannot progress and callus will not form. In this instance, healing has to be **direct**, meaning that bone is laid down primarily, without a fibrocartilage precursor, resulting in **intramembranous ossification**. Importantly though, this direct healing process is very different between cortical and cancellous bone.

Absolute stability in cortical bone

The functional unit of cortical bone is the Haversian canal or osteon and the cell type that remodels it is the **osteoclast** via 'cutting cones'. The reason that cortical bone has to be 'cored out' is because of its density. It is not porous, like cancellous bone, which would allow blood vessels to grow right into damaged or attenuated sections. In order for cortical bone to be remodelled, a hole has to be drilled out from within and then replaced in concentric layers by an 'entourage' of osteoblasts. This process of remodelling is a constant, on-going process in all areas of Haversian bone and can be harnessed to treat fractures.

However, in order for fractures to be healed by this so-called 'primary' or 'osteonal' mechanism, three fundamental conditions have to be present:

- **Absolute stability**: there must be virtually no strain at all (<2%) at the fracture site.
- **Perfect reduction**: the bone ends must be touching, in order for the cutting cones to pass across. Osteons cannot form across fibrous tissue gaps.
- **Viable bone ends**: there has to be a blood supply to bring the osteoclast precursors (haematopoetic cell lineage) and osteoblast precursors (MSCs) to the fracture site. Devitalized (non-bleeding) bone ends are unlikely to heal by this mechanism.

What if there is a small gap at the fracture site?

If the gap between the bone ends is small (<500 µm), then **gap healing** can occur. Here, surface osteoblasts lay down sequential layers of bone on the fractured bone ends (rather like periosteum on the surface), thereby closing down the gap between the two fragments (**Figure 31.2**). If the blood supply is good, allowing gap healing on both sides, then the gap is closed down, the two fronts meet in the middle and cutting cones are free to pass across the fracture site and deliver a strong repair. As the gap increases to **greater than 500** µm, the likelihood of this osteoblast gap healing becomes increasingly unlikely.

Absolute stability in cancellous bone

Cancellous/trabecular bone does not contain osteons and therefore it cannot heal by the same direct method as cortical bone. **Direct cancellous healing** is poorly explained in existing textbooks and is described using confusing terms, including 'endosteal callus', 'intramembranous osteogenesis' and 'creeping substitution'.

The approximated ends of cancellous bone provide an ideal scaffold of porous bone surface into which blood vessels can grow directly, worming their way into the cancellous spaces between trabeculae. Following this revascularization, osteoblasts then lay down new layers of bone, directly on top of the old trabeculae, thus progressively bridging the fracture site. This allows devitalized bone (as found in some metaphyseal fractures or autologous bone graft) to be incorporated back into the metaphysis of healthy vascularized bone. The process of direct revascularization, followed by 'bony in-growth' only occurs in cancellous bone, since cortical bone is too densely packed to allow penetration of the blood vessels into the trabecular system, and without a blood supply, the osteoblasts cannot proliferate.

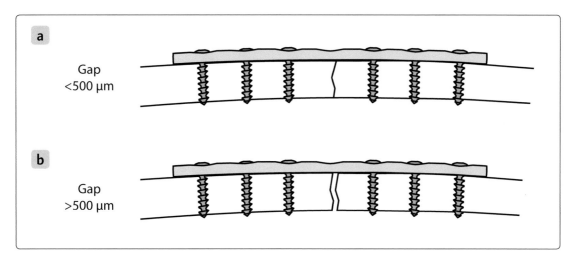

Figure 31.2 Gap healing. Diagram demonstrating the difference in healing between varying 'bone gaps in the presence of absolute stability'. The diagram in (b) shows a large gap, which in the presence of absolute stability, produces no callus and the osteoblasts are unable to bridge the gap, resulting in a non-union. In (a) the gap is small (‹50–500 µm) and therefore 'gap healing' can occur. Osteoblasts migrate over the fracture surface and produce sequential layers of bone until they meet in the middle. Then the bridge can be remodelled by osteoclasts in the form of cutting cones.

Summary

To summarize, in absolute stability conditions, devitalized cortical bone has to be remodelled via cutting cones to form new osteons. Devitalized cancellous bone can be populated by direct blood vessel invasion and subsequent cell migration onto the existing trabecular scaffold, upon which new bone is laid down directly. Importantly, these are both forms of direct bone healing, using intramembranous ossification, since there is no fibrocartilaginous intermediate stage.

Relative stability

This can be defined as providing a fracture with mechanical conditions that allow greater than 2% strain, when subjected to functional loading. Rather than encouraging direct healing, the ambient strain (movement) stimulates fracture gaps to form **callus**.

Following any fracture, a haematoma forms around the fracture site, which organizes and recruits a host of cells, inflammatory mediators and new vessels. These cells organize the haematoma into a mass of granulation tissue. If the granulation tissue is subject to strain, the cell population that proliferates is of fibroblastic and then chondroblastic lineage. Fibrocartilage is formed, which later undergoes a process of calcification, producing **soft callus**. The biomechanical function of this soft callus is to reduce strain by stiffening the fracture site, such that bone can then be laid down in its place. This reduction in strain occurs in two ways:

- By increasing the cross-sectional area of the fracture (increases the original length).
- By increasing stiffness. If strain remains high, precursors for woven bone will not kick into action and proliferation of fibrous tissue ensues, culminating in a fibrous non-union.

Once woven bone has formed (hard callus), replacing the fibrocartilage, the fracture is said to have 'united'. Remodelling is a secondary process, which takes many months and is directed by osteoclastic resorption, taking the form of osteons in the cortices and Howship's lacunae in the metaphyses.

The fixation device chosen by a surgeon has a critical bearing on the mode of fracture healing. The device chosen to treat a particular fracture must maintain adequate reduction, whilst providing favourable biomechanics and ideally allowing early function of the affected limb. This is known as **optimizing the strain environment** and is a critical consideration when planning any fracture treatment, whether it be operative or non-operative.

Elastic modulus

How stress and strain affect a fracture site is discussed above. This has to be considered differently from their effect on biomaterials.

The stiffness of a structure is calculated by its ratio of stress to strain, calculated numerically as the 'modulus of elasticity'. The greater the modulus of elasticity, the stiffer the structure is. Since stress can either be in the plane of the biomaterial (so-called 'normal stresses' i.e. tension/compression) or oblique to it (shear or rotational forces), there is a **Young's modulus** for tension/compression and a **shear modulus** for shear stresses. These are both types of elastic moduli. Note that a third modulus, **bulk modulus**, applies to volumetric strain and is not considered further in this chapter.

Elastic properties/phase

Initially as stress is applied to a structure, such as a regular dynamic compression plate, strain will increase in a linear fashion, i.e. the plate will bend. If the stress is removed the plate will return to its original shape. During this phase, the degree the plate bends is directly proportional to the force applied to it and therefore it is said to follow Hooke's Law. The elastic modulus is calculated by measuring the gradient of the stress–strain curve in this elastic phase. The **limit of proportionality** is the point at which the linear proportionality is lost, i.e. Hooke's Law is no longer obeyed and the stress–strain graph stops being a straight line. However, importantly the material will continue to exhibit elastic properties for a short time before reaching its **elastic limit**, which is therefore the limit at which elastic properties are still displayed. Beyond this, if the deforming force is removed completely, there will still be some degree of permanent deformation.

Plastic properties/phase

The **yield point** signifies the onset of the plastic phase, which is characterized by **irreversible deformation** of the material, i.e. the original shape of the material/plate is no longer recoverable. Within the plastic phase, two discrete changes are seen: **work hardening**, whereby the material becomes paradoxically harder, followed by **necking**, whereby the strain increases spontaneously without any need for further stress to be applied. Different materials have different limits in the amount of stress that can be loaded on them. This is known as the ultimate stress or ultimate failure. Superseding it will cause the material to fail.

1. **Elastic limit:** the point on the stress–strain curve at which a material stops exhibiting elastic properties, i.e. deformation stops being entirely reversible.
2. **Yield point:** the point on the stress–strain curve at which the material demonstrates plastic deformation, i.e. deformation is permanent. This is very fractionally later in the curve than elastic limit but the two values are virtually inseparable for most materials.
3. **Limit of proportionality:** a magnitude of stress applied to a material after which the stress–strain relationship is no longer linear but does still follow elastic properties.
4. **Ultimate strength:** the maximum stress a material can withstand before ultimately failing (or fracturing).

Broadly speaking, cortical bone can tolerate around 2% of strain and cancellous bone around 10% before either type of bone begins to fail. The average Young's modulus for cortical bone is around 20 GPa and that of cancellous is around 1.0 GPa. These figures are significantly dependent on the density and orientation of the trabeculae in cancellous bone and the orientation/organization of Haversian systems for cortical bone. A 25% decrease in bone density, for example, will lead to approximately a 45% decrease in stiffness and in strength, explaining in part why osteoporotic bone fractures so much more easily than the healthy equivalent. Conversely, paediatric bone has a lower Young's modulus and ultimate stress values than adult bones. This means that for a given stress, immature bone will deform further than mature bone. However, immature bone is also much less brittle, meaning that there is much more capacity for plastic deformation prior to failure. For this reason, paediatric forearm fractures commonly fail by bending, whereas healthy adults will just break.

Anisotropy

A material that is completely uniform in its response to stress (i.e. its modulus is constant, whether it is subjected to shear or tension) is termed **isotropic**. An example of this would be woven bone; a homogenous material made up of randomly orientated mineralized collagen fibres.

Conversely, when a material has an organized internal structure, it will respond differently to varying modes of stress. It is therefore **anisotropic**. An example is lamellar bone, whose collagen fibres are laid down in specific orientations, either within the Haversian systems or the trabeculae, to resist the incumbent forces subjected on it.

Mature, lamellar bone can therefore be considered an anisotropic material: it exhibits directional dependence of physical properties. The clinical significance of the anisotropy of bone is that it can resist different types of forces to different degrees. Broadly speaking, cortical bone resists compressive forces best of all (elastic modulus of 18 GPa), followed by tensile forces (12 GPa) and is weakest at resisting shear forces (3.3 GPa). The mechanical properties of cancellous bone are both more varied and complex as trabecular orientation and density influence its stiffness. The elastic modulus of cancellous bone ranges from 0.1 to 3.5 GPa (**Figure 31.3**).

Area and polar moments of inertia

Moments of inertia describe the ability of a structure to resist changes in angular velocity about an axis of rotation, or put more simply, the ability of an object to resist displacement.

The **area moment of inertia** or 'second moment of area' pertains to a beam or plate's ability to **resist bending or deflection**. Importantly, the resistance to bending of a plate is proportional to the 3rd power of its thickness (i.e. its thickness cubed). So doubling the thickness of a 2 mm plate increases its stiffness to bending by eight times.

The **polar moment of inertia** describes the **resistance to torsion of a cylindrical object** (e.g. an intramedullary [IM] nail) about its longitudinal axis. The resistance to torsion of a nail is proportional to the 4th power of its radius (r^4), so doubling the radius of a 2 mm Kirschner (K-) wire increases its torsional rigidity by 16 times! Therefore, small increases in diameter yield a big increase in stiffness. This relationship also applies to the bending of a nail.

Regarding nails:

- For a given diameter, a solid structure is stronger at resisting bending and rotational forces than a hollow one (however there is clearly more material in the solid one).
- The greater the wall thickness of a hollow structure, the stronger it is.
- In a hollow cylinder with a set mass, the further the material is distributed from the axis of rotation (i.e. the centre of the cylinder), the greater its rigidity and ability to resist deforming forces. Therefore, if hollow and solid cylinders are constructed by **using the same amount of material**, the hollow one will be stronger because it has a greater diameter.

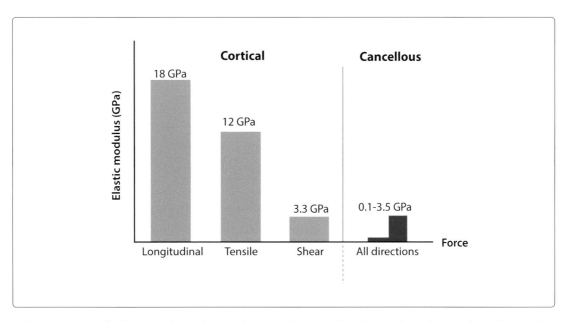

Figure 31.3 Lamellar bone is anisotropic, whether cortical or cancellous. Its elastic modulus and overall strength vary depending on the type of force it is subjected to. This is because it has an organized internal structure in terms of the orientation of the lamellae and indeed the collagen fibres within them.

When selecting IM nails, reaming up to an extra 1–2 mm diameter of nail size will have a significant effect on its strength. Some early IM nails used either a cloverleaf or slotted design to increase their flexibility and ease of passage, prior to the routine introduction of reaming. These designs were indeed more flexible than simple cylinders but were also weaker and prone to fracture, following which they could be devilishly difficult to get out due to bony in-growth around the slots!

With regard to cortical bone strength, the thickness of a cortex affects its ability to load. As bone ages, the periosteal thickness ceases to expand but the endosteal diameter continues to do so, hence the cortical thickness reduces. The area and polar moments of inertia, and therefore the bone strength, decrease with age. This is made worse by the age-related changes in trabecular bone and accelerated in osteoporosis.

Viscoelasticity

A viscoelastic material is one that has different mechanical properties, depending on the **rate of loading**. Almost all structural materials in the body are viscoelastic (including cortical and cancellous bone, tendons, ligaments, articular cartilages, meniscus and intervertebral discs).

There are three specific mechanical properties that are present in any viscoelastic material:

- **Creep**: when a constant stress is applied and maintained, strain (therefore deformation) will increase over time. Put another way, a material will **stretch out over time**, when subjected to a constant deforming force (e.g. the handle of a plastic bag containing heavy shopping gets longer and thinner as you walk home. If the bag is heavy enough, the handles may creep so far that they start 'necking' and then failing – resulting in tins of beans rolling down the street…).
- **Stress relaxation**: if strain is applied and held constant, a resisting stress will be felt immediately but will decrease over time. Put another way, a material that is stretched and held at the new length will accommodate ('**get used to**') that new length, such that the force required to hold it there reduces, e.g. stretching out a lump of bread dough or plasticine requires force to elongate it but increasingly little force to then hold it at its new position.
- **Hysteresis**: if a stress is applied and released, the stress–strain cycles are not reversible, i.e. energy is dissipated within bone.

All of the body's structural tissues demonstrate these three features of viscoelasticity. In addition, viscoelastic biomaterials are **more rigid when they are loaded rapidly**.

If a bone is **loaded relatively slowly**, it can dissipate some of that force (stress relaxation) by microscopic fractures 'slipping' along cement lines and defects in the bone. If the force is removed before the bone breaks, these micro-fractures can then be repaired by the on-going osteoclastic remodelling process. However, if the bone is further loaded slowly until it breaks, much of the energy of the loading process will be dissipated by the time it actually fractures (i.e. the bone 'creeps'). So when loading is slow, relatively **simple fracture patterns** are seen, with minimal comminution.

In the presence of a high-energy injury, where **force is applied very rapidly**, the bone does not have time to dissipate the force being applied and therefore it has to 'store' that energy by deforming (bending, stretching, twisting, i.e. elastic movements). When it finally breaks, the overall energy release is greater because the bone hasn't had time to stress relax, which results in **more comminuted** (exploded) fracture patterns.

Remember, Energy = ½ mass × velocity^2, so when a bone breaks, it's not so much the **size** of the force being applied (½ mass) that decides the energy transfer/comminution, but rather the **speed** with which it is applied (velocity^2).

If an elephant sits on your leg and breaks your tibia, because the rate of loading is relatively slow, it is likely that a simple fracture pattern will result even though the elephant is very heavy. If you are hit by a car bumper at 50 mph, the loading is very rapid and a comminuted fracture pattern is more likely because the bone had no time to stress relax before it fractured.

Casts, splints and functional braces

Casts, splints and braces have been used to treat fractures for thousands of years. They work by applying pressure or restriction upon the soft tissues and thereby the underlying bones/joints.

Casts and splints

Casts and splints may be used for **neutralization** by stopping movement (bending, torsion, compression, etc) and therefore preventing fracture displacement; for example, casting following an undisplaced waist of scaphoid fracture. By immobilizing the joints above and below, the intervening fractures can be immobilized. Equally they can control fractures by applying **three-point fixation**, such as following paediatric forearm fractures. Joints can be either immobilized completely or blocked in one direction or other to prevent an unwanted movement, e.g. a foot drop splint, or an extension block splint following flexor tendon repair.

Functional braces

Functional braces have a different mechanism of action. They apply **hydrostatic pressure** to a muscle compartment, which then approximates the underlying bone to line up. The advantage of this is that the joints and muscles can be **rehabilitated and moved** even before the fracture has healed, e.g. a humeral brace for a mid-shaft fracture. However, this technique is dependent on the brace applying some degree of constant pressure on the soft tissues and therefore the patient needs to be counselled to keep Velcro straps tight to **prevent the splint slackening off** and losing its control of the underlying bone.

Wires and pins

A single K-wire can provide stability in fracture alignment in good quality bone, although multiple K-wires are typically required to provide translational and rotational stability. They can be used to provide permanent fixation or used as part of another fixation method, either temporary or permanent.

K-wires are a versatile element of the orthopaedic armamentarium and are particularly useful in both paediatric fractures and as intraoperative temporary forms of fixation. They come in several types:

- Size: range from 0.6 mm to 3.0 mm.
- Ends: single- or double-ended.
- Points: diamond, trocar or spade points.
- Threads: fully, partially or not at all.

The main drawbacks of K-wires are their **relatively limited strength** and holding power in bone, their potential to cause **thermal injuries**, particularly if they are inserted under power through hard cortical bone and their risk of **wound infections**. Trocar-ended wires have the greatest holding power but the worst thermal characteristics. Thermal damage can be mitigated by introducing wires in a pulsed fashion. This is particularly important when the wires are planned to remain in place long term, as with fine-wire circular frames.

Half pins are used for external fixation and skeletal traction. There is considerable variety in the type of half pins available:

- Size: range from 3 mm to 6 mm diameter.
- End: threaded or trocar-tipped (Steinman pin).
- Geometry: conical or straight. Conical half pins are designed to increase their interference fit as they are inserted. The caveat is that they should not be over-inserted and then backed-off, since this results in them loosening.
- Coating: hyaluronic acid (HA) coated or plain.
- Tip: self-tapping and/or self-drilling.
- Threads: variable length and at various points along the pin, e.g. the Denham pin has a central threaded section for applying skeletal traction.

Screws

Screws are the workhorses of internal fixation. A screw consists of **head** (with drive mechanism), **shaft, thread** and **tip** (**Figure 31.4**). Each part is considered below.

Head

The head acts as both an attachment for a driver and as a stop to engage the substrate (bone, plate, nail etc). **Hex** and **star** drives are the most commonly used drive designs.

Conventional screw heads are **hemi-spherical**, which allows them to be inserted at differing angles and enables them to be used in dynamic compression mode with a plate. When putting screws directly into bone (e.g. in a forearm fracture), the entry hole should ideally be countersunk, both to prevent prominence and more importantly to spread the area of contact of the screw head, preventing point-loading that could cause an iatrogenic fracture of the bone end. **Locking screws** come in many different designs, some with **threaded heads** that engage with the plate and others with **locking end-caps** that fit over the top to lock them.

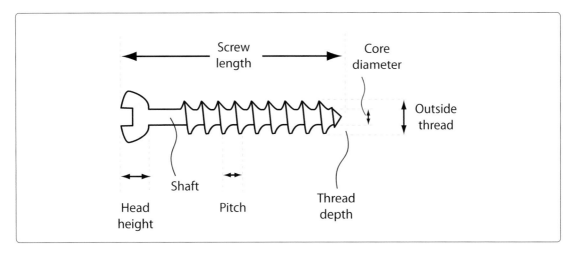

Figure 31.4 Parts of a screw.

Shaft/thread

A conventional screw has a solid central core (measured as the **core diameter**), which determines its torsional strength. The helical surface which surrounds the core provides the thread of a screw, and thus the **outside thread diameter** or **size** of the screw. The **pitch** is the distance between each thread. The shorter the distance, the finer the pitch and the higher the pullout strength. The **lead** of a screw is the distance travelled with each 360° turn. If a screw has a single thread, the pitch is the same as the lead. The shaft of the screw is the smooth part between the head and the thread. The **thread is the helical part** and the **screw length is defined as the distance between the head and the tip of the thread**.

Screw stability

The stability of a screw depends on factors related to the screw itself or the bone it is inserted into (*Table 31.2*):

- Screw factors:
  - Length: **longer screws** have greater pullout strength, as their holding power is related to the number of threads engaged in bone.
  - Diameter: the **larger the diameter**, the greater the pullout strength. Furthermore the stiffness of a screw is determined by the fourth power of its diameter (see moment of inertia). Thus a 6 mm screw is approximately five times stiffer than a 3 mm screw, and can resist up to 16 times the amount of shear forces during its insertion.
  - Thread depth: the **greater the thread depth**, the greater the bone volume in contact with the screw, hence the greater the pullout strength.
  - Pitch: the **smaller the pitch**, the greater the pullout strength
- Bone factors:
  - Density: broadly speaking, a higher bone density will increase pullout strength.
  - Cortical thickness: the greater the thickness, the greater the pullout strength. If two cortices are crossed, the strength further increases.

Table 31.2 Factors leading to optimal screw biomechanics

Core diameter	Increasing the core diameter increases the tensile strength, meaning the screw is more likely to resist fatigue failure
Outer thread diameter	Increasing the outer thread diameter and reducing the core diameter increases the pullout strength but dramatically reduces the strength of the screw (by a factor of r^4)
Thread density	Increasing the thread density increases the pullout strength
Bone density	Denser bone with thicker cortices or increasing the number of cortices will increase the pullout strength
Pilot holes	An optimum pilot hole to screw diameter ratio of 85–90% increases strength Smaller holes mean high levels of torque are required to insert the screw, which may cause radial cracking of bone Larger holes reduce the interface pressure and therefore the holding strength

Screw failure

A screw may fail either by breaking or by losing its grip on the surrounding bone. In a conventional compression screw (e.g. through a plate) there are two forces at work, which are equal and opposite. As the head comes down onto the plate, a tensile force is created between the head (which is stopped on the plate) and the screw threads (which are engaged in the bone and trying to advance). This is counterbalanced by a shear force at the bone–'screw-thread' interface. As the screw is tightened, both of these forces increase equally, matching each other. If the screw head is over-turned, the tensile stress in the screw exceeds the ultimate strength of the bone–'screw-thread' interface and stripping occurs, leading to sudden loss of the previous tensile force in the screw and hence the pressure on the plate.

In a locking screw, there is no tensile vs. shear force interaction. Once the screw is locked in the plate, it sits completely neutrally within the bone until the whole construct is loaded, at which point a combination of compressive and shear forces at the screw–bone interface are transmitted directly to the plate via the locking mechanism. When loaded to failure, locking screws tend either to fracture at their neck, or they cut out of the bone, often creating extensive fracture lines in the process.

Alternatively, if small loads are repeatedly applied over a long period of time, a screw itself may fatigue and then ultimately fail. Equally, micro-fractures or osteolysis at the bone–screw-thread' interface may occur, either due to infection or repeated overloading, causing loosening.

Plates

Plates are strips of metal or biomaterial containing holes that typically accept screws, pegs or blades (either in locking or non-locking modes). Numerous designs exist and increasingly they are constructed to be anatomically specific to one particular bone region.

As with all orthopaedic implants, plates can be used to deliver either absolute or relative stability to a fracture site, depending on how they are applied.

Plating in 'absolute stability' mode

This mode of plating is typically chosen in situations where an anatomic reduction is highly desirable. The usual indications include:

- **Intra-articular fractures**: in which the surgical aim is for perfect joint congruity to be restored and held rigidly, preventing articular malreductions that, if present, may lead to poor joint function and secondary osteoarthritis. Examples include fixing a fractured medial malleolus, tibial plateau, olecranon or patella. In this mode, callus is inhibited and bone heals via **direct cancellous healing**.
- **Diaphyseal/metaphyseal fractures** that are intimately linked to joints: making their reduction integral to the normal articular function. Examples include diaphyseal forearm fractures where malreduction results in reduced forearm rotation, and ankle fractures that involve a significantly displaced fibular shaft, since malreduced unstable ankle fractures or diastases lead to irreversible ankle arthrosis. In this mode, callus is also inhibited but cortical bone heals via **direct osteonal healing**.

Absolute stability has two important elements, an anatomic reduction and compression between the fragments. Applying a plate in 'compression' may be considered a misnomer as the plate itself is in tension, and it is by virtue of Newton's Third Law (action and reaction are equal and opposite), that the underlying bone is compressed.

Importantly, by imposing absolute stability on a fracture, the surgeon is also defining the mode of healing. Fracture callus will be inhibited by the lack of movement; cortical bone will heal by direct osteonal healing and cancellous bone will heal by direct cancellous healing (see earlier). Also, because the fracture surfaces are compressed together, the bone itself will transmit some of the force across it when the limb is loaded. This 'load sharing' means that the whole plating construct is somewhat more robust, because the plate/screws themselves are not transmitting the entire force going through the limb.

Compression across fracture sites using plates can be achieved in several ways:

- Lag technique (**Figure 31.5**), either by over-drilling or by using a partially threaded screw. This can be augmented by a **neutralization plate**, which prevents the fracture rotating around the compression screw.
- Dynamic compression (**Figure 31.6**), using conventional screws and eccentric drill-holes.
- Pre-bending plates, used in non-locking mode in diaphyseal fractures. This allows compression of the far cortex as the plate is brought down onto the surface.
- Screws placed *outside* of the plate can be used with either the articulated tensioning device or a Verbrugge clamp to apply heavy compressive force to a fracture site.
- Plates can be used to provide compression across fracture sites or to neutralize forces across compressive lag screws. When employed in this manner, plates are considered 'load sharing devices' as both plate and bone bear load. A plate placed at the apex of a metaphyseal fracture can act as a **buttress** or **antiglide** plate (**Figure 31.7**), effectively creating an axilla into which the leading spike of cortical bone gets trapped, converting a shear force into a compressive one by trapping and compressing the apex.

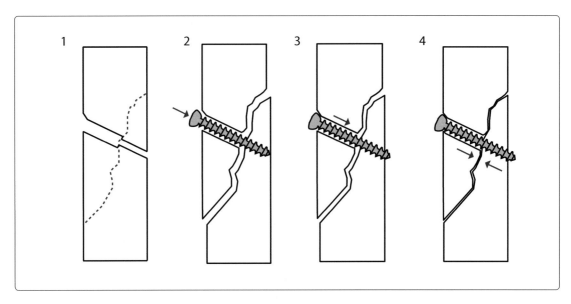

Figure 31.5 This diagram illustrates a lag screw used to compress an oblique fracture, and demonstrates the drill holes for a subsequent screw. By over-drilling the proximal cortex, a lag screw is able to compress across the fracture site.

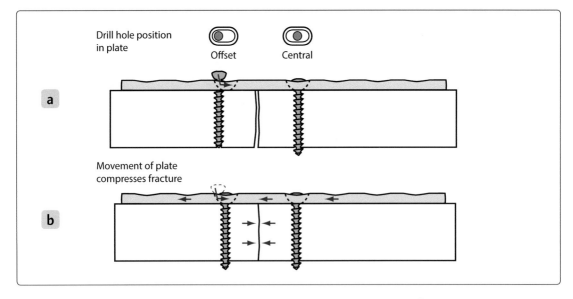

Figure 31.6 This diagram illustrates how a plate can be used to compress across a fracture site. a: A screw is prepared in an eccentric manner. Whilst the screw is driven into the pilot hole, the head abuts on the plate causing it to displace in a manner in which compression is achieved at the fracture site (b).

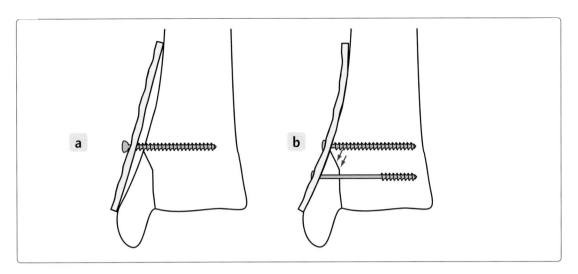

Figure 31.7 An example of an antiglide plate. a: A fully threaded screw at the proximal apex of the fracture brings the under-contoured plate down onto the medial malleolus, effectively 'trapping' the fracture apex and compressing the fracture line; b: a further screw directly across the fracture prevents translation beneath the plate and may add to the compression.

- When placed on the convexity of a fracture, plates can act as a tension band, such that when loaded, they lead to compression at the other side of the bone (the concavity) (**Figure 31.8**). Good examples include plating the posterior wall of the acetabulum or the radial border of the radial shaft. By placing a plate on the side of the fractured bone that is under tension, the whole construct may be up to 200 times stronger, compared to a plate applied on the side of the bone under compression.

Plating in 'relative stability' mode

This is generally chosen in situations where pinpoint accuracy of reduction is less important and callus formation (i.e. speedy union) is desirable. A plate can be used in **bridging mode**, so that when it is loaded, there is some degree of movement at the fracture site, which leads to healing by callus formation. Crucially, the plate is transmitting the majority of the force through the limb in this scenario, which is why it bends and deflects when loaded. The benefit of this mode of healing is that callus forms relatively quickly, the fracture heals and the plate becomes redundant. The downside of this fixation strategy is that the plate has much more work to do, taking on a **load-bearing role** and it is therefore more prone to fatigue fracture.

The use of angle-stable locking screws in the treatment of comminuted metaphyseal fractures (where a plate is used in bridge mode) has certainly improved the performance of plates because of their hold in metaphyseal bone, even in the presence of osteoporosis, is much greater than with conventional (non-locking) screws.

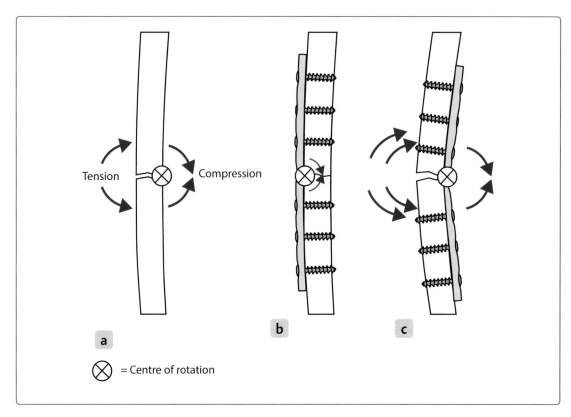

a

b

c

⊗ = Centre of rotation

Figure 31.8 a: A fractured radius, which, because of its radial bow, tends to open up on the radial side (tension) and hinge/rotate on the ulnar cortex (a). By applying a plate on the radial side, a tension band is created, effectively moving the centre of rotation from the ulnar side to the radial cortex (b). Now when the bone is loaded, this centre of rotation causes compression at the fracture site. Applying a plate on the ulnar side of the radius (c) leaves the hinge point where it is so that when loaded, the fracture will tend to distract on the radial side. Indeed putting the plate on the concavity in this way may even cause gapping on the other side when the fracture is compressed.

How does a non-locked (conventional) plate work?

When non-locking screws secure a plate, the plate is squeezed down onto the bone surface, creating a **frictional force** between the bone and plate. When the limb is loaded, shear forces are generated between plate and bone. Provided the frictional force remains greater than the shear force (generated from load being applied across a construct), it will remain stable. The size of the frictional force (see equation below) is dependent upon two things: the **coefficient of friction** (which is constant) and the force generated between plate and bone, which in turn comes from the **torsional forces** generated by each of the screws.

$Fr = \mu N$

Where:

Fr = resistive forces of friction

μ = coefficient of friction for the two surfaces in question

N = normal or perpendicular force pushing the two objects together

Therefore, the ability of a non-locked plate to resist loading is directly related to how much the screws can be tightened. Unfortunately, this direct pressure causes localized osteonecrosis immediately beneath the pate (see section on screws above), although this has never been shown to correlate negatively with bone healing.

When screwing into healthy cortical bone, the frictional force generated is very high, much higher than the shear forces generated by physiological movement (e.g. when applying a dynamic hip screw to the proximal femur). However, in osteoporotic or metaphyseal bone, the force may not be so great and this is where the use of locking screws is an attractive alternative.

How does a locked plate work?

A plate secured by locking screws has fundamentally different biomechanics. It does not rely on the frictional force between implant and bone and therefore the quality of screw 'bite' is not relevant. In a locked system, because angle-stable screws have the effect of 'trapping' large areas of bone between them, in order for them to be pulled out they would have to take a large section of bone with them, since they would all have to cut-out simultaneously. This is in contrast to non-locked screws, which can all loosen and fail individually, by angulating in their holes.

In essence, locked screws are powerful because they all act together as a single bone-holding construct with no movement between the bone, plate or screws. Non-locked systems rely on friction generated between plate and bone, which is usually sufficient in the diaphysis, but in the metaphysis it may not be.

In reality, most modern plating systems allow either locked or non-locked screws into any plate hole, giving the surgeon a choice. Non-locked screws are good for pulling the plate down onto bone, gaining fixation in healthy cortical bone or lagging specific fragments together. Locked screws are good for gaining stability in cancellous bone but they are not good as reduction tools or for lagging.

How do plates fail?

- Plate bending: stress on a plate that exceeds the elastic limit will lead to the plate bending.
- Plate fracture: cyclical bending forces above the fatigue limit will ultimately lead to failure of a plate. Bending forces below the fatigue limit can continue indefinitely.
- Construct pullout: non-locked screws tend to loosen and fail individually by toggling in their screw holes, whereas locked screws have to either pull-out *en masse* or fracture out of the bone in which they are embedded.
- Screw head failure: screw drives (hex or star) become threaded when over-tightened or tightened with the screwdriver at an inappropriate angle, making further tightening impossible.

Plate strength

The strength of a plate is governed by two main variables:

Cross-sectional area of the plate

The **area moment of inertia** (see above) defines a plate's resistance to bending, and so its stiffness is therefore related to the third power of its thickness. In other words, if the plate thickness is doubled, the stiffness is cubed.

Given 'stress = force per unit area' and screw holes are areas of reduced metal cross-section, they represent areas of increased stress in a plate and therefore increased weakness. Furthermore, the hole(s) immediately adjacent to a fracture site are subject to the highest strain and therefore represent the area most likely to fail should the plate be repeatedly loaded beyond its **fatigue limit**. Conversely, filling an empty screw hole offsets some of the increased stresses.

Material

This affects both strength and rigidity. The two most commonly employed materials are steel (elastic modulus of 200 GPa) and titanium (elastic modulus of 110 GPa).

How many screws and where to put them?

For conventional non-locking plate constructs, the AO group states that in a small (3.5 mm) fragment application (e.g. a forearm fracture), a minimum of three bicortical screws are required either side of the fracture to give adequate stability. In the large (4.5 mm) fragment application (e.g. a humeral shaft), a minimum of four bicortical screws are required either side of the fracture. Adding further screws increases the torsional rigidity, but there is little mechanical gain beyond 8–10 screws.

For locking plate constructs, the overall strength is not governed by frictional interference with the bone and therefore the biomechanics are very different. Whilst there are no clear 'rules' as to how many screws should be used, the principles of external fixation are often applied, since locking plates can be thought of as so-called **internal fixators**. Therefore, surgeons are increasingly using the near-far principle, by choosing long plates with wide separation between top and bottom screws; effectively gaining strength from the lever arm generated by well separated screws. Therefore, the **separation of screws** appears to be almost as important as the number used.

For both locked and non-locked constructs, the smaller the working length of the fixation (i.e. the distance between the closest two screws either side for the fracture), the more rigid it will be. As described above, rigidity defines the mode of fracture healing and therefore the surgeon has to consider carefully how they place screws in each clinical context. For example, where absolute stability is required for direct osteonal or cancellous bone healing (e.g. an intra-articular fracture), screws can be placed very close to the fracture, since this provides the maximal rigidity. Where a bridging plate is required, for relative stability to encourage callus formation, several screw holes should be left unused around the fracture site, so that when it is loaded, some movement occurs. To achieve both 'empty holes' for flexibility in the plate and wide screw separation to give strength to the construct, very long plates may be required.

Intramedullary nails

IM nails were originally developed as an elegant solution to the treatment of diaphyseal fractures of the femur and tibia. Since the original, non-locked Kuntscher nail was developed in the 1930s–1940s, numerous design modifications have been made and the indications for nailing have been extended to include metaphyseal fractures. Specific IM devices now exist for the humerus, olecranon, forearm, fibula, clavicle and ribs. There are even retrograde nails for the tibia and distal radius in early trials.

Nail design

In the past, nails with clover-leaf and slotted cross-sections were commonly used because they were flexible enough to pass down an unreamed medulla. They were however, also dramatically weaker at resisting torsional forces and had a lower fatigue resistance when compared with the cylindrical nails used today.

The use of interlocking screws in IM nails provides axial and rotational stability by controlling torsional and axial loads. This is particularly useful in unstable fractures and proximal or distal fractures. The disadvantage of locking screws is that holes act as stress risers in the nail and therefore represent the weakest part of it; fractures occurring most commonly just proximal or distal to the screw holes. The risk is actually increased the closer the screw holes are to the fracture site, particularly if the hole is left unfilled.

In the majority of applications, nails are **relative stability constructs**. This means that when the limb is loaded, they allow some movement at the fracture site and therefore promote the formation of callus. Just how much movement takes place is governed chiefly by three factors:

- The **fracture configuration/comminution**.
- The **diameter of the nail**.
- The **working length of the nail**.

Fracture configuration

Not only are nails strong devices, they also sit in a mechanically advantageous IM position. This means that when they are used for a simple transverse or short oblique diaphyseal fracture, they effectively force the fragments to reduce as the nail is passed, with just rotation needing to be adjusted. In this scenario, with the fracture effectively reduced and the limb loaded, the forces across the fracture site are shared between bone and nail (so-called **load sharing**), effectively increasing the longevity of the nail. In more comminuted fracture patterns that are not axially stable, the nail has to transmit all the forces applied to the limb, so-called **load bearing**.

Nail diameter and stiffness

The cylindrical nature of nails makes them structurally strong devices, more so than plates, for a given amount of metal. Whilst the resistance (stiffness) to bending of a plate is governed by the **area moment of inertia**, the stiffness of a nail in torsion is governed by the **polar moment of inertia** (see above).

Given that a nail's area and polar moment of inertia are both proportional to the fourth power of its radius, small increases in diameter create a huge increase in stiffness. Choosing an 11 mm instead of a 10 mm diameter nail, for example, will increase its ability to resist loading by around 3–4 times.

Role of reaming

- By reaming up the canal and increasing its diameter, it allows a slightly larger (but much stronger – r^4) nail to be passed.
- This in turn may allow slightly larger (but much stronger – r^4) locking bolts to be inserted, which are more resistant to breaking (auto-dynamization).

- Remember, just a **1 mm increase in locking bolt diameter** from 4 mm to 5 mm **increases the strength by 2.5 times**.
- The larger the diameter of the nail, the better control it has over the fracture reduction. Small diameter nails allow 'play' at the fracture site, particularly near the metaphyses where the medulla widens.
- IM reaming effectively destroys all centrifugal (inside-to-out) blood flow through bone. Whilst this would seem to be detrimental to fracture healing, it appears to have a paradoxical stimulatory effect on the periosteal blood supply, which proliferates and effectively reverses the blood flow to become centripetal (outside-to-in).
- It has been speculated that reaming also creates 'autologous bone graft' at the fracture site, although this theoretical model of enhancement has never been proven scientifically.

Working length

The working length of a nail is the distance between the **closest proximal and distal statically locked bolts** (**Figure 31.9**). Increasing the working length allows greater strain at the fracture site and *vice versa*.

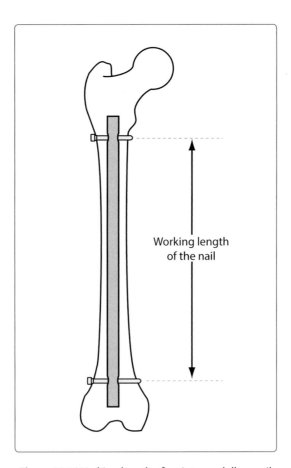

Figure 31.9 Working length of an intramedullary nail.

The role of dynamization

Locking screw holes typically include the options of either **static** or **dynamic** locking. The dynamic option (an oval hole) allows axial displacement (shortening) of a fracture site without allowing rotation. In this way, the fracture site can be compressed without allowing rotational shear forces, which are generally inhibitory to fracture healing. **Compression nailing** is one purposeful application of this, whereby an axially stable diaphyseal fracture (e.g. transverse tibia fracture) is nailed and locked via the dynamic hole, after which a grub screw is sent down onto the dynamic locker, forcing the fracture to shorten and thus compress the fracture site. However, with this fracture pattern, most surgeons still choose to simply 'back-slap' the nail once distally locked, in order to oppose the fracture surfaces.

Tension bands

Tension band devices can be used to treat fractures that are under compression at one cortex and tension at the other. Examples include long bones that are significantly bent, such as the radius (radial bow) and the femur (anterior bow). In these, the tension side, and therefore the place where a tension band should sit, is the convexity (outside) of the curve. The concavity is the compression side. Another example is bones that tend to fracture (and therefore displace) around a centre of rotation, such as the olecranon and patella.

In principle, a tension band **converts a tensile force into a compressive force by translating the centre of rotation of a fracture to instead sit at the tension band**. This is demonstrated diagrammatically on the I-beam construct and the fractures illustrated below (**Figures 31.10, 31.11**). The key to understanding the principle is to appreciate that the fractures in question displace around a **centre of rotation**. The tension band has the effect of **translating** that centre of rotation from the compression side to the tension side of the fracture.

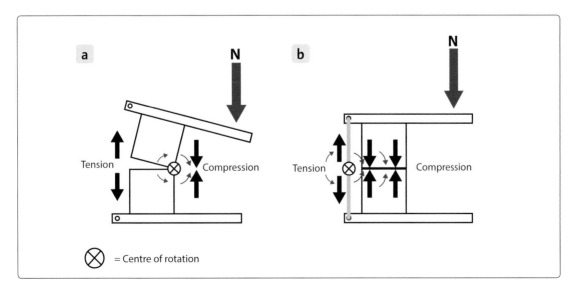

Figure 31.10 Principles of tension band fixation. A force (N) causes one side of the construct (a) to be under tension by rotating around the other side of the block (the compression side). The force causes a turning moment about the labelled centre of rotation. By applying a tension band (b), the centre of rotation of the construct is moved to the tension band, such that both cortices of the bone are now under compression, providing a favourable healing environment.

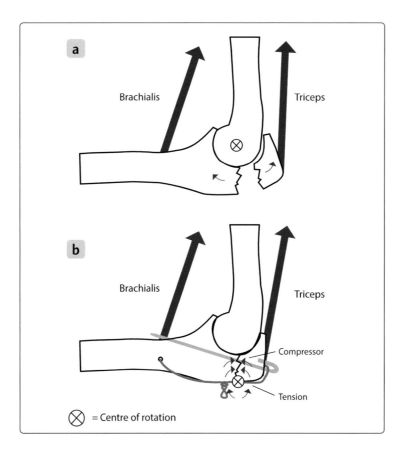

Figure 31.11 Example of an olecranon fracture tension band wire system. In (a), the triceps and brachialis muscles pull on the proximal ulna, causing tensile forces at the fracture site, as the olecranon fragment rotates around the trochlea centre of rotation. In (b), a tension band wire is placed on the dorsal side of the fracture, thereby translating the centre of rotation from the centre of the trochlea to the dorsal cortex. Now when triceps pulls, the olecranon fragment rotates around the dorsal cortex, effectively compressing the whole fracture line. In this way, the tension band converts a tensile force across the fracture site into a compressive one. The longitudinal K-wire is not part of the tension band effect but it does provide a 'railroad' over which the fracture compresses and prevents rotation or translation of the olecranon fragment.

Viva questions

1. What is a screw?
2. What is the difference in the way locking vs non-locked plates work?
3. Tell me about this intramedullary nail.
4. Can you draw how tension band wiring works for an olecranon fracture of the elbow?
5. What size K-wires do you use for fixation of paediatric supracondylar elbow fractures? Why?.

Further reading

Perren SM, Cordey J. *The Concept of Interfragmentary Strain*. Berlin Heidelberg New York: Springer-Verlag, 1980.

Appendix Common Bone Disorders

Peter Bates, Prakash Jayakumar and Manoj Ramachandran

A detailed understanding of the breadth of disorders affecting bone is vital for the orthopaedic surgeon. In this appendix, some of these disorders (excluding fractures) are covered in detail in systematic note form, allowing the reader to review rapidly the pertinent facts. The following definitions are worth committing to memory:

Metabolic bone disease: generalized disorder of skeletal homeostasis.

Osteopenia: radiological appearance of decreased bone density. The term is neither a disease nor a diagnosis, and implies no aetiology.

Osteoporosis: a disease characterized by low bone mass per unit volume (density) of normally mineralized bone matrix leading to bone deficient in quality, structural integrity, enhanced bone fragility and increased low-velocity fracture risk.

Osteomalacia: increased, normal or decreased mass of insufficiently mineralized bone.

(For definitions of abbreviations, please see Abbreviations, pp. vii–xii.)

Disorders of calcium metabolism

Hypercalcaemia

- Hypercalcaemia is much more common than hypocalcaemia and caused by **primary hyperparathyroidism** and **malignancy** in > 90% of cases.
- More common in elderly females.
- Incidence: 25–30/100,000.

Causes

1. Primary hyperparathyroidism

Aetiology

- Solitary parathyroid adenoma (80%).
- Diffuse parathyroid hyperplasia (15%).
- Multiple parathyroid adenomas (4%) (part of MEN Type 1/2a – see below).
- Parathyroid carcinoma (1%):
  - hyperparathyroidism–jaw tumour syndrome (extremely rare; hyperparathyroidism associated with maxillary/mandibular tumours).

Effects

- **Plasma calcium** is **high** from all three sources (gut, kidney, bone).
- **Plasma phosphate** is **low** due to increased renal excretion.
- Result is **bone resorption** and **inadequate repair** (due to lack of phosphate).

2. Malignancy

- Humoral hypercalcaemia of malignancy:
  - ectopic secretion of **PTH-related protein**;
  - especially squamous lung carcinoma.
- Primary solid tumours with bone **metastases**:
  - e.g. breast, bronchus, thyroid, kidney (renal cell carcinoma), prostate, oesophagus;

- prostaglandin and cytokine-related effects (e.g. IL-1, IL-6, TNF-α) via activation of osteoclasts locally at metastatic skeletal lesions, leading to resorption and osteolysis.
- Primary haematological malignancy:
  - myeloma involves clonal plasma cells that resorb bone via cytokine-related effects;
  - lymphomas can synthesize $1,25(OH)_2$ D3.
- Osteoclastic trigger factors may be produced by tumours.

3. Other

Excessive PTH secretion

- **Secondary hyperparathyroidism**:
  - physiological compensatory hypertrophy of all the parathyroids leading to excess PTH as an appropriate response for low calcium;
  - e.g. in dietary vitamin D deficiency, renal osteodystrophy in chronic renal failure;
  - PTH levels are raised and calcium levels are low or normal.
- **Tertiary hyperparathyroidism**:
  - development of parathyroid hyperplasia after prolonged primary hyperparathyroidism and autonomous activity of glands secreting excess PTH;
  - e.g. in renal failure;
  - plasma calcium and especially phosphate are raised;
  - treatment includes parathyroidectomy.
- Ectopic PTH secretion (very rare).

Excess Vitamin D activity

- Granulomatous disease (granulomas synthesize $1,25(OH)_2$ D3): sarcoidosis, TB.
- Exogenous vitamin D analogues/excess.
- Lymphoma.

Excess calcium intake

- Metabolic: milk-alkali syndrome

Endocrine disease

- Hyperthyroidism / thyrotoxicosis.
- Addison's disease.

Drugs

- Thiazide diuretics.
- Vitamin A.
- Lithium administration (chronic).
- Steroid administration.

Miscellaneous

- Long-term immobility.
- Familial:
  - Familial hypocalciuric hypercalcaemia;
    - Autosomal dominant; chromosome 3 gene mutations;
    - Usually asymptomatic;
    - Defect in calcium-ion-sensing G-protein-coupled receptor in kidney and parathyroid leading to poor renal clearance of calcium despite hypercalcaemia;
    - PTH levels normal/slightly raised, urinary calcium low.
  - MEN syndromes:
    - MEN I (Wermer syndrome): pancreatic and pituitary tumours, parathyroid hyperplasia;
    - MEN IIa (Sipple syndrome): thyroid medullary carcinoma, bilateral phaeochromocytomas, parathyroid hyperplasia;
    - MEN IIb: thyroid medullary carincoma, phaeochromocytoma, marfanoid body habitus, mucosal neuroma;
    - MEN II FMTC: thyroid medullary carcinoma.

Clinical features

May be **asymptomatic**.

Bones: bone pain mainly due to excessive bone resorption; 5–10% have bone lesions.

Stones (renal): kidney stones, renal colic, polyuria, nocturia, haematuria, polydipsia, dehydration.

Groans (gastrointestinal): abdominal pain, constipation, anorexia, nausea, vomiting, peptic ulceration.

Psychic moans (central nervous system): confusion, stupor, malaise, depression.

Other effects: stiff joints, myopathy, hypertension, corneal/ectopic calcification, chondrocalcinosis.

Investigations

Bloods:
- High calcium.
- High PTH.
- Low phosphate.
- Hypochloraemic acidosis.
- Elevated alkaline phosphatase (severe PT bone disease).
- Serum TSH (hyperthyroidism).
- Cortisol (Addison's disease).
- Hydrocortisone suppression test (malignancy, vitamin D-mediated hypercalcaemia, sarcoidosis).

Urine:
- High phosphate.
- 24-hour urinary calcium (familial hypocalciuric hypercalcaemia).

Protein electrophoresis:
- Myeloma.

ECG:
- Decreased Q-T interval.

Imaging:
- X-rays:
  - predilection for **cortical bone** (cancellous sparing);
  - **osteopenia**;
  - **subperiosteal erosion** (especially radial borders of proximal phalanges and tufts of distal phalanges; also seen at the medial end of clavicle, femoral neck and upper tibia);
  - **chondrocalcinosis** and **metastatic calcification** of soft tissues;
  - osteitis fibrosa et cystica, or **brown tumours** (fibrous marrow changes);
  - **pepper-pot skull** (diffuse multiple areas of resorption);
  - **loss of lamina dura around the teeth** is specific;
  - abdominal X-rays: renal calculi, nephrocalcinosis.
- **DEXA**.
- **US**, high resolution **CT**, **MRI**, **radioisotope scanning** using 99mTc-sestamibi (adenomas).

Histology:
- Brown tumours: contain increased giant cell population and fibrous tissue with haemosiderin staining.
- Osteoblasts and osteoclasts active on both sides of trabeculae (as in Paget's disease), with widened osteoid seams.

Treatment

- Treat underlying cause.
- Emergency:
  - rehydrate 4–6 L normal saline (saline diuresis);
  - IV bisphosphonates (pamidronate/zoledronate) (inhibits osteoclastic activity).
- Avoid high calcium/vitamin D intake and encourage exercise.
- Loop diuretics with or without dialysis (severe cases).
- Chemotherapy in malignancy, e.g. mithramycin.
- Calcium-sensing receptor blockers e.g. cinacalcet (parathyroid carcinoma, dialysis patients).
- Surgery:
  - parathyroidectomy is sometimes indicated:
    - renal involvement and impaired renal function;
    - bone involvement and reduced cortical bone density;
    - marked hypercalcaemia >3.0 mmol/L;
    - patients <50 years old;
    - previous acute episode of hypercalcaemia.

Hypocalcaemia

- High phosphate, low PTH, low vitamin D levels and dysfunction in calcium homeostasis can lead to hypocalcaemia.
- **Chronic kidney disease** is the commonest cause.
- Hypocalcaemia post thyroid/parathyroid surgery is common but usually transient.

Clinical features

Acute
- **Neuromuscular irritability**:
  - tetany;
  - seizures;
  - cramps/circumoral numbness.
  - Chvostek's sign (tapping over parotid gland in region of facial nerve causes twitching of the ipsilateral facial muscles);
  - Trousseau's sign (carpopedal spasm if brachial artery occluded with blood pressure cuff above systolic pressure for 3 minutes).
- **Neuropsychiatric features**:
  - anxiety;
  - depression;
  - psychosis;
  - papilloedema (severe).
- ECG shows prolonged Q-T interval.

Chronic
- Cataracts.
- Fungal nail infections.

Causes

1. Renal osteodystrophy (chronic kidney disease)

A group of disorders of bone mineral metabolism seen in chronic renal failure.

Aetiology

High-turnover renal bone disease
- **Uraemia** and **phosphate retention** from glomerular dysfunction.

- **High plasma phosphate** leads to hypocalcaemia by:
  - impairing synthesis of 1,25 $(OH)_2$ vitamin D3 by inhibiting renal 1α hydroxylase;
  - (note that synthesis of the renal vitamin D metabolite is also directly impaired by tubular damage in renal failure);
  - direct lowering of calcium, which stimulates PTH secretion;
  - direct stimulation of PTH secretion.
- Low serum calcium produces **secondary hyperparathyroidism** (and ultimately hyperplasia of the chief cells of the parathyroid gland and **tertiary hyperparathyroidism**).
- As renal function deteriorates, acidosis exacerbates the negative calcium balance.

Low-turnover renal bone disease
- Slowed bone formation and turnover (**adynamic** lesion of bone).
- Slowed mineralization (osteomalacia).
- **Aluminium deposition** (impaired renal excretion) produces osteomalacia:
  - inhibition of proliferation and differentiation of osteoblasts;
  - inhibition of PTH release from parathyroid gland.
- **No secondary hyperparathyroidism**.

Effects

- Hypocalcaemia:
  - rickets or osteomalacia;
  - osteoporosis.
- Slipped upper femoral epiphysis in children.
- Secondary hyperparathyroidism:
  - osteitis fibrosa et cystica (bone-marrow replacement by fibrous tissue);
  - osteosclerosis (20% of cases):
    - from secondary hyperparathyroidism and increased osteoblast activity;
    - lucent and dense bands in the spine ('rugger-jersey spine').

- metastatic calcification: calcium and phosphate solubility may be affected, producing ectopic calcification in the conjunctivae, blood vessels, skin and periarticular tissues.
- Amyloidosis:
  - as a result of beta-2 microglobulin from chronic dialysis;
  - clinical effects include pathological fractures (from amyloid deposits – amyloidomas), arthropathy, CTS;
  - diagnosis made on histology by staining amyloid pink with Congo red stain.

Investigations

Bloods
- Raised serum urea and creatinine.
- Normal to low serum calcium and high phosphate.
- Raised alkaline phosphatase (osteoblasts) and high PTH levels.

Tetracycline-labelled bone biopsy.

Treatment

- Predominantly medical.
- Adjust serum phosphate to normal:
  - reduce dietary phosphate (less milk, cheese and eggs);
  - phosphate binders, e.g. calcium carbonate.
- Adjust serum calcium to normal:
  - increase calcium absorption with $1,25(OH)_2 D3$;
  - calcium supplementation;
  - suppress secondary hyperparathyroidism with $1,25(OH)_2 D3$ (or may require parathyroidectomy). Alpha-hydroxylated derivatives preferred due to shorter half-life;
  - chelate bone aluminium in cases of aluminium retention (with desferrioxamine).
- Manage chronic renal failure with dialysis or renal transplant.

2. Hypoparathyroidism

Aetiology
- Commonly iatrogenic following neck exploration surgery, (para) thyroidectomy ('hungry bone' syndrome).
- Congenital deficiency (DiGeorge syndrome) (rare):
  - familial, associated with learning difficulties, cataracts, calcified basal ganglia.
- Idiopathic (rare):
  - autoimmune condition associated with vitiligo and cutaneous candidiasis.
- Severe hypomagnesaemia (rare).

Effects
- Decreased PTH leads to low plasma calcium and high plasma phosphate.
- Alkaline phosphatase normal.
- Parathyroid antibodies (present in idiopathic hypoparathyroidism).

Clinical features
- Of hypocalcaemia.
- Vitiligo, hair loss.

Treatment
- Vitamin D analogues, e.g. alfacalcidol.
- Magnesium (in hypomagnesaemia induced functional hypoparathyroidism).

3. Pseudo-hypoparathyroidism (PHP) – resistance to PTH

Aetiology
- Rare hereditary disorder due to failure of target cell response to PTH.
- Signalling abnormality:
  - Gsα-protein (GNAS1) mutation which is normally coupled with PTH-receptor;
  - cAMP defect.
- PTH receptor abnormality.
- Lack of necessary cofactors, e.g. magnesium.

Effects

- Increased PTH but low calcium.
- Increased phosphate.
- Normal or increased alkaline phosphatase.
- Note: In pseudo pseudo-hypoparathyroidism, the same gene defect and clinical features as in PHP are present but biochemistry is normal and there is a normal response to PTH.

Clinical features

- Features common to all forms of PHP including Albright hereditary osteodystrophy, include:
- (use the mnemonic **BORESSS**):
  - **B**rachydactyly: short first, fourth and fifth metacarpals and metatarsals;
  - **O**besity;
  - **R**educed intelligence;
  - **E**xostoses;
  - **S**kull X-rays show basal ganglia calcification;
  - **S**ubcutaneous ossification/calcification;
  - **S**hort stature.

4. Vitamin D deficiency, osteomalacia and rickets

Definition

Osteomalacia is **deficient** or **impaired mineralization** of bone matrix (osteoid). **Rickets** is the **juvenile form**, with impaired mineralization of cartilage matrix (chondroid), affecting the physis in the zone of provisional calcification.

Aetiology

The common causative factors in all aetiologies are inadequate serum calcium and phosphate levels to allow mineralization of newly formed osteoid/chondroid. This is usually due to a lack of Vitamin D availability or defect in its metabolism.

At risk: elderly, Asian women, housebound.

Dietary deficiency
- **Deficient intake**
  - calcium or vitamin D deficiency;
  - dietary chelators (phytates in chapattis, oxalates in spinach);
  - phosphorus deficiency (aluminium-containing antacid abuse);
  - inadequate synthesis in skin (lack of sunlight exposure).
- **Gastrointestinal malabsorption**:
  - post-gastrectomy;
  - biliary disease;
  - intestinal defects;
  - short bowel syndrome, coeliac disease, small intestinal Crohn's disease.

Defective 25-hydroxylation
- Chronic cholestasis, e.g. primary biliary cirrhosis.
- Anticonvulsant therapy, e.g. phenytoin, phenobarbital.
- **Defective 1α-hydroxylation**
- **Chronic kidney disease**.
- **Renal tubular defects**
  (loss of phosphate):
  - renal tubular acidosis:
    - inherited (PEX gene mutation):
      - proximal (bicarbonate wastage);
      - distal (H+ gradient defect).
    - acquired: ureterosigmoid anastomosis;
    - phosphaturia.
- **Fanconi's syndrome** (multiple renal tubular defects leading to aminoaciduria):
  - inherited, e.g. cystinosis;
  - acquired, e.g. multiple myeloma;
  - phosphaturia.
- **hypophosphataemic vitamin D-resistant rickets/osteomalacia (Dent's disease)**:
  - most common form of rickets;
  - X-linked dominant (mutation in PEX gene);
  - impaired renal tubular reabsorption

of phosphate;
- characteristic deformity of bilateral symmetrical anterolateral femoral and tibial bowing;
- normal glomerular filtration rate but reduced vitamin D response;
- radiographs resemble ankylosing spondylitis, with ligamentous calcification and ossification (enthesiopathy);
- phosphate replacement and high-dose vitamin D3 necessary.
- **hereditary vitamin D-dependent rickets (Type I and II)**:
  - very rare;
  - clinically severe rickets with alopecia totalis, epidermal cysts and oligodontia;
  - inherited defect of 1.25(OH)2 vitamin D3 hydroxylation:
    - VDDR Type I:
      - renal 1α-hydroxylase deficiency;
      - autosomal recessive (chromosome 12q14; p450c1 α gene mutation);
    - VDDR Type II:
      - end-organ insensitivity to $1,25(OH)_2$ vitamin D3;
      - abnormality in nuclear receptor.

Inhibitors of mineralization
- **Fluoride.**
- **Aluminium.**
- **High-dose bisphosphonates.**
- **Heavy-metal overdose.**

Other
- **Renal osteodytrophy** (see above).
- **Hypophosphatasia**:
  - autosomal recessive disorder of phosphate synthesis (alkaline phosphatase gene mutation);
  - due to low levels of alkaline phosphatase;
  - increased urine phosphoethanolamine

is diagnostic;
- trend towards distinguishing hypophosphatasia as a clinical entity separate from osteomalacia.
- **Oncogenic tumour-induced hypophosphataemic osteomalacia**:
  - haemangiopericytomas, non-ossifying fibroma, fibrous dysplasia, neurofibromatosis;
  - excess FGF-23 production by tumours.
- **Chronic alcoholism.**

Pathology

Rickets
- Elongation of growth plates with abnormal arrangement of chondrocytes.
- Calcification is delayed.
- Vascularization is impaired.

Osteomalacia
- Bone biopsy characterization.
- Increased osteoid width (>15 µm).
- Increased mineralization lag time.
- Osteoid seams are unable to take up double tetracycline labelling.
- Changes of secondary hyperparathyroidism.

Clinical Features

General
- Retarded bone growth and short stature.
- Pathological fractures (Looser's zones on compression side).
- Symptoms of hypocalcaemia (see above) – vague bone and muscle pain.
- Proximal myopathy (vitamin D receptors present in skeletal muscle).

Focal, from top to bottom
- Craniotabes (thin deformed skull) at birth, neonatal rickets.
- Delayed fontanelle closure and frontal and parietal bossing.
- Dental disease.
- Enlargement of costochondral junction ('rickety rosary').
- Harrison's sulcus (indentation of lower

ribs at diaphragm insertion).
- Centrally depressed 'codfish vertebrae', dorsal kyphosis ('cat back').
- Bowing of the knees ('sabre shin').
- Waddling gait.

Investigations

Bloods
- Increased serum alkaline phosphatase (commonest abnormality; Note: elevated during pubertal growth spurt).
- Increased PTH; therefore, low/normal calcium and low phosphate.
- Low vitamin D levels (except in VDDR).
- Increased serum FGF-23 in tumour-associated osteomalacia.

Plain X-rays

Rickets
- Physeal increase in height and width (continues to grow but cannot mineralize).
- Metaphyseal cupping, flaring and jagged appearance.
- Small ossific nuclei.
- Coxa vara.
- Flattening of the skull.

Osteomalacia
- Looser's zones (microscopic stress fractures on concave border of long bones).
- Milkman pseudo-fracture on compression side of long bones (fractures that have healed but not mineralized).
- Biconcave vertebral bodies – can lead to severe kyphosis.
- Thin cortices; indistinct, fuzzy trabeculae.
- Triradiate pelvis.
- Signs of hyperparathyroidism.

Bone biopsy (trans-iliac)
- Widened osteoid seams.
- Double tetracycline labels abnormal.

Treatment

Treatments are aimed at correcting the cause and restoring calcium and phosphate levels to normal so that mineralization can occur.

- Vitamin D and vitamin D-metabolite formulations.
- Calcitriol/alfacalcidol (in defective 1α-hydroxylation).

5. Other causes of hypocalcaemia

- Acute pancreatitis.
- Massive transfusion (citrated blood).
- Low plasma albumin, e.g. chronic liver disease, malnutrition.
- Malabsorption, e.g. coeliac disease.
- Drugs.
- Phosphate therapy, calcitonin, bisphosphonates.

Disorders of bone mineral density

Osteoporosis

WHO definition, 1994: a skeletal disease characterized by **low bone mass per unit volume** and **deterioration** of the **micro-architecture** of bone tissue, with a consequent increase in bone **fragility** and susceptibility to **low-trauma fractures** (vertebral most common).

Diagnosis

Estimation of BMD is measured against the population mean in young healthy adults:

- **Normal** BMD is within 1 SD of that mean.
- **Osteopenia** is considered 1–2.5 SD below the mean peak bone mass.
- **Osteoporosis** is considered >2.5 SDs below the mean (T-score ≤-2.5) peak bone mass.

The **T-score** is the number of SDs below the mean for a sex- and race-matched healthy young adult population (aged 25–35 years).

The **Z-score** is the number of SDs below the mean for an age-, sex- and race-matched young adult population.

Rationale

- Inverse relationship between BMD and fracture risk in postmenopausal women and older men.
- Definition not applicable to younger women, men or children.
- Fracture risk doubles with reduction in bone density for every 1 SD.

These values are guidelines rather than diagnostic standards. It is important to differentiate between osteomalacia and osteoporosis (*Table A.1*).

Epidemiology

- Remaining lifetime risk osteoporotic fracture: 1 in 2 women and 1 in 3–5 men aged 50 years.
- Caucasian and Asian races higher risk.
- Healthcare burden est. £1.8 billion/year (UK).
- Osteoporotic hip fracture: 50% never reach previous functional capacity, 25% mortality within 1st year after fracture.

Risk factors

BMD-dependent
- Female sex.
- Ethinicity:
  - northern European and Far Eastern descent are at greater risk than black people and Polynesians.
- Family history and genetic factors:
  - single most significant influence on peak bone mass;
  - collagen type 1 A1 gene;
  - vitamin D receptor gene;
  - oestrogen receptor gene.
- Gastrointestinal /nutritional:
  - GI disease (malabsorption);
  - low calcium intake and absorption are strongly associated with fracture risk;*
  - vitamin D insufficiency;
  - anorexia nervosa leads to amenorrhoea.
- Environmental/lifestyle:*
  - excessive exercise leading to amenorrhoea at a relatively young age reduces peak bone mass;

Table A.1 Osteoporosis versus osteomalacia

	Osteoporosis	Osteomalacia
Definition	Bone mass decreased, mineralization normal	Bone mass variable, mineralization deficient
Age of onset	Elderly, postmenopausal	Any age
Aetiology (examples)	Idiopathic, age-related, endocrine abnormality, disuse, alcoholism, calcium deficient	Vitamin D deficiency, abnormality of vitamin D pathway, hypophosphatasia, renal failure
Symptoms	Pain when fractures occur	Generalized bone pain
Laboratory tests	Serum Ca normal Serum PO$_4$ normal ALP normal Urinary Ca high or normal	Serum Ca low or normal (high in hypophosphatasia) Serum PO$_4$ low or normal ALP elevated (unless hypophosphatasia) Urinary Ca normal or low (high in hypophosphatasia)
Bone biopsy	Tetracycline labels normal	Tetracycline labels abnormal

ALP: alkaline phosphatase; Ca: calcium; PO$_4$: phosphate.

- immobilization/sedentary lifestyle: mechanical loading inhibits resorption;
  - breastfeeding.
- Drugs:
  - chronic corticosteroid therapy;
  - excessive thyroxine;
  - anticoagulants, e.g. heparin;
  - anticonvulsants, e.g. phenytoin;
  - chemotherapy;
  - calcineurin inhibitors, e.g. cyclosporin;
  - antiandrogens, GnRH analogues;
  - proton pump inhibitors.
- Chronic disease:
  - COPD;
  - chronic kidney disease;
  - chronic liver disease.
- Endocrine disease (*Table A.2*):
  - Cushing's syndrome;
  - hyperparathyroidism;
  - hyperthyroidism;
  - diabetes mellitus;
  - hypogonadism.
- Other diseases:
  - mastocytosis;
  - multiple myeloma;
  - osteogenesis imperfecta;
  - rheumatoid arthritis.

BMD-independent
- Aging:
  - normal aging process in which men and women are almost equivalent;
  - with each decade, there is a 1.4–1.8-fold increased risk.
- Oestrogen deficiency:*
  - oestrogen blocks the action of PTH on osteoclasts and marrow stromal cells, thus preventing accelerated bone loss;
  - oestrogen levels in women may fall below those in age-matched men following menopause;
  - early menopause confers greater risk.
- Low BMI ($<19 \text{ kg/m}^2$).*
- Environmental/lifestyle:*
  - smoking;
  - alcohol.
- Drugs:
  - glucocorticoid therapy.
- Rheumatoid arthritis.
- Clinical factors:
  - previous fragility fracture (wrist, hip, vertebrae);
  - loss of height, kyphosis;
  - osteopenia or loss of vertebral morphology on plain X-ray;
  - strong family history of hip fracture or osteoporosis;
  - falls risk.*

* modifiable risk factors

Table A.2 Biochemical changes in conditions affecting calcium metabolism

CONDITION	Serum calcium	Serum phosphate	Serum alkaline phosphatase
Osteoporosis	Normal	Normal	Normal
Osteomalacia	May be normal	May be reduced	Increased
Paget's disease	May be increased in fracture	Normal	Increased
1° Hyperparathyroidism	Increased	Reduced	Normal
2° Hyperparathyroidism	May be normalized	Normal	May be increased
Hypoparathyroidism	Reduced	Increased	Normal

Pathophysiology

- Osteoclastic bone resorption is greater than osteoblastic bone formation leading to net loss of bone mass as well as micro-architectural change.
- Peak bone mass is achieved between 20 and 30 years in both men and women.
- Consolidation occurs up to approximately 40 years.
- Age-related bone loss occurs after 40 years and is accelerated in women around menopause, lasting 5 to 10 years.

The two major determinants in the development of osteoporosis are:

- peak bone mass (3rd decade, influenced by genes, nutrition, sex hormone status and physical activity);
- rate of bone loss thereafter.

Histology

- **Cancellous bone**: trabeculae are thinned and decreased in number. Some are lost completely. This loss of bony struts leaves adjacent areas unsupported and therefore significantly weakened.
- **Cortical bone**: decreased size of osteons and enlargement of marrow space. The cortices of long bones become thinner with age, while the overall bone diameter expands.

Clinical features

- Fracture symptoms – pain, swelling, deformity:
  - vertebral crush fracture (1 in 3 symptomatic; typical 'wedge-compression' type):
    - kyphosis (dowager's hump);
    - loss of height;
    - abdominal protruberance;
  - proximal femoral fracture;
  - distal radius fracture (Colles').

Investigations

Plain X-ray
- More than 30% bone loss is required to be seen on X-ray, making subjective osteopenia an insensitive test.
- Old wedge fractures may be seen in the thoracolumbar spine:
  - anterior wedging;
  - centrally depressed 'codfish' vertebrae.

Blood tests
- FBC, ESR, biochemistry, bone profile, thyroid function.
- PSA, testosterone and gonadotrophin levels in men.
- Serum PTH (hyperparathyroidism).
- 25(OH)-D3 levels (vitamin D body stores).
- Plasma electrophoresis (multiple myeloma).
- Testosterone.

Bone biomarkers
- Serum bone-specific alkaline phosphatase (osteoblast activity).
- Serum osteocalcin (bone matrix protein).
- Collagen degradation products in urine (bone resorption):
  - telopeptides, i.e. amino-terminal cross-linked telopeptides of collagen I (NTx), carboxy-terminal cross-linked telopeptides of collagen I (CTx);
  - pyridinolines.

Urine
- 24-hour urinary calcium.
- Urinary free cortisol (Cushing's disease).

Trans-iliac bone biopsy
- Tetracycline-labelled biopsy to exclude osteomalacia, e.g. in young osteopenic patients and in chronic renal failure.

Bone mineral density (g/cm²) assessment
DEXA

- Gold-standard clinical test for osteoporosis diagnosis and its response to treatment.
- Only investigation applicable to the WHO T-score definition of osteoporosis when carried out on the proximal femur and lumbar spine (most predictive of fracture).
- Measures axial bone density (i.e. mineral per surface area, not volumetric density).
- Twin X-ray beams of different energies are passed through the chosen bone and their emerging strength is measured.
- Low radiation, accurate, quick, simple to perform.
- Caution: artefactual elevation of spinal values from osteophytes, spinal deformity and vertebral fractures in elderly.
- According to current treatment guidelines from the British Orthopaedic Association:
  - if over age 75 years and one insufficiency fracture, start treatment;
  - if under age 75 years and one insufficiency fracture, order DEXA scan;
  - scanning also recommended for patients on corticosteroids.

Other indications for DEXA scanning:

- Radiographic osteopenia.
- Body mass index below 19 (kg/m²)
- Maternal history of hip fracture.
- BMD-dependent risk factors.

Other indications for treatment

- Glucorticoid therapy (start treatment without delay).

Quantitative CT

- The vertebra is scanned alongside an artificial phantom, and the two are compared.

- Measurements are taken from the centres of T12 to L4, and a mean is calculated.
- Provides true volumetric assessment of BMD and distinction between cortical and cancellous bone.
- Precision and accuracy are good, but cost and radiation dose are much higher than DEXA.

Quantitative US

- Usually calcaneum.
- Non-invasive, inexpensive, portable, no ionizing radiation.
- Experimental; used in screening prior to DEXA and not used to diagnose osteoporosis.

Risk assessment

- BMD measurements of hip and spine have a low sensitivity; age and history of previous fracture are 2 important risk factors independent of BMD measurements.
- WHO 'Fracture Risk Assessment Tool' (FRAX):
  - algorithm for calculating 10-year 'absolute' fracture risk for each individual;
  - based on independent clinical risk factors ± BMD values;
  - treatment thresholds based on clinical and cost-effectiveness;
  - patients with higher BMD plus clinical risk factors may have greater fracture probability than those with lower BMD without clinical risk factors, e.g. fracture risk may be greater in an older woman with osteopenia than a younger woman with osteoporosis.

Prevention

- Lifestyle modification: avoid smoking, excess alcohol, drug abuse.
- Nutrition: maintain adequate balanced diet.

- Exercise: load-bearing exercise in young women and gentle exercise in elderly may improve protective responses to falls.
- Falls prevention: physical therapy, home assessment, hip protectors.
- Monitor: patients on corticosteroid treatment and with strong family history.

Treatment

- Aim to reduce risk of fractures by **preventing bone loss** or **stimulating bone formation**.
- Fracture at one site increases risk of subsequent fracture at any site, thus treatments with antifracture efficacy at all major fracture sites, i.e. spine and hip are preferred.
- **Bisphosphonates** and **strontium ranelate** are first-line agents in majority of post-menopausal women with osteoporosis.

Preventing bone loss

Bisphosphonates

- See Chapter 4.
- Synthetic analogues of bone pyrophosphate that inhibit osteoclasts and adhere to hydroxyapatite.
- Traditional bisphosphonates, e.g. alendronate, risedronate (given weekly) shown to increase BMD, dramatically reduce fragility fractures and reduce vertebral fractures in men with osteoporosis.
- Newer bisphosphonates may be given less frequently, e.g. ibandronate (every 3 months) and zoledronic acid (once a year).
- Overall, reduce hip fracture rate by up to 50%.
- Caution: chronic kidney disease (reduced GFR), women of childbearing age, osteonecrosis of the jaw (rare), subtrochanteric hip fractures (rare; young, active patients on therapy).

Calcium and vitamin D

- Decreases bone resorption but does not increase bone mass or density.
- Minimum RDA should be achieved:
  - RDA calcium = 1200–1500 mg;
  - RDA vitamin D = 1000 IU;
  - Adding 500 mg Ca and 700 IU vitamin D reduces fractures (non-vertebral including hip fractures) by 50% over 3 years in people over age 65 years;
  - calcium and vitamin D supplements are advised in patients with low calcium intake, vitamin D insufficiency and those on bone protective medication.

Selective oestrogen receptor modulators (SERMs), e.g. raloxifene

- Activates oestrogen receptors in bone, acting like oestrogen to prevent BMD loss but may enhance menopausal symptoms, so not indicated within 5 years of menopause.
- Good evidence for vertebral but not hip fractures.
- Reduces oestrogen receptor positive breast cancer when used for up to 4 years.
- Use in women with low thrombotic risk.

Oestrogen therapy (HRT)

- Helps to decrease bone resorption and slow progression of osteoporosis, but does not increase bone mass, i.e. prevention not treatment.
- Should be initiated within 6 years of menopause.
- 2nd line option due to cardiovascular side-effects and breast malignancy, except in post-menopausal women having high fracture risk and peri-menopausal symptoms.

Calcitriol (1,25-$(OH)_2$D3)

- May reduce vertebral fracture rates.
- Side-effects, e.g. hypercalcaemia, hypercalciuria.

Calcitonin

- See Chapter 4.
- Inhibits osteoclastic resorption in the short term, but bone mass stabilizes in the long term.
- May reduce vertebral fracture rates and decrease pain associated with compression fractures of spine.
- Significant side-effects are a problem, e.g. nausea, flushing, vomiting, antisalmon antibodies.

Stimulating bone formation

Physical activity.

Strontium

- See Chapter 4.
- Two stable strontium atoms linked to ranelate, an organic acid.
- Increases bone formation and decreases bone resorption (weakly).
- Excellent for reducing risk of both vertebral and non-vertebral fractures.

Recombinant human parathyroid peptide 1-34 (teriparatide)/PTH

- See Chapter 4.
- Anabolic agents that stimulate bone formation.
- Licensed in subcutaneous form for women with post-menopausal osteoporosis.
- Reduces likelihood of both vertebral (by 65%) and non-vertebral (by 53%) fractures in post-menopausal women with osteoporosis. No data on hip fractures.
- Caution: PTH linked with development of bone tumours (in rats) with long-term use (>2years), avoid in patients with risk of developing osteosarcoma, i.e. Paget's, previous bone irradiation therapy.

Sodium fluoride

- Stimulates osteoblastic activity but not shown to reduce fracture rate (although slow-release fluoride may be better).

- Significant side-effects are a problem, e.g. gastrointestinal symptoms, distal tibial stress fractures as bone formed may be abnormal.

Combination therapy

- 2 antiresorptive agents/1 antiresorptive agent plus 1 anabolic agent.
- Larger increases in BMD compared with monotherapy but not shown to confer a greater reduction in fractures.

Osteopetrosis (marble bone disease)

- A group of disorders characterized by increased bony sclerosis loss of medullary canal caused by impaired osteoclast function.
- Bone density increased throughout skeleton but fractures and infections occur more easily.
- Raised acid phosphate level.
- Stem cell transplant therapy.

Types

- Autosomal recessive infantile or 'malignant' form is most severe:
  - renal tubular acidosis due to carbonic anhydrase deficiency;
  - gene mutation encoding chloride channel action (required for osteoclast activity).
- Autosomal dominant benign form (Albers–Schönberg disease).

Histology

- Osteoclasts lack the ruffled border required for effective resorption.
- Marrow spaces filled with necrotic calcified cartilage.

Paget's disease of bone

Paget's disease of bone (osteitis deformans) is a focal disorder of bone remodelling.

Epidemiology

- Age >40 years: 3% prevalence.
- Age >80 years: 10% prevalence.
- Epidemiologically difficult to define as most individuals are asymptomatic.
- Strong geographical prevalence (high in UK and USA; rare in Scandinavia and Asia), especially mining communities, e.g. Lancashire, UK.
- Familial history (15–30% of cases).
- Genetic links: increased incidence in HLA-DQw1; nuclear factor kappa ($NF_\kappa B$); sequestosome p62 (activates $NF_\kappa B$), osteoprotegerin and 6Cl2 (antiapoptotic gene).
- No racial differences in incidence.
- Slight male preponderance.

Aetiology

- Potentially **viral** (paramyxovirus, e.g. measles, respiratory syncytial virus, canine distemper virus): osteoclasts in pagetic lesions contain viral-like, nucleocapsid inclusion bodies. Altered expression of c-fos oncogene supports this theory.
- **Genetic** predisposition: chromosome focus for familial expansile osteolysis, an analogous disease, has been found.

Pathophysiology

Phases

Use the mnemonic 'LAB'.

- **Lytic** phase: initial phase involves **increased osteoclast size and number**, leading to **increased bone resorption**. An osteoclastic resorption 'front' is seen, usually near the metaphyseal region of a long bone or osteoporosis circumscripta in the skull.
- **Active** phase: this is followed by a **compensatory increase** (up to 40 times) in **disorganized osteoblastic woven bone formation**, i.e. accelerated, chaotic process of bone turnover, remodelling and deposition, leading to areas of sclerosis and areas of relative osteopenia. Concurrently, there is increased **local blood flow** and **fibrous tissue formation** in adjacent bone marrow. Both osteoclastic resorption and osteoblastic bone formation occur in the same area of bone.
- **Burnt-out** phase: a dense mosaic pattern of bone is seen, with little cellular activity.

Overall, formation exceeds resorption resulting in new, structurally abnormal bone that is weaker, prone to deformity and increased risk of fracture.

Histology

- Multiple resorbing and forming surfaces are characteristic with mosaic appearance.
- The chaotic process produces disorganization of collagen fibrils, making the matrix brittle and susceptible to pathological fracture and deformity.
- The marrow becomes fibrous, with scanty marrow cells.
- Fracture healing in pagetic bone is slower than normal.

Clinical features

- Usually **asymptomatic** (95%).
- Monostotic 17%, polyostotic 83%.
- **Bone pain** unrelated to activity, and often worse at night, especially spinal or pelvic.
- **Secondary osteoarthritis** in joints affected by Paget's disease in supporting bone.
- **Deformity** e.g. bowing of long bones, enlargement of the skull ('tam-o'-shanter' or large soft beret).
- **Affected sites** (in order of frequency): pelvis, lumbar spine, femur, thoracic spine, sacrum, skull, tibia.

Complications

- **Pathological fracture**, e.g. femoral neck.
- **Nerve compression**: cranial nerve (CN) VIIIth – conductive hearing loss due to temporal bone enlargement; also CN II, V, VII involvement, basilar invagination, spinal stenosis, cauda equine syndrome (exacerbated by 'steal syndrome'), hydrocephalus.
- **Vascular shunting** and increased bone blood flow – high output cardiac failure and myocardial hypertrophy.
- **Gout** – increased nucleic acid turnover.
- **Leontiasis ossea**.
- **Osteosarcoma** of pagetic bone – suspect this when a previously asymptomatic lesion becomes painful; 1% cases, 30-fold increase compared to normal population.

Investigations

Laboratory tests

- Raised serum alkaline phosphatase (marker of osteoblast activity).
- Raised serum acid phosphatase (marker of osteoclast activity).
- Raised urine hydroxyproline and collagen derived cross-linked peptides (marker of collagen turnover).
- Normal serum calcium and phosphate.

Plain X-rays

Early

- Lytic areas in any bone.
- Metaphyses of long bones – candle-flame areas of porosis (flame or arrow sign).
- Osteoporosis circumscripta in the skull.

Later
- **Cortices** become **thickened**, sclerotic and irregular.
- **Loss** of **corticomedullary differentiation** (dedifferentiation).
- **Loss** of **normal bony architecture, coarse trabeculae**.
- **Widened bones** and bowing.

- Disease progression from one end of a bone (usually proximal).
- **Fissure fracture** (on the convex side of long bones).

Bone scintigraphy

- Hot spots seen in areas of active Paget's disease (occasionally with cold areas centrally due to necrosis).
- Only 65% of lesions seen on bone scan will be seen on X-ray.
- Unable to distinguish between Paget's and sclerotic metastatic carcinoma (esp breast/prostate).

Indications for medical treatment of Paget's disease

- Bone pain and deformity.
- Before orthopaedic surgery (e.g. arthroplasty) in order to reduce bleeding.
- Pagetic spinal stenosis or nerve entrapment.
- Prevention of fracture or deformity in severe osteolytic cases and in young patients.
- Secondary high-output cardiac failure.

Treatment

- Bisphosphonates (alendronate/ etidronate/risedronate/ibandronate/ pamidronate [iv]/zolendronate [iv; potent]):
  - mainstay of medical treatment, taken for 2–3 months before elective surgery;
  - new bone formation after therapy is lamellar not woven, i.e. normalization of bone turnover.
- Calcitonin: not used frequently.
- Open reduction and internal fixation for fractures.
- Osteotomy or arthroplasty for secondary degenerative joint disease.
- Neurosurgery for cranial/spinal disease.
- Wide excision/limb salvage/amputation for osteosarcoma.

Malignant sarcomatous change

- Up to 30 times increased risk of osteogenic sarcoma (1–6% of all patients with Paget's disease).
- Usually in diffuse, long-standing, polyostotic disease.
- 50% are osteogenic.
- Less commonly, fibrosarcoma, chondrosarcoma and giant-cell tumour.
- Prognosis very poor.

Osteonecrosis (ON)

Definition

- Death of the cell population within a segment of bone following loss of blood circulation, i.e. aseptic avascular or ischaemic necrosis of bone.
- Organic and inorganic components of the matrix are unaffected, but the cells die.

Aetiology

- Idiopathic (40%): half of these are bilateral.
- Arterial disruption: fracture (acute or stress fracture), dislocation or infection.
- Arteriolar occlusion: thrombosis, embolism, Caisson disease (nitrogen bubbles from acute decompression during deep sea diving), haemoglobinopathies, e.g. sickle cell.
- Vessel-wall damage: vasculitis (SLE), irradiation.
- Capillary occlusion from fatty infiltration.
- Steroid treatment: >30 mg prednisolone for >30 days carries 37% risk, 80% bilateral.
- High alcohol intake: 20%.
- Gaucher's disease:
  - marrow cavity packed with Gaucher's macrophages filled with cerebroside.
- Pancreatitis.
- Hyperlipidaemia.

- Other: renal transplant, haematological malignancies, diabetes, Cushing's disease, sepsis, inflammatory bowel disease.

Pathology

The actual mechanism of ischaemia leading to ON is not understood fully in most cases. Proposed mechanisms include:

- **Intraosseous hypertension**: 'compartment syndrome of bone' – increased pressure found within bones with early ON, but it is not clear whether this is a cause or effect.
- **Abnormal extra-osseous blood flow**: loss of trans-cortical blood flow has been demonstrated in pre-radiographically-defined ON.
- **Fat embolism**: resulting from a fatty liver, disruption of depot or marrow fat, or coalescence of plasma lipoproteins. This mechanical blockage leads to a release of prostaglandins and subsequent intravascular thrombosis.
- **Fat-cell abnormalities**: fat-cell hypertrophy and fatty marrow overload have been demonstrated in animal studies.

Necrosis

- Dead bone is indistinguishable from live bone, both structurally and radiologically.
- Up to 1 week, there are no histological changes.
- During the second week, all cell types show evidence of necrosis. Cell death in the fatty marrow causes release of lysosomes and saponified free fatty acids from dead lipocytes.
- Increased water content follows, which is visible on MRI (normal marrow has little water).

Repair

- Initial inflammatory response with in-growth of blood vessels and chemotaxis of mesenchymal cells within the first few weeks.
- **Creeping substitution** (as with bone graft incorporation): new vessels revascularize the dead bone, growing into the spaces between trabeculae (cancellous) and into the old Haversian canals (cortical). Mesenchymal cells follow and differentiate into osteoblasts and osteoclasts.
- **Cancellous bone**: osteoblasts lay down new woven bone on to the scaffold of existing (dead) trabeculae. Osteoclasts then remodel these. The initial laying down of new bone produces an increased density seen on plain X-rays at 6–12 months.
- **Cortical bone**: following revascularization, osteoclasts follow blood vessels and resorb the old (dead) Haversian canals. Osteoblasts follow these new channels and form new osteons. Repair and revascularization advance from the vascular margins. The initial resorption leads to weakening of the bone and decreased density for up to 18 months before osteoblastic repair and return of strength.

Structural outcome

- Necrotic bone has no initial loss of strength, merely a loss of cell population.
- The absence of cells renders the bone unable to respond to normal, daily micro-trauma from loading.
- Repeated micro-stress fractures do not heal, leading to progressive collapse of the loaded bone.
- In subchondral bone, this collapse produces loss of joint congruency and early degenerative change.
- Subchondral bone around the peripheries (cortical) undergoes initial resorption, which weakens the bone further.
- **Crescent sign**: appearance of a sclerotic margin below the joint surface, representing subchondral collapse from repeated microtrauma in non-healing bone.
- **Hawkins sign (talus)**: subchondral radiolucency or mottled area, which represents the wave of revascularization and initial resorption before new bone formation. Implies good prognosis.

Clinical features

- **Age**: 20–50 years (average 38 years).
- **Site** (descending order of frequency):
  - femoral head;
  - medial femoral condyle;
  - humeral head;
  - talus;
  - lunate (Keinbock's disease);
  - capitellum (Panner's disease);
  - metatarsal heads (Freiberg's infraction);
  - tarsal navicular (Kohler's disease).
- **Symptoms**:
  - slow insidious onset of pain, starting initially on exercise and later at rest/at night;
  - pain may subside after 6–8 weeks;
  - pain may precede X-ray changes by many weeks;
  - early sign in the hip is loss of internal rotation.

Investigations

X-rays: Ficat and Arlet staging

- **Stage 0–1**: no changes seen.
- **Stage 2**: osteopenia and sclerosis.
- **Stage 3**: subchondral collapse (crescent sign).
- **Stage 4**: secondary osteoarthritis.

Magnetic resonance imaging

- Ischaemic marrow changes evident before bone scan changes.
- T1: decreased signal from ischaemic marrow, appearing like a single band.
- T2: second high signal line is seen within that seen on the T1 views (double-line sign).
- High sensitivity (100%) and specificity (98%).

Bone scan

- Initial cold area seen before revascularization (2–3 weeks).
- Becomes hot after revascularization, but only on affected side of the joint – both sides suggests OA.

Single photon-emission computed tomography (SPECT)

- Three-dimensional isotope scanning technique.
- Sensitive for early ON and gives a three dimensional image.

Staging

Modified Ficat

- **Stage 0**: preclinical, not seen on any imaging modality (first few days).
- **Stage 1**: pre-radiological, clinical loss of internal rotation, visible on MRI.
- **Stage 2**: moderate, decreased range of motion, some early osteopenia or sclerosis on plain X-ray but femoral head still spherical. Bone scan and MRI positive.
- **Stage 3**: moderate/severe, flattened head with crescent sign of subchondral collapse.
- **Stage 4**: severe, secondary degenerative changes.

Steinberg

- Same as above for Ficat stages 0–3.
- Added stages 4–6, subdivided into mild, moderate and severe.

Association Research Circulation Osseous (ARCO)

- Stages 0–4 described.
- Subdivisions based upon area of femoral head involved and amount of depression.

Treatment options (some controversial)

- Protective weight-bearing: minimal demonstrable benefit.
- Core decompression: evidence to suggest benefit in early Ficat stages (1–2).
- Proximal femoral osteotomy: technically demanding and may compromise later hip arthroplasty.
- Vascularized bone grafts.
- Vascularized pedicle flaps.
- Trapdoor procedures.
- Arthrodesis (rarely indicated).
- Hip arthroplasty (resurfacing or total).

Inflammatory arthritis

- Group of disorders where the common feature is **synovial inflammation**:
  - rheumatoid arthritis (RA);
  - seronegative spondyloarthropathy:
    - ankylosing spondylitis (AS);
    - psoriatic arthritis;
    - reactive arthritis (e.g. Reiter's disease, sexually acquired);
    - post-dysenteric reactive arthritis;
    - enteropathic arthritis (e.g. ulcerative colitis, Crohn's disease).
  - post-viral arthritis;
  - crystal arthritis;
  - Lyme arthritis.
- Classically causes early morning and post-rest pain and stiffness.
- Usually raised CRP, ESR and normochromic, normocytic anaemia.

Rheumatoid arthritis

- Autoimmune disorder characterized by chronic symmetrical polyarthritis with systemic involvement.
- Mainly peripheral joint synovitis associated with non-articular features.

Epidemiology

- 0.5–1% of world population.
- Peak onset 30–50 years.
- Female preponderance.
- Especially in Pima Indians.

Aetiology

- Gender/sex hormones: pre-menopausal women (F3:M1), post-menopausal (F=M).
- Familial: high incidence in first-degree relatives, mono- and dizygotic twins.
- Genetic: HLA-DR4 (50–75%), HLA-DRB1, Class II MHC genes.

Immunology

- Chronic synovial inflammation is caused by **immune dysregulation** and **maintenance of inflammation**.
- Initial triggering antigen is unknown but leads to on-going activity of T-cells, macrophages, fibroblasts, mast cells and local production of immune complexes and rheumatoid factor (RhF) autoantibodies.
- T-cells:
  - activity increased;
  - produce interferon, IL-2 and -4.
- Macrophages:
  - stimulation via IgG Fc receptors;
  - produce cytokines (IL-1, IL-8, TNF-α, G-CSF), chemokines (MIP) and MCP.
- Fibroblasts:
  - produce cytokines (IL-6).
  - synovial fibroblasts produce factors modulating formation of ectopic lymphoid tissue in synovium, i.e. VCAM-1, supports B lymphocyte survival and differentiation, DAF, prevents complement-induced cell lysis) and cadherin-II (mediates cell to cell interactions).
- Activated mast cells:
  - release histamine and TNF-α.

Pathology

- Widespread persisting synovitis (inflammation of joint synovial lining, tendon sheaths, bursae).
- Normal synovium contains thin lining layers of fibroblast-like synoviocytes plus macrophages overlying loose connective tissue.
- Pathological synovium ('pannus') contains a proliferation of synoviocytes forming hyperplastic, thickened, 'boggy' tissue in 'folds and fronds' with disorganized lymphoid follicles and marked vascular proliferation affecting joint margins.
- Inflammatory cells transit through and into joint fluid via tissue and/or through highly permeable blood vessels and synovial linings.
- Cartilage destruction is caused **directly** by cytokine action on chondrocytes and **indirectly** by blocking normal channels of nutrition.
- Juxta-articular osteoporosis is caused directly by local cytokine and fibroblast action on underlying bone and indirectly by joint disuse.

RhF

- Circulating autoantibodies produced by synovial plasma cells with the IgG Fc portion as their antigen.
- Self-aggregate into immune complexes, activating complement and stimulate inflammation (normally transient, pathologically persistent with higher affinity).
- IgM, IgG, or IgA involved.
- IgM RhF most commonly used in clinical testing:
  - seropositive in 70% of patients with polyarticular RA;
  - prognostic not diagnostic, pre-dating onset of RA, indicating level of activity.
- Seronegative RA patients have more limited pattern of synovitis.

Anti-CCP antibodies

- CCPs distinguish early RA from transient polyarthritis.
- RhF alone indicates persistence.
- RhF plus anti-CCP more specific predictor of greater joint damage, earlier development of erosions, greater long-term disability and earlier conversion to chronic destructive synovitis.
- Indicates early, aggressive treatment with DMARDs.

Clinical presentation

- **Palindromic** (5%) (acute monoarticular attacks lasting 24–72 hours).
- **Transient** (self-limiting lasting <12 months with no permanent joint damage).
- **Remitting** (lasting several years before remission).
- **Slowly progressive** (70%) – most typical form, chronic, persistent evolving over weeks to months, relapsing and remitting over years.
- **Rapidly progressive** – high disease velocity over years, severe damage, usually seropositive plus anti-CCP.

Symptoms and signs

Articular features

- Morning pain, stiffness and swelling of small joints of the hands and feet, wrists, elbows, shoulders, knees and ankles.
- Wrist and hand manifestations:
  - flexor tenosynovitis;
  - CTS;
  - MCP joint ulnar deviation and volar subluxation;
  - PIP joint Boutonnière deformity;
  - PIP joint Swan-neck deformity;
  - ulnar styloid dorsal subluxation;
  - extensor tendon rupture (usually ring/little finger drop).
- Foot and ankle manifestations:
  - MTPJ swelling;
  - hammer-toe deformity;
  - ulcers and callouses over MT heads and dorsum toes;
  - flat medial arch (mid- and hindfoot RA);
  - valgus deformity ankle.
- Cervical spine manifestations:
  - atlantoaxial/upper cervical instability;
  - pyramidal and sensory signs;
  - spinal cord compression;
- 90% polyarthritis;
- 10% monoarthritis of knee or shoulder or CTS.

Non-articular features

- Juxta-articular soft tissues:
  - subcutaneous nodules (elbow, fingers, Achilles tendon);
  - bursitis (esp. olecranon);
  - hand flexor tenosynovitis;
  - trigger finger;
  - wrist extensor tenosynovitis.
- Lungs – pulmonary/pleural nodules, effusion, pneumoconiosis [Caplan's syndrome], serositis, fibrosing alveolitis, obstructive bronchiolitis, infective lesions, e.g. TB).
- Heart and peripheral vessels – pericarditis, endocarditis, myocarditis, coronary artery and cerebrovascular atherosclerosis.
- Vasculitis – immune complex deposition in arterial walls, uncommon; Raynaud's syndrome.
- Eyes – scleritis, scleromalacia perforans, episcleritis, sicca/Sjögren's syndrome (dry eyes, dry mouth).

- Nervous system – sensorimotor polyneuropathy, moneuritis multiplex, 'glove and stocking' sensory loss due to vasculitis of vasa nervorum, compression neuropathy, e.g. CTS.
- Haematological – anaemia (commonly normochromic, normocytic), lymphadenopathy, splenomegaly and neutropenia (Felty's syndrome).
- Kidneys – amyloidosis, nephroticsyndrome, renal failure.

Diagnosis

- Bloods:
  - anaemia;
  - ESR/CRP raised.
- Serology:
  - RhF (70%);
  - anti-CCP (earlier in disease, indicator of progression in early disease);
  - ANA (30%).
- Radiographs: erosions.
- MRI.
- Joint aspirate.

Criteria for the diagnosis of rheumatoid arthritis (American College of Rheumatology [ACR], 1988 revision)

- Morning stiffness >1 hour.*
- Arthritis of three or more joints.*
- Arthritis of hand joints and wrists.*
- Symmetrical arthritis.
- Subcutaneous nodules.
- Positive serum RhF.
- Typical radiological changes (erosions and/or periarticular osteopenia).

* For 6 weeks or more; 4 or more criteria necessary for diagnosis.

Treatment

Non-operative

- **Analgesia, NSAIDS and coxibs:**
  - night pain, morning stiffness symptom control;

- COX pathway.
- **Corticosteroids:**
  - early use slows disease velocity and may induce remissions;
  - intra-articular/intramuscular.
- **DMARDs:**
  - reduces rate of progressive joint damage in early and late disease;
  - **traditional DMARDs**, e.g. sulfasalazine, methotrexate, leflunomide:
    - early, aggressive use (especially with RhF plus anti-CCP positive patients);
    - slow-acting via cytokine inhibition; 20–50% improvement.
  - **biological DMARDs**, e.g. TNF-α blockers – etanercept, adalimumab, infliximab:
    - TNF cytokine superfamily produced by activated macrophages and T-cells play key role in joint inflammation;
    - rapid acting. Slows or stops erosion in 70% of patients and heals in a few;
    - in combination with methotrexate.
- Other biological agents:
  - rituximab (B-cell ablation);
  - anakinra (IL-1 antagonist);
  - abatacept;
  - tocilizumab (anti-IL-6):
    - rapid acting. 70% improvement in 20% patients;
    - in combination with methotrexate.
- Other agents:
  - e.g. gold, hydroxychloroquine, penicillamine, azathioprine, cyclosporin.
- Physical and occupational therapy.

Operative

- Surgical synovectomy.
- Excision arthroplasty, e.g. ulnar styloid, MT head.
- Total joint arthroplasty.

Complications

- Ruptured joint capsule, e.g. Baker's cysts.
- Tendon rupture.
- Septic arthritis (most commonly *S. aureus*).
- Spinal cord compression (AA or upper cervical spine).
- Amyloidosis (rare; RA is the commonest cause of secondary amyloidosis).
- Pharmacological treatment side-effects.

Prognosis

Factors indicating poorer prognosis:

- Clinical
  - female;
  - insidious onset;
  - progressively increasing peripheral joint involvement and disability.
- Bloods:
  - high CRP/ESR;
  - normochromic normocytic anaemia within 3 months of onset;
  - high titres of RhF and anti-CCP antibodies;
  - HAL-DR4, HLA-DRB1 positive (HLA-DRB1 plus RhF indicates 13 × increased risk of bony erosions in early disease).
- Imaging:
  - early erosive damage.

Seronegative spondyloarthropathies

- Group of inflammatory joint disorders linked to Class 1 HLA antigens (**increased HLA-B27**).
- Spine and peripheral joint involvement.
- Non-spinal complications:
  - acute anterior uveitis (all types);
  - iriitis (AS);
  - costochondritis (all types);
  - cutaneous lesions (reactive arthritis);
  - nail dystrophy (psoriatic arthritis, reactive arthritis);
  - aortitis (AS, reactive arthritis).

Ankylosing spondylitis (AS)

- Inflammatory disorder of the spine and sacroiliac joints affecting young adults.
- HLA-B27 present > 90% Caucasians with AS.
- HLA-DR1, HLA-B60 also linked.

Epidemiology

- Worldwide (1% men; 0.5% women in Caucasian populations).
- 2.5M:1F.
- High incidence in North American Haida Indians.
- High heritability (spinal and sacroiliac disease [90%]; monozygotic twins [70%] dizygotic twins [25%]; HLA-B27 positive offspring have 30% risk of developing AS).

Pathology

- Lymphocyte and plasma cell infiltration.
- Enthesitis (local bony erosion at attachments of intervertebral and other ligaments).
- Syndesmophytes (persistent enthesitis and healing with new bone formation).
- Bony ankylosis (facet joints, SI joints and costovertebral joints).

Clinical features

- Episodic sacroiliitis during late teens to early twenties.
- Pain (buttocks, lower back) and stiffness (Schoeber's test positive), especially in mornings, relieved by exercise.
- Retained lumbar lordosis during flexion (early), dorsal kyphosis and paraspinal muscle wasting (late).
- Non-spinal complications including peripheral joints, e.g. hip fixed flexion deformity.

Diagnosis

- Morning stiffness >30 minutes.
- Back pain at rest that improves with exercise.

- Nocturnal back pain during second half of night.
- Alternating buttock pain.

3 of 4 criteria necessary for diagnosis

Investigations

- Bloods: ESR/CRP raised.
- HLA-testing: high HLA-B27.
- X-rays:
  - SI joint erosions and marginal sclerosis;
  - thoracolumbar junction end plates loss of definition, 'blurring';
  - erosions at superior and inferior end plate corners of vertebral bodies ('shiny corner' sign or Romanus lesion);
  - 'bamboo spine' – calcification intervertebral ligaments + facet joint fusion + bridging syndesmophytes.
- MRI: useful to determine pre-radiographic sacroiliitis.

Treatment

- Early diagnosis and preventative morning exercises (spinal mobility, posture, chest expansion).
- Medical:
  - analgesia and NSAIDs;
  - local steroid injection;
  - methotrexate (peripheral arthritis);
  - TNF-α blockers.

Prognosis

Excellent with early exercise regime and analgesia.

Psoriatic arthritis

- Arthritis and enthesitis in association with psoriasis or family history of psoriasis.
- 5–10% psoriasis patients develop arthritis (variety of patterns exist).
- HLA-B27 (50% only); no serological marker.

Clinical features

- DIP joint arthritis: typically involving nail dystrophy.
- Pauciarticular:
  - cutaneous lesions;
  - IP joint synovitis;
  - tenosynovitis ('sausage finger') or toe (dactylitis).
- Seronegative symmetrical polyarthritis: similar to RA.
- Arthritis mutilans (5%):
  - marked periarticular osteolysis;
  - shortening ('telescopic fingers').
- Uni- or bilateral sacroiliitis/cervical spondylitis (15%).

Investigations

X-rays – central joint erosions not juxta-articular ('pencil-in-cup').

Treatment

NSAIDs, local intra-articular corticosteroid injections, sulfasalazine, methotrexate, cyclosporin, anti-TNF.

Reactive arthritis

- Arthritis caused by a sterile synovitis that occurs post-infection.
- 1–2% incidence in patients post-acute dysentery/sexually acquired infection (non-specific urethritis [male], non-specific cervicitis [female]).
- HLA-B27 positive males – RR = 30–50.

Aetiology

- *Salmonella*/*Shigella* spp. (bacillary dysentery).
- Post-streptococcal arthritis (both reactive and septic arthritis).
- *Yersinia enterocolitica.*
- *Chlamydia trachomatis*/*Ureaplasma urealyticum* (NSU).
- Gonococcal arthritis (both reactive and septic arthritis).
- Brucellosis (both reactive and septic arthritis).

Pathology

- Bacterial antigens or DNA present within inflamed synovium of affected joints.
- HLA-B27 increases susceptibility but is not obligatory for disease.

Clinical features

- Acute, asymmetrical, lower limb arthritis.
- Onset after a few days to weeks post-infective episode.
- Enthesitis (plantar fasciitis, Achilles tendon).
- Sacroiliitis/spondylitis.
- Sterile conjunctivitis, acute anterior uveitis.
- Skin lesions (circinate balanitis, keratoderma blenorrhagica, nail dystrophy).
- Reiter's disease (urethritis, arthritis, conjunctivitis).

Treatment

- Cultures and antibiotics.
- Education.
- NSAIDs and local corticosteroid injections, methotrexate, sulfasalazine, TNF-α blocking agents.

Prognosis

- Recovery within 6 months (70%).

Enteropathic arthritis

Synovitis occurring in ulcerative colitis and Crohn's disease (10–15%).

Pathology

Selective mucosal leak of antigens triggering a synovitis?

Clinical features

- Asymmetrical arthritis of lower limb joints.
- HLA-B27 associated sacroiliitis or spondylitis (5%).

Treatment

- Standard treatments for inflammatory bowel disease.
- NSAIDs, intra-articular corticosteroid injections, sulfasalazine, TNF-α blocking agents (infliximab).

Crystal arthritis

Gout and hyperuricaemia

Inflammatory arthritis associated with hyperuricaemia and intra-articular deposits of sodium urate crystals.

Epidemiology

- Increasing in developed countries (0.2% Europe, USA).
- 10M:1F, especially in middle-aged males.
- Hyperuricaemia (serum uric acid >2 SD from mean: 420 μmol/L men; 360 μmol/L women).
- Especially in Maoris.

Associations

- Diuretic use.
- OA.
- Age.
- Obesity.
- High-protein diet, high alchohol intake, high fructose intake.
- Combined hyperlipidaemia.
- Diabetes mellitus.
- Hypertension and ischaemic heart disease.
- Family history.

Aetiology/pathogenesis

- Uric acid is the final product of purine metabolism.
- Imbalance between purine synthesis, dietary purine ingestion and uric acid excretion by kidneys (66%) and intestine (33%).

- **Uric acid synthesis (increase)** (10%):
  - increased **purine synthesis** *de novo*:
    - hypoxanthine–guanine phosphoribosyltransferase (HGPRT) reduction;
    - phosphoribosyl-pyrophosphate synthase overactivity;
    - glucose-6-phosphatase deficiency with glycogen storage disease type 1.
  - **increased purine turnover**:
    - myeloproliferative disorders;
    - lymphoproliferative disorders;
    - carcinoma;
    - psoriasis.
- **Uric acid excretion (impaired)** (90%):
  - chronic kidney disease (CKD);
  - drugs (diuretics, low-dose aspirin);
  - hypertension;
  - primary hyperparathyroidism;
  - hypothyroidism;
  - lactic acidosis (exercise, starvation, alcohol);
  - glucose-6-phosphatase deficiency;
  - lead toxicity.
- Acute gout caused by release of proinflammatory cytokines and complement activation by polymorpholeucocytes on ingesting sodium urate crystals.

Clinical features

- Acute sodium urate synovitis – gout.
- Chronic polyarticular gout.
- Chronic tophaceous gout.
- Urate renal stone formation.
- Pain, swelling, redness over joints (1st MTP joint [75%] other joints [25%]).
- Crystal cellulitis.
- Tophi (cutaneous white deposits, ears, fingers, Achilles tendon).

Investigations

- Serum urate raised.
- Serum urea and creatinine.
- Joint fluid microscopy.
- X-rays: periarticular deposit halos and 'punched-out' bone cysts.

Treatment

- NSAIDs/coxibs (acute attacks; caution: renal impairment).
- Corticosteroids intra-articular or intramuscular, e.g. methylprednisolone.
- Colchicine: inhibits microtubule formation limiting polymorphic nuclear leucocyte release of pro-inflammatory factors; alternative in patients with renal impairment/history of peptic ulceration.
- Dietary advice: reduce alcohol intake especially beer, reduce cholesterol, reduce purine rich foods, e.g. fish, spinach.
- Allopurinol:
  - xanthine oxidase blocker;
  - use for frequent, severe attacks, renal impairment, NSAID or colchicine intolerance at least 1 month after acute attack.
- Febuxostat: non-purine analogue inhibitor of xanthine oxidase.
- Uricosuric agents: benzbromarone, probenecid, losartan.

Pseudogout (pyrophoshate arthropathy)

- Calcium pyrophosphate deposits in hyaline and fibrocartilage.
- Crystal deposit-induced acute synovitis of joints.

Epidemiology

- More common in elderly women.
- Associated with haemochromatosis, hyperparathyroidism, Wilson's disease, alkaptonuria.

Clinical features

Painful, swollen knee and wrist.

Diagnosis

- Pyrexia.
- Raised WCC.
- Joint fluid microscopy: rhomboidal, weakly positive birefringent crystals.
- X-ray: appearance of chondrocalcinosis.

Treatment

- Joint aspiration.
- NSAIDs, colchicine, intra-articular corticosteroid injection.

Index

Note: page numbers in *italics* refer to figures and tables.